Planning, Markets and Hospitals

Improving access to hospital services has been a goal of public policy in Britain for over seventy years, but the means by which this goal is to be attained have changed significantly over time. Drawing substantially on original research, *Planning, Markets and Hospitals* represents a systematic attempt to assess the strengths and weaknesses of different forms of planning and coordination of hospital development.

The book encompasses an era which began with a mixed economy of hospital provision in the inter-war period, incorporating some embryonic public-private partnerships. There ensued, after 1948, a period of hierarchical planning, symbolised by the 1962 Hospital Plan. Frustrations with the problems of implementing this Plan led ultimately to the re-emergence of pro-competitive solutions to hospital development, exemplified by the 1991 NHS reforms and the subsequent Private Finance Initiative. Despite these important changes, however, the book shows that there were also substantial continuities in terms of regulatory and steering mechanisms in the hospital service.

Planning, Markets and Hospitals makes a fresh contribution to enduring debates about planning and regulation of health care, about the governance of welfare services and about the appropriate role for voluntary, commercial and charitable provision of services. It reinterprets previous histories of hospital policy and questions whether current policies will reconcile competing goals of equity and choice.

John Mohan is Professor of Geography, University of Portsmouth. He has published widely, in academic and professional journals, on historical and contemporary geographies of health and health care.

Planning, Markets and Hospitals

John Mohan

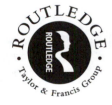

London and New York

First published 2002
by Routledge
11 New Fetter Lane, London EC4P 4EE

Simultaneously published in the USA and Canada
by Routledge
29 West 35th Street, New York, NY 10001

Routledge is an imprint of the Taylor & Francis Group

© 2002 John Mohan

Typeset in Times by Taylor and Francis Books Ltd
Printed and bound in Great Britain by St Edmundsbury Press,
Bury St Edmunds, Suffolk

British Library Cataloguing in Publication Data
A catalogue record for this book is available from the British Library

Library of Congress Cataloging in Publication Data
Library of Congress data for this book have been requested

ISBN 0–415–19607–8 (pbk)
      0–415–19606–X (hbk)

Contents

Illustrations

Abbreviations

AHA	Area Health Authority	*HSJ*	*Health Service Journal*
ARM	Annual Representative Meeting (of the BMA)	*HSSJ*	*Health and Social Service Journal*
BG	Board of Governors (of teaching hospitals)	KWS	Keynesian Welfare State
		LCC	London County Council
BHA	British Hospitals Association	MPU	Medical Practitioners' Union
BHSSJ	*British Hospital and Social Service Journal*	NCB	National Coal Board
		NHS	National Health Service
BMA	British Medical Association	NHSE	National Health Service Executive
BMJ	*British Medical Journal*		
CB	County Borough	NPHT	Nuffield Provincial Hospitals Trust
CC	County Council		
CDSC	Capital Development Sub-committee (of Newcastle RHB)	NTDC	New Town Development Corporation
		PAI	Public Assistance Institution
CPAG	Capital Prioritisation Advisory Group	PESC	Public Expenditure Survey Committee
CSA	Commissioner for the Special Areas	PFI	Private Finance Initiative
		RAWP	Resource Allocation Working Party
DGH	District General Hospital		
DHA	District Health Authority	RCCS	Revenue Consequences of Capital Schemes
DHSS	Department of Health and Social Security		
		RHA	Regional Health Authority
EMS	Emergency Medical Service	RHB	Regional Hospital Board
HCHS	Hospital and Community Health Services	RSP	Regional Strategic Plan
		RVI	Royal Victoria Infirmary, Newcastle-upon-Tyne
HMC	Hospital Management Committee		
		SMA	Socialist Medical Association
HSB	Health Services Board		

Preface and acknowledgements

The research that underpins this book draws on a number of projects, and some indication of its provenance is appropriate. My initial work on this topic was at postgraduate level, in the form of an investigation of geographical aspects of the planning of hospital services under the NHS. This concentrated mainly on the first three decades of the NHS and consisted largely of local case studies in NE England, albeit making some reference to broader debates. Some publications resulted from that project, but the present book broadens its scope considerably. The immediate stimulus to it arose from work on the geography of the NHS reforms and specifically on the tension between planning and markets posed by those reforms. At about the same time I became involved in work on the historical development of the pre-NHS hospital services. These contrasting periods were connected by the question of how – indeed whether – it was possible to regulate and plan a system driven by competitive pressures. Moreover, and from my own specific disciplinary background, the uneven impacts of these processes was noteworthy. In between the 1930s and the 1990s, the era of state planning of hospital services had arrived, symbolised by the establishment of the NHS and the 1962 Hospital Plan. The broad outlines of a project examining the rise and fall of hospital planning therefore took place. The book therefore allows different forms of regulation to be examined in a relatively long-term historical perspective, and it also seeks to integrate work on the development of national policies with an analysis of their local impacts.

Though this means that the book covers considerable ground, a corollary was restriction of its scope in important ways. First, it does emphasise the physical construction of hospitals, and it can be argued that this is one-dimensional, in that the capacity of a health-care system is also determined by the availability of skilled staff, the quality of management, the possibility that technological change will facilitate delivery of treatment outside hospitals, and the presence or absence of primary and community care. However, hospitals will continue to be needed in some form and a focus on the different ways in which their provision has been organised allows evaluation of the strengths and weaknesses of arrangements for the delivery of welfare services.

Second, choice of the Newcastle region logically meant a focus on England, for which I apologise to readers interested in developments elsewhere in the UK. I would justify choice of this region on several grounds. It is relatively self-contained in terms of hospital provision, with only small cross-boundary flows. It contained examples of all that was good and bad about pre-NHS hospital provision, but it also incorporated areas which by any standards were underserved. It had seen embryonic public–private partnerships in the 1930s, and the range of public policy measures designed to modernise the region's infrastructure in the post-war period also made it a valuable case study. A case could probably be made for other RHBs though, as other commentators have pointed out, we need to avoid the 'distorting prism of London' through which NHS policy is often viewed. The alternative to a regional focus would have been an issue-based organisation, around such themes as the difficulty of providing services in rural areas, but this would have been at the expense of the coherence given by a focus on one region.

Although moving to Portsmouth had the unfortunate side-effect of increasing the distance between author and archives, it also provided the opportunity to research and write the book. Among a generally tolerant and supportive group of colleagues, I am particularly grateful to successive Heads of Department, Mike Taylor and Kelvyn Jones, for their support. However, I am especially indebted to two individuals at Portsmouth: Graham Moon has been a constant source of constructive criticism and advice and also found time to comment on most of the book in draft form, while the book would never have appeared at all without Margaret Fairhead, who typed it with formidable speed and accuracy, and cheerfully coped with reconstructing the ruins of previous drafts.

The book draws on projects which have received funding from a number of sources, principally ESRC, the Leverhulme Trust and the Nuffield Foundation. It is based on archival sources relating to the formulation of policy both nationally and locally, and I should particularly like to acknowledge the cooperation of the former Northern RHA in granting access to records in advance of their opening under the usual thirty-year rule. However, I have followed convention by not quoting directly from material still subject to such restrictions. The primary archival material is held in a number of locations and I am grateful to the staff of all of them for their assistance: Tyne and Wear Archives Service; the Public Record Office; Durham County Record Office; Northumberland County Record Office; Newcastle City Library Local History Section; and Churchill College Archives, Cambridge. Several libraries have been particularly helpful; as well as the Frewen Library, Portsmouth, thanks are due to the British Library of Political and Economic Science, the King's Fund, and the London School of Hygiene and Tropical Medicine.

I am grateful to Mrs M. Pater for permission to quote from the papers of John Pater, which are held at Churchill College, Cambridge. Every effort has been made to trace other copyright holders.

A number of individuals have contributed to the development of the ideas herein either through joint projects or more generally through exchanging ideas and publications. I am especially grateful to Rodney Lowe for a number of timely suggestions. Others who have helped along the way include Ross Barnett, Tim Blackman, Paul Bridgen, Barry Doyle, Mark Exworthy, Martin Gorsky, Ben Griffith, Ray Hudson, Gerry Kearns, Roger Lee, Allyson Pollock, Martin Powell, David Price, Geof Rayner, Humphrey Southall, Jon Sussex and Charles Webster. Versions of some chapters were presented at seminars in London, Portsmouth and Oxford, and at conferences of the ESRC Whitehall programme, the Society for the Social History of Medicine, the Social Policy Association, and the Institute of British Geographers. The bulk of the book is original to this volume although parts of Chapters 2 and 3 draw on an article previously published in *Social History of Medicine* and on an Office of Health Economics monograph. I am grateful to the editors of *Social History of Medicine* and to the Office of Health Economics and the Association of Chartered and Certified Accountants for permission to use the material in this book.

Finally, three generations of my family have contributed enormously to the completion of this book. Fortunately that is not a comment on the length of time it has taken to finish it! Instead it is an acknowledgement of my parents, Jim and Anna Mohan, for their unstinting support and encouragement (accompanied by bemused tolerance if not amused scepticism). It is also an acknowledgement of generous offers of accommodation on the part of my parents, in Newcastle, and my brother, Tom Mohan, in London; this was essential to completion of the archival work for this project. My greatest debt, with apologies for protracted absences and distracted presences, is to Ellie, Jennifer and Clare, who have lived with this book and its disruptive consequences for far too long.

John Mohan
November 2001

1 Planning, markets and welfare

Debates about hospital policy and the welfare state

In 1962 Enoch Powell launched the Macmillan government's *Hospital Plan for England and Wales* (Ministry of Health 1962a). After nearly 14 years of the NHS, it appeared that at long last a committed effort would be made to improve the quality of hospital accommodation throughout the service and provide new facilities where they were most needed. In England and Wales the plan envisaged spending £500 million over 10 years, which would enable the provision of 90 new and 134 substantially remodelled hospitals. There was a parallel plan for Scotland. The result would be a national network of District General Hospitals (DGHs) of 600–800 beds, serving catchments of between 100,000–150,000 people. 'Bed norms' – ratios of the numbers of beds needed to population – were to be used to equalise the distribution of the hospital stock. The Plan also envisaged a role for facilities offering different levels of specialisation. The most complex services would be available in teaching hospitals; the DGHs would provide the normal range of general hospital treatment; and, though some 700 hospitals were to close, there was still to be a place for smaller hospitals, either in rural areas or as support hospitals, offering less interventionist care than the DGHs. A fuller outline of the Plan is given in Chapter 6, but Powell took the opportunity to present it as an (unparalleled) initiative, declaring that the government were planning hospital provision on a scale unimagined anywhere else, 'certainly not this side of the Iron Curtain'.

The reference is apt, and ironic; by 1989, Conservative spokesmen were drawing legitimacy for the NHS reforms from the collapse of state socialism, and arguing that the time had come to sweep away an era of 'monolithic, oppressive overplanning'. The implication was that such arrangements might have been appropriate in straitened post-war circumstances but their *raison d'être* had been undermined by economic and social changes. Henceforth, the future of individual hospitals would, it appeared, be determined by their competitiveness and managerial efficiency. Yet barely two decades before the national plan, conversely, it was asserted that the nation was not yet ready for full state ownership and control, and that some form of public–private mix could secure access to health services.

This book therefore offers a study of the development of policy towards the provision of acute hospital services, and this focus is deliberate. There have been for many years debates about the place of the hospital in health care delivery systems and about the contribution of hospitals to population health and wellbeing. Most contemporary opinion and policy now inclines towards health services led by prevention and primary care, the aim being to minimise hospitalisation. Nevertheless, for most of the twentieth century it was, as Fox (1986) suggests, a central aim of policy to make hospital care as widely available as possible, even if the mechanisms whereby that was to be achieved were the subject of much dispute (Webster 1990). This study is therefore using acute hospital policy as a lens through which to examine broader debates about the organisation of welfare services. It does not, as a consequence, consider psychiatric provision or services for people with learning disabilities, and it makes but passing reference to debates about relationships between acute and community care. It attempts to cover both national policy and its local impacts, thereby complementing the regional studies of Pickstone (1985) and Rivett (1986).

The book pivots around the 1962 Hospital Plan, because in one sense this was the zenith of an era of faith in state management, and also the end of it: a few years after its launch it was already being referred to as the hospital 'building programme'. The Plan has generally had a good press but has been subject to little critical analysis. Most texts on the NHS devote little space to it, presenting it in a positive light – and it is certainly true that by comparison with the inaction that preceded it, the Plan was a great advance (Chapter 5). The only book devoted to the Plan (Allen 1979) was written before the papers on its formulation became available, and the present book draws on primary sources and seeks to put the Plan in a broader historical context. Admittedly with the advantage of a further two decades of hindsight, it is possible to see the Plan as part of what Finlayson (1994) has termed the 'moving frontier' between state, market and community. Consideration of the problems of the pre-war hospitals demonstrates the strengths and weaknesses of that embryonic mixed economy of welfare, and helps to demonstrate the need for a coordinated national policy. This seemed to have arrived with the 1962 Plan, but analysis of its foundations shows that these were somewhat 'shaky' (to quote the then Permanent Secretary at the Ministry of Health: Fraser 1964), raising doubts as to its coherence. Examination of its implementation, which has had relatively little attention, perhaps helps understand more clearly why pro-market arguments began to gain ascendancy in the 1980s; there was much potential for frustration, in a time of economic turbulence, which contributed to disaffection with the idea of 'planning' and to a turn towards more competitive, localist solutions (as in the 1991 reforms). These, in their turn, have been shown to have their limitations, requiring relaxation of the emphasis on competition as a primary steering mechanism for hospital development. The latest developments in hospital policy provide a further justification for this study. The

1962 Plan envisaged laying out, according to national norms, a system of hospitals for each of the constituent regions of the NHS; thus, hospitals and beds were provided according to (simplistic) criteria of need. The Private Finance Initiative (PFI) of recent years has been criticised for emphasising financial viability, not population need, and for considering only issues relating to individual hospital developments rather than system-wide criteria (Chapter 9). There are some relevant (if not precise) parallels here with the pre-NHS era, in which hospital developments often proceeded in isolation from one another, with consequences in terms of duplication and inefficiency.

This brief chronological outline suggests that if we are to put efforts at hospital planning in their context we need to examine both their antecedents and consequences. We need to know more about the inadequacies of and frustrations with the pre-war system, which contributed to demands for nationalisation; we also need to know more about the technical weaknesses of the Plan and the difficulties of pursuing it, as well as about the efforts to replace planning with internal markets and private finance. There has been a tendency, from both ends of the political spectrum, to present a partial view of events. Thus, advocates of state planning invoke the maldistribution and inequity of the pre-NHS system, possibly at the expense of its positive features, such as mobilising public involvement. Conversely, the inflexibilities and delays of state planning have been inflated into a generalised pro-market critique, neglecting the very real improvements in access to care under state provision. Others contend that there is a case for attempting to fuse the best features of both: the ability of the state to promote an equitable distribution of services, combined with the flexibility and responsiveness of the private or voluntary sectors (Ham 1996; Bosanquet 1999). Whether services were delivered by state, market or voluntary provision would be a matter of indifference. On this view, networking and partnerships would be the order of the day and policies would be judged in instrumental terms – 'what matters is what works', in currently fashionable jargon. The historical and contextual approach adopted here allows these diverse claims to be adjudicated perhaps more comprehensively than has previously been the case. I hope, in addition, that the book contributes to debate about some broader themes in the analysis of developments in the welfare state.

The history charted here resonates with three important themes in welfare policy, which can be thought of as operating at three interlocking scales. First, there are macro-level arguments, about the boundary between public and private provision of services, about the degree of convergence between states on the appropriate balance between them, and about the relationship between these issues and broader economic and social changes. Second, there are debates about the appropriate scale of organisation of services, encapsulated in Fox's (1986) contentions that a regional form of organisation was a consensus matter, but also evident in ongoing arguments about the character and powers of sub-national units in the NHS, and in debates about the extent to which hospitals should be accountable to their local communities. Third, there are micro-level arguments about how to govern the individual components of the system: should one rely on hierarchy and bureaucracy to transmit commands from centre to periphery, or should one, instead, trust to market forces, which send unambiguous signals to individual agents regarding desirable courses of action? Related to this latter point, it has been argued that there has been a transition in the way the state operates, encapsulated in the phrase 'from government to governance'.

State, market and community: understanding the shifting boundary between public and private provision

At the macro-level of political economy key issues concern the boundary between the public and private sectors, and the effects of contemporary economic and social changes on arrangements for delivering welfare. The boundary between public and private has been a 'moving frontier' (Finlayson 1994). Study of welfare state development has been prone to the identification of 'convergence' between states; regardless of political differences, the 'logic of industrialism' led inexorably towards large-scale hierarchical organisation of services, financed and provided by the state (Pierson 1998). There is a body of evidence in support of this contention. After all, states as diverse as the Soviet Union, the UK and the USA all appeared to have converged on hierarchical and regional forms of organisation of hospital provision. Such similarities led Flora and Heidenheimer (1981: 23) to suggest that because non-democratic and non-capitalist societies had established similar institutions, the welfare state was 'a more general form of modernisation'. More specifically, commentators have identified correspondences and temporal coincidences in forms of state intervention. Thus one rather glib explanation of the 1962 Hospital Plan was the diffusionist view that 'French-style economic planning spread across the channel' (Rodwin 1984). And Moran (1992), while not subscribing to a view of an inexorable convergence, nevertheless noted a tendency for hospital provision to become the responsibility of the state. Similar contentions about convergence are evident in respect of the NHS reforms, which were sometimes presented as an inevitable development, in which the NHS simply mimicked global trends from 'centralised institutions towards networks ... (and) from hierarchic top-down models to looser constellations' (Day and Klein 1989: 9).

These easy generalisations have been questioned by historians, who have challenged the implication that there was anything inevitable about a progression from a pre-war patchwork of voluntarist initiatives to the sunlit uplands of collectivism. Johnson (1996: 244–5) shows, for example, that most social risks have been met, most of the time, through a range of public or private sources, and that the 'redistributive intent and performance of any particular welfare structure was not a function of its location on the public/private axis' (p. 245). Harris (1992: 117) likewise points out that there is nothing inevitable about large-scale organisation; it is manifestly not the case that all societies have eliminated localism, pluralism and voluntarism in welfare delivery. Changes in the boundary between public and private sectors, and changes in policy within the public sector, have not always been in a predictable direction.

Instead of simply drawing attention to broad similarities in the welfare state, the contribution of Marxist theories has been to show how particular arrangements for welfare delivery are compatible (or not) with trends in capitalist economic development. Social scientists have drawn on the French 'regulationist' school of political economy, whose distinctive contribution is its emphasis on how capitalism, as a system of production, is stabilised by various social and institutional structures, including the welfare state. They focus in particular on the way in which the 'Fordist' era of mass production came to develop particular institutional arrangements for welfare delivery (Jessop 1991a, 1991b, 1992, 1995). The 'Fordist' era was allegedly charac-terised by mass inflexible production of standardised commodities and by strong vertical integration within large firms. The Keynesian welfare state (KWS) developed in parallel, offering a basic level of service to the great bulk of the population whose incomes did not permit them to purchase services privately. Only through state intervention could the problems of market failure, which had been evident in the inter-war years, be resolved. The KWS thus socialised the costs of welfare provision, but in doing so within tight fiscal parameters, it was only able to offer a basic, standardised level of service. Nevertheless, providing health, education and housing in this way helped stave off working-class demands for greater intervention, and appeared to be broadly compatible (affordable) with the post-war devel-opment of capitalism. Public ownership helped ensure this to the extent that it was a very effective way of containing costs. Standardised services seemed compatible with a broadly homogeneous society that was yet to experience post-war social differentiation. Bureaucratic and hierarchical, the NHS arguably began to develop some of the trappings of Fordism: one author rather superficially compared hospitals to 'factories in the Green Belt' (Murray 1991). There were also attempts to plan and organise hospital services, involving attempts at standardisation and system-building. These were initiated (Chapter 6) in response to heightened perceptions of economic decline in the late 1950s, the aim being to improve productivity in the public services, but the extent to which they were implemented was vari-able. Hence the extent to which the NHS became subject to 'Fordist' principles is questionable (and it could be argued that even to the extent that it was, the NHS has been (by European standards) unusually centralised, and therefore exceptional: Moran 1992).

Subsequent events have transformed the socio-economic landscape against which the KWS had been established. In terms of the organisation of produc-tion, although commentators disagree on many details, there seems to have been agreement that large-scale mass production of standard commodities has been superseded by small-scale, flexible production, organised not through vertically integrated corporations, but through dense and overlapping links between small firms. There are corresponding changes in the socio-economic structure as well; whereas Fordism was characterised by the mass-collective worker and a largely homogeneous working class, post-Fordism is said to exhibit a much more diverse and segmented social structure. For some writers these trends have had further correlates in patterns of consumption and political affiliation, leading to an enhanced consumerism rather than an unquestioning acceptance of centrally provided services, and to a progressive dealignment from traditional political affiliations. The effect is to undermine faith in the state as a provider of welfare, producing a much more pluralistic welfare system (Burrows and Loader 1994).

At the same time the globalisation of production is held to impose unbudgeable constraints on state intervention, although again the implications for welfare are disputed, with some writers contending that governments have rather more scope for manoeuvre than they wish to admit (compare Hay 1998; Taylor-Gooby 1997; Pierson 1998). These sets of developments lead to efforts to reorient the public sector towards the goals of innovation and competitiveness. Thus, rather than improve productivity through large-scale capital investment, state structures are reorganised in ways designed to inculcate flexibility and entrepreneurship (Jessop 1991a, 1995) and regulatory structures are 'hollowed out' (Jessop 1993).

On the face of it such a sequence might appear a fairly accurate description of events relating to hospital policy. As shown in Chapters 5 and 6, from the early 1950s there were concerns about the productivity of the NHS, the perceived need for scale economies and efficiency-raising capital investment, and the possibility of standardisation. In later decades there is more emphasis on diversification, choice, flexibility and localism, both within the NHS and through the growth of the private sector. However, does one have to buy the whole explanatory package here? Could the latter developments result from political pressures, seeking an ideological rationale for scaling back public expenditure in a restrictive economic climate? Could they merely reflect the exercise of preferences by a more diverse, consumerist population? The argument developed is that the strands in hospital policy are simply too diverse to be captured by an overarching logic founded on transitions in the organisation of production.

This, in turn, takes us into the terrain of arguments about the transition from an era of modernity to one of post-modernity. This issue is relevant because of the way the Hospital Plan might be thought to exemplify a commitment to the Enlightenment goals of instilling reason and order into human affairs. In attempting to root out small, inefficient relics of a bygone age, replacing them with a network of modern, efficient general hospitals, distributed according to a rationalist logic rather than the chance or choice of their founders, the Plan appeared eminently modernist (Chapter 6). However, for its critics, modernism is also associated with centralised and totalitarian, ultimately dehumanising, efforts to control social life, notably with respect to architecture and urban planning. In rejecting this, postmodernists celebrate diversity, difference, eclecticism and decentralisation, against the homogenising and centralising tendencies of modernism (Carter 1998).

There have been times at which these ideas seemed highly relevant to hospital policy. Though they would not necessarily have acknowledged a modernist/postmodernist dichotomy, critics of the Hospital Plan lamented its perceived homogenising tendencies, warned of the threat these posed to community effort (Chapter 6), and argued for decentralisation which would promote innovation and responsiveness. More generally the welfare state's universalistic and egalitarian aspirations have been criticised from both right and left. Proposals to re-engage communities in fundraising for and managing hospitals have therefore been welcomed as recognition of diversity and community identity, but critics would warn against neglecting structural inequalities in the ability of communities to initiate such developments (Taylor-Gooby 1997; Taylor 1998).

These arguments are helpful in placing hospital policy in its broader context – for example, in drawing attention to the process of regulatory trial-and-error that goes on as welfare states seek to come to terms with broader changes. But the applicability of such macro-scale theoretical abstractions to specific policy initiatives is questionable. In particular, the distinctive character of policy-making in medical care must be acknowledged. Tuohy (1999) makes relevant contributions here. Providing health care involves an asymmetric relationship between patient and doctor; the patient has little information, it is difficult to evaluate the product, and the costs of error are high. Medical professionals, being largely in control of information, have a substantial power base from which to resist change (Tuohy 1999: 11; see also Elston 1991; Cawson 1982). This can be overcome only when influences external to the health arena coalesce to bring it about. It means there is a considerable degree of path dependence in health-care policy; even ostensibly radical innovations, grand designs or blueprints become substantially diluted in practice (Chapter 9). This is why Tuohy (1999) suggests that health policy has an 'accidental logic'; it is why Harrison and Wood (2000) contend that what we see in health policy is less the unproblematic rolling-out of plans than the 'manipulated emergence' of policies whose outlines can be only dimly seen at first.

'Hierarchical regionalism' and the governance of health care

Below these macro-scale arguments, there are debates in hospital policy regarding the administrative structures through which national policy goals are to be realised on the ground. These essentially revolve around the necessity for, and the character of, the regional tier of management, and the key author in this context is Fox (1986).

Fox's work draws comparisons in the development of hospital policy between the USA and the UK. He discerns common ground between the two (while noting some differences) in terms of a commitment to 'hierarchical regionalism'. This is characterised as a 'particular logic of organisation based on a theory of how medical knowledge is discovered and disseminated' (p. ix). There are three key assumptions here. First, the causes of, and cures for, sickness are usually discovered in teaching hospitals or medical schools. Second, this knowledge is then disseminated down hierarchies of investigators, institutions and practitioners that serve particular geographical areas. Third, the goal of health policy should be to stimulate the creation of hierarchies in areas that lack them, and make existing ones operate more efficiently. By the second decade of the twentieth century, it was seen as 'self-evidently correct' that hierarchical regionalism (a descriptive, not judgemental, phrase, in Fox's words) was the appropriate *modus operandi* for the delivery of hospital care. It was hierarchical because the relative status of medical personnel was determined by their knowledge and skill, and by the complexity of the tasks they performed. Their workplaces should therefore relate to one another as an orderly pyramid. It was regional because it was believed that large geographical areas (whether or not coterminous with political jurisdictions) were the 'proper units for which to plan, administer and evaluate medical care'.

This is a reasonable description of the organisation of hospital care, but as an explanation of how policies develop it is limited. Regionalism meant such different things to different people and interest groups that it is hard to sustain Fox's view that it was a consensus matter. Webster (1990) points out the extent of opposition to regionalism from a range of sources, and criticises Fox for ignoring the conflicts between the various proposals for and proponents of regionalism. More generally, Webster is highly critical of Fox's contention that regionalism had settled the question of how hospital services were to be organised: 'if the logic of science was so compelling', why did it take so long to establish regionalism (p. 133)? The reason, of course, is that proposals for regionalism confronted vested interests which blocked, or sought to subvert, change (Chapters 3 and 4). Only with determined political intervention was regionalism instituted. Fox presents the outlines of a plausible case, because there certainly was extensive debate about forms of organisation which would secure coordination above the level of an individual hospital, but he underplays the conflicts over the issue. It might, nevertheless, be argued that, by the time of the Hospital Plan, there was much more agreement than in the inter-war years. The goal of policy by then was to establish hierarchies around DGHs, with referral links up to regional specialities located in teaching hospitals, and links down to satellite hospitals for less-intensive forms of treatment. The issue then becomes one of the extent to which such a blueprint has been followed through. Hospital policy has been characterised by trade-offs between professional considerations (for instance the availability of adequate specialist support, or the need (to satisfy training requirements) for a threshold level of patient throughput, social issues (such as accessibility), and economic questions (affordability and economies of scale). In combination these interacted with local loyalties to individual institutions to blur the neat outlines of top-down blueprints.

Two related questions flow from this. The first concerns the kind of 'regional' structures most appropriate to hospital development. There have consequently been debates about definitions of what counts as 'regions', how they were to be delimited, and what roles and powers they were to have. Second, there have been debates about accountability, and the relationships between hospitals and their communities. A persistent criticism of the NHS has been that, by taking the hospitals out of local control, public participation in the running of the service was limited from the start. This criticism arose in slightly different forms, in relation to both the Hospital Plan and the 1991 NHS reforms: opponents of both saw in them the danger of an administrative logic severing hospitals from their communities. The issue resurfaced in debates about the post-reform rationalisation of London's hospitals and also in opposition to PFI developments. Should the contribution of an institution be evaluated in terms purely of its place in an administrative hierarchy, or of its 'success' (or otherwise) in attracting contracts? Or should a broader set of criteria hold sway? This might in turn raise questions about democratic input into decisions on hospital closures, and about just who runs institutions. These issues are at the heart of various recent proposals to transfer hospitals to community 'ownership' (Ham 1996; Bosanquet 1999), involving much greater local fundraising and management. However, such localism also raises questions about the criteria by which the trajectory of hospital development is to be determined.

Steering mechanisms: markets, hierarchies and networks

The third theme considered relates to the criteria by which decisions are taken about the future of individual units within the hospital system. One way in which this has been conceptualised is in terms of a move from markets, to hierarchies, to networked forms of organisation. This would suggest, very schematically, that prior to 1948 hospital development was a function of market forces; that this was superseded on the Appointed Day by a rational and hierarchical system of planning; when that system collapsed it, in turn, was superseded by markets; in turn, when they once again failed, they were replaced by a hybrid, networked form of organisation.

There are at least two key issues that follow from this very bald caricature of the actual situation. They will be explored in more depth as the book proceeds. They relate to the sense in which these organisational forms exist independently of one another and in a pure form, and second to the senses in which any such organisational form can be said to have 'failed' and thus become ripe for overthrow.

Taking the case of markets, first of all, many analysts hold that markets do not exist in a pure form independent of broader social and institutional contexts. This means that market forces are modified and kept in check, in various ways. It might be said that the pre-NHS hospital system 'approximated to a market' (Webster 1995), since the availability of consultant staff at hospitals depended on the prospects for private practice in any given locality. However, in the inter-war years there were various proposals and attempts to regulate market forces, and there were also hesitant moves in the direction of 'networks', in the form of varying degrees of collaboration between voluntary and municipal hospitals (Chapters 2 and 3). Indeed there were even proposals to create, in the wartime years, a mixed economy of welfare not without resemblance to the arrangements eventually adopted after 1991 (Chapter 4).

The era of 'planning' and hierarchical organisation might at first appear more clear-cut. One can identify a start date (1948, though some might go for the establishment of the EMS (Emergency Medical Service) in 1938), and a high point (the Hospital Plan, which appeared to map out a clear blueprint for the future trajectory of development). But when did the era of 'planning' terminate? The word 'Plan' was quietly dropped in published revisions; insiders contend it was dead within 3 years of being launched; others might argue for the oil crisis, which led to swingeing cutbacks (Chapter 7); alternatively a case might be made that old-style planning was going on as late as 1991 (Chapter 8). It very much depends on how one defines 'planning'. The term implies vision, strategy, rationality, giving orders and having the capacity to carry them out. Very obviously, the process of hospital development did not live up to these ideals, and part of the aim of the book is to evaluate the rather exaggerated claims for the coherence of the 1962 Plan. It is helpful here to refer to statements about what planning can, and cannot, achieve in a political context. Small (1990: 125–7) argues that planning adopts a 'mode of rationality that emphasises the instrumental and the technical'. This serves to narrow the terms of debate, because policy is preoccupied with predicting from the existing state of affairs and there is reluctance to question fundamental assumptions. Debate takes place in a language that is specialised, ambiguous and arcane: Parston (1980: 159) talks of statements 'so vaguely drafted that they are too good to be critically questioned'. This is the terrain of Edelman's (1971) pioneering exploration of the symbolic uses of political language, but it has links to Alford's (1975) analysis, which shows how the structures and language of policy debate serve to marginalise certain interest groups. On this view, planning is a communicative process which risks being neither comprehensible nor sincere (Small 1990), but one which ends up claiming more than it can actually deliver. There is certainly evidence that this is the case in the context of the 1962 Plan. There were also constraints on the Plan's implementation, resulting from its dependence on many influences and variables, from the state of the economy to the agreement of doctors and planners on local hospital configurations; planning was thus a long way from the exercise of hierarchical, bureaucratic authority.

The same might, of course, be said for markets – and indeed for what many claim to be their successor: networked forms of organisation. The argument that the post-1991 internal market was in fact a tightly managed one has become standard currency (e.g. Light 1997; Paton 2000) because it was established within constrained parameters by a government that could not afford the risk of market failure. The Conservative government thus had to soften their pro-market rhetoric. The problem was somewhat more difficult for Labour because they continued to operate the market while denying that they were doing so. This meant asserting a language of cooperation, partnerships and networks, while simultaneously imposing central targets and relying on quasi-commercial criteria to allocate capital. The emphasis on collaboration, partnership and so on is welcome to the extent that it signals efforts to avoid the worst consequences of competition. But whether this represents a truly novel form of organisation is questionable (Chapter 9).

It is therefore one aim of the book to consider the extent to which this 'markets–hierarchies–networks' periodisation is a valid characterisation of events in the hospital sector. From these introductory comments, what we are likely to find is the co-existence of elements of each rather than failure, and the supersession of one by another. This is because it is arguable that neither 'pure' markets nor 'pure' hierarchies have really been tried; to what extent, therefore, can they be said to have 'failed'? Various suggestions have been made. The pre-NHS system was found wanting for its lack of comprehensiveness and inequity – but this may be judging it by *post hoc* collectivist criteria. Conversely, the question of government failure has, Le Grand (1991) suggests, received less attention than market failure. Some commentators (e.g. Offe 1984) point to the gap between the intentions and outcomes of state intervention, and to the consequent loss of legitimacy, and argue that these are an inevitable consequence of the contradictory pressures on the capitalist state. Le Grand's (1991) elements of failure are more narrowly drawn – relating to inefficiencies and inequities of state intervention – and the degree to which these are tolerable is ultimately a political judgement. The question of failure might, instead, be rephrased as one of whether policies are *deemed* to have failed. Thus, drawing on arguments based on a linguistic turn in political and cultural theory, the real value of periodisations such as these may be to define innovations with respect to their opposite. Rhetorical antitheses thus create discursive space in which novel solutions seem feasible and indeed inevitable. It was thus in the interests of pro-market advocates to exaggerate the extent of hierarchical bureaucracy in the NHS; it was certainly in the interests of new Labour to make a case that the internal market had failed and that what was needed was a 'third way' (Paton 2000). We need to look beneath the surface of such apparently straightforward rhetorical devices.

From governance to government ... and back again?

The historical account given here covers a period in which social scientists have first of all developed, and then moved away from, explanatory models which stress the power of government to achieve its aims. This is not just a matter of rejecting ideal-typical models of political systems, or of policy-making. Instead it might better be seen as an acknowledgement that the era has passed in which states appeared to wield considerable power. Discussion has thus moved from govern*ment* to govern*ance*.

External circumstances have forced a reappraisal of constraints on state power, especially in the context of an open international economy. Marxists emphasised the irreconcilable nature of demands placed upon the state, while the new right pointed to the epistemological impossibility of planning: governments could never hope to process all the information needed in order to steer the economy. For these and other reasons, political scientists began to question the validity of the centralist – or 'Westminster' – model of policy-making. In this model, Britain is seen as a unitary state, in which substantial power is vested in the executive, especially when backed by a strong Parliamentary majority (Gamble 1990: 407). The implication is that strong hierarchical authority can be exercised. However, Rhodes (1997) argues that this view needs to be qualified. He speaks of a 'differentiated polity' in which the exercise of power relies on networks of relationships between institutions and organisations on which the central state is ultimately dependent. In this view, the activities of central government departments require the sanction of various institutional mechanisms for coordinating policy (Rhodes 1992: 76). These mechanisms include Cabinet and its associated committees, but a key constraint on individual departments, which has been crucial for decisions on hospital expenditure, has been the Treasury (Lowe 1998: 43–5). *Primus inter pares* among government departments, it often seems to be the case that the baleful gaze of the Treasury 'orthodoxy' has led to automatic dismissal of proposals for additional expenditure. Understanding the exchanges between the Treasury and the Ministry of Health is important because it demonstrates the tensions which developed between providing services in a decommodified form and the economic orthodoxy espoused by the Treasury, against which the Ministry of Health was judged (see Chapter 6).

Rhodes goes on to suggest that even when departments have obtained support for their policies, they are still dependent on agencies to achieve their goals. Power is thus relational, not an object or a quantum of resource. It 'depends on relationships between actors and not on command'. Even an apparently hierarchical exercise like the Hospital Plan (Chapter 6) depended on the competence of health boards, their relationships with the Ministry and local authorities, the strength of medical lobbies, and the state of the building industry. Power is not just exercised in high-profile confrontation and negotiation, but in 'every situation and relationship [in which] actors develop strategies and alliances in order to exchange resources and achieve goals' (M. Smith 1998: 67–8). The power of actors and institutions varies according to policy, tactics and context, and commentators therefore suggest that we should replace analyses of the hierarchical exercise of power by governments, with discussions of the allocation of resources through interactions within self-organising networks. This is summarised as a shift from government to governance.

Etymologically, governance refers to the 'modes and manner of governing, government [refers] to the institutions and agents charged with governing, and governing [refers] to the act of governing itself' (Jessop 1998: 30). Uses of the term governance need not be confined to the activities of the state; the term could refer to any mode of coordination of interdependent activities. The term has become fashionable because of new debates about ways of governing. Critiques of state failure, and the march of privatisation, led to talk of the 'new public management' in which, in Osborne and Gaebler's (1992) formulation, the task of government was one of 'steering not rowing': policy decisions (steering) are taken by government, but service delivery (rowing) can be done by any organisation, and preferably not by bureaucracies. In the place of sovereign authorities there is a multiplicity of actors at various levels. Command bureaucracies are replaced by a range of service providers (public, private, voluntary) which relate to one another in complex ways. What matters is not who delivers services; 'what counts is what works' in New Labour's pragmatic phraseology.

It follows from this that the state has lost several functions. It has been 'hollowed out' (Jessop, 1993). Powers have been displaced upwards (e.g. to the EU) and downwards (e.g. to regional or local authorities) This has reignited arguments about the respective role of regional and local tiers of authority in the NHS. Functions are carried out by alternative delivery systems (agencies, private contractors). Delivery of services may entail interactions between many organisations. However, just as state failure may result from the limitations of bureaucracy, so the new public management may have its own limitations. The separation of purchasing and providing responsibilities in the NHS has given freedoms to agencies which may be used in ways which are self-interestedly rational but collectively dysfunctional (Chapter 9). In turn this may give rise to demands for new forms of regulation. Moreover, governance would appear to imply decentralisation, but new Labour can hardly be characterised as a 'hands-off' government in respect of the NHS.

Many commentators have been impressed by the apparent novelty of these developments – consider the vigour of debates about public–private partnerships in urban policy, for example – but in the case of hospital provision they may represent a reversion. Inter-war hospital policy – insofar as there was one – surely involved arrangements which carry familiar echoes of current debates about governance. These include emphases on the supervisory role of the Ministry of Health, reliance on voluntary cooperation and/or public-private collaboration, and some financial instruments (the processes whereby loans for new hospital development were sanctioned) (Chapter 3). Much wartime debate concerned how better arrangements might be devised for the governance of the inherited patchwork of services (Chapter 4). Before the state could be 'hollowed out' at the end of the twentieth century, therefore, it first had to be filled out in the post-war period (Lowe and Rollings 2000: 100). The relative success or failure of these diverse steering mechanisms is a key theme of this book.

A final insight may be provided by Foucauldian and other accounts of relationships between civil society and the state. Against arguments which suggest that the public is excluded from control of services by their technical complexities, some contend that the era of governance has the potential for greater citizen engagement, by opening up scope for community control of welfare services. Hirst (1994) takes this further in his radical proposals for a pluralist welfare system (see also Hirst's (1999) exchange with Stears (1999)).

This progressive vision is challenged by others for whom new 'govern-mentalities' (ways of thinking about governing) are emerging. Specifically, more responsibilities are devolved to individuals and communities, and as a result new relationships emerge between government and forms of self-government. New freedoms are thus allocated to individuals and communities, who become autonomous actors who are deemed responsible, through their individual choices, for their own welfare. Rose (1996) sees this as the 'governance of the social': the impersonal, paternalistic and bureau-cratic state is transformed into a 'supervisory' state. While the state still provides resources, it also signals to communities that they must develop their own strategies for self-help and self-management. Government seeks to act upon individuals through their supposed allegiance to particular communities (Murdoch 1997: 112). State intervention thus becomes much more selective; 'discourses of community, locality and diversity ... [are used] to promote a profound shift in state–society relations' (Murdoch 1997: 116–17). The success of neoliberal parties in recent years is thus to be explained in terms of re-establishing a sphere of freedom in which the 'language of the entrepreneurial individual predominate(s) over almost any other in evaluations of the ethical claims of political power and programmes of government' (Rose and Miller 1992: 200). The result (see Chapter 9 on charitable initiative and commercial hospitals) may be a more localist and less egalitarian pattern of services. The key point about governmentality is that it enlists individuals and communities in a strategy for delivering welfare which may be neither progressive nor participatory.

Geography, 'place' and health care

Geography ought to feature more strongly in accounts of the welfare state than it actually does. This is not so much an attempt to plant a flag on academic territory, but more a recognition of the universalising aspirations of the welfare state. These have not been realised and thus differences in the availability of care provide an important channel by which 'social inequality permeates the NHS' (Townsend *et al.* 1992: 81). More generally Powell (1995) contends that territorial justice and accessibility are neglected in Le Grand's (1982) classic evaluation of the degree of equality in the welfare state.

When geographers initially took an interest in the distribution of hospital services they did so from a quantitative, rather technocratic standpoint. Mayhew's (1986) study of the historical development of the London hospital system is a good example. He obtained data on hospital location and bed provision for all hospitals within an arbitrary (50 km) radius of Charing Cross. Via a range of complex mathematical techniques he then assessed the relationships between hospital development and population distribution. Similarly Cowan (1963, 1965, 1967, 1969) attempted to derive a theory of hospital location *post hoc*, as it were, from an examination of their existing pattern. He found a 'strong correlation' between the location of public (local authority) hospitals and 'cemeteries, burial grounds, gasworks and other indicators of low land values' (Cowan 1965: 418). He also attributed the spatial pattern of the voluntary hospitals to the iron laws of the market. Central locations facilitated the attraction of voluntary support and minimised travel time for consultants. Similarly the location of mental hospitals was explained in terms of their large land requirements and the importance of therapeutic sites. A weakness of these analyses, however, was the treatment of all sorts of different institutions purely as points on a map. Thus, 2,000-bed psychiatric hospitals, 1,000-bed teaching hospitals, and 50-bed cottage hospitals were treated as logically equivalent except in terms of size. Yet the underlying processes producing these patterns of services varied considerably. Hospitals could have been located in a particular place for very different reasons: the *ad hoc* localism of the voluntary system; the spatial separation of the rural asylums; the need to avoid bomb damage, which produced some dispersal of capacity via the wartime EMS; and the (constrained) rationality of public sector planning. And alternative ways of delivery treatment or administering health care might have had rather different locational outcomes.

This might be viewed as counterfactual speculation but the point is that alternatives were possible. Neither Cowan nor Mayhew raise such issues. Other work has contributed much to debates about the influence of accessibility on the utilisation of health services, which has been an important technical issue in debates about resource allocation (Royston *et al.* 1992; Sheldon *et al.* 1994). The accessibility consequences of strategies for community hospital development were also a key focus of work by Haynes and Bentham (1979).

Such approaches clearly help evaluate the degree of equity in a pattern of service provision, and may even offer broad criteria by which to plan services. However, *explaining* the evolution of systems of hospitals requires a rather different approach, which seeks to reconstruct the opportunities and constraints affecting decisions. Most examples in this book are drawn from the area served by the Newcastle Regional Hospital Board (RHB) and its successor authorities. Given its social and economic history there were some rather obvious constraints on hospital development. In much of this region subsidence resulting from coal mining affected many potential sites. Second, local authority policies, and those of other public and private agencies, often meant either that desirable locations were unavailable or that they could not be developed in a way conducive to hospital provision. The National Coal Board (NCB) effectively had priority in determining land-use patterns; if workable coal reserves existed, they could veto development. More generally, even where plots of land were available, hospital authorities were not permitted to acquire and retain them indefinitely and so site availability was a key consideration. Hospital projects could move up and down the planners' pecking order because a lease expired or because a site became available. Hospital authorities had no priority claims on land. It was said that, when local authorities ceased to be responsible for hospital provision, 'hospitals went to the bottom of the queue for land requirements'.[1] Public bodies, such as local government, or New Town Development Corporations, were reluctant to 'sterilise' large areas of land pending a proposal finding its way into the NHS's capital programme. These are narrowly technical considerations up to a point, but arguments about hospital siting raise wider questions about the priorities of state agencies and the relationships between them.

Constraints were also imposed by the pre-existing settlement pattern. Here the legacy of industrialisation in the region left its mark. Outside the principal industrial estuaries, the region was characterised by a dispersed pattern of small settlements usually built to house the labour force of the local mine, steelworks or shipyard. This meant that for facilities which served a larger population, such as general hospitals, arguments would invariably arise about where best to locate them. South East Northumberland was a case in point. The towns of Ashington, Blyth, Morpeth and (from the 1960s) the new town of Cramlington, were all regarded as too small individually for a general hospital but the area required more than the scattered cottage or accident hospitals which it had inherited. Nonetheless the first 30 years of the NHS were marked by continual, though inconclusive, discussions about how best to serve this population. Populations and hospital catchments were vigorously disputed, but issues were never satisfactorily resolved, perhaps because of the political problems attending major reconfigurations of services.[2]

There is a tendency here to present geography simply as a matter of physical constraint but recent developments in the social sciences suggest that, instead, geography is crucial to contextually sensitive explanations of social phenomena. The implication is not just that policies need to be spatially sensitive, or that policies do not just roll out unproblematically over space. Rather, the socio-economic landscape against which policies are implemented is crucial to an understanding of policy development. Tuohy (1999: 18–19) captures something of this in suggesting that a feature which is important to understanding health policy is its 'essentially local base'. Economies of scale are not feasible beyond a certain level so the delivery of services is decentralised and characterised by local monopoly or oligopoly. Moreover, relationships between medical practitioners, hospitals and local institutional structures may become 'embedded' through routine. This is likely to have effects on policy outcomes, as can be seen from an examination of the NHS reforms; for example, close local ties between purchasers and providers served to limit the amount of change that took place (Chapter 9). Tuohy's point also implies that local contextual circumstances may play a crucial role in determining the trajectory of service development. Vociferous medical and political lobbies, cohering around either a perceived threat to, or a novel vision of, service development, are one obvious illustration (Chapter 7). Alternatively, the socio-economic landscape, against which reforms in the welfare state are played out, may itself be influential. For example, one plausible interpretation of recent developments in British social policy is as a strategy designed selectively to appeal to particular socio-economic groups concentrated in particular regions (Jessop *et al.* (1988); Mohan (1998) applies these arguments to the NHS). It is also arguable that some proposals for greater state intervention in hospital provision emerged in the inter-war period in locations where voluntarism and self-help were most severely challenged (Chapter 3).

These comments suggest the importance of a geographical approach which is sensitive to the 'difference that space makes' (Sayer 1985) to the operation of social processes. There has been a tendency in the NHS to see events through the 'distorting prism' of London (Day and Klein 1991). This book tries to redress that through a rather different prism by focusing on the Newcastle Regional Hospital Board and its successor authorities. This is a quite distinctive context. The industrial legacy has been noted. In addition, the distinctive character of local politics, and the perception that a major modernisation of the region's infrastructure was desirable, came to shape public policy in specific ways which had ramifications for the development of health service policy. This can be traced to wartime statements, in the Hospital Surveys and elsewhere.

First, recognition of the dependence of much of the region on the coal industry led to awareness that future planning proposals 'ought not to be too rigid'. Thus:

> the future prospects of industry in the North East are still uncertain, and the possibility that there may be important changes in the size of the population in some areas must be taken into consideration in any reorganisation of the hospital services.
>
> (Pepler and Macfarlane 1949: 4)

Inter-war discussions of the collapse of coal-mining in West Durham had led to proposals for selective disinvestment in – even demolition of – mining villages and, as a corollary, spatially concentrated public sector investment in locations deemed to possess growth potential (Hudson 1989). The objective was to assemble pools of labour of sufficient size to attract new inward investment. Plans for hospital services therefore had to take account of, and be coordinated with, those of other state agencies such as New Town Development Corporations (NTDCs)[3] (see Chapters 5 and 7).

The assumption that a spatially selective pattern of infrastructural investment was essential to the region's future prosperity was one which cut across political divides, and led to protracted disputes over hospital investment. Most obviously, projects moved up and down the agenda of the hospital authorities not solely according to relative need but also depending on the importance of a particular locality to economic development. The perceived need to modernise the infrastructure of Teesside, which was seen as a crucial growth point for the region, is a case in point, but a corollary was that other locations slipped down the list of priorities. Elsewhere, prominent regional politicians promoted a vision of Newcastle as a modern regional capital with an infrastructure to match. Their interests converged with those of the Medical School and the University on an alternative to the RHBs strategy for the city, provoking a dispute which ran for several years (Chapter 7). The formulation of a regional strategy was influenced to a substantial degree, then, by the quite specific political circumstances obtaining in the region, and the associated consensus on how best to modernise the infrastructure.

The interactions between national hospital policy and its local outcomes are, therefore, a key theme of this book. The intention is to show that just as an historical approach is necessary to put social policies in their temporal context, so too a geographical approach is necessary to fully comprehend how policies work out in their spatial context.

Outline of the book

The broad approach taken is chronological and in some – but not all – respects the periodisation used is determined by key events. First, the legacy of services inherited by the NHS is considered; an attempt is made to assess the adequacy of services and consider evidence as to whether the public-private mix may be deemed to have failed (Chapter 2). Various responses to inter-war difficulties are reviewed (Chapter 3) and this throws light on substantial differences of opinion about how best to secure improved access to health care, as well as illuminating the strengths and weaknesses of 'partnership' arrangements. Chapter 4 switches attention to wartime debates about the future organisation of health care, drawing extensively on Ministry of Health papers. The purpose here is to assess whether or not the various wartime proposals could have worked, and whether there were realistic alternatives to nationalisation.

Three chapters then trace events leading to the formulation of the 1962 Hospital Plan. The focus of Chapter 5 is on criteria used for the allocation of capital in the public sector. Whereas previous commentaries have emphasised the low political priority given to the NHS, and the relative weakness of health ministers, there is evidence that the Ministry of Health had difficulties in demonstrating to a sceptical Treasury what returns would be achieved by building hospitals. The consequence was a minuscule capital programme and the implications of this for hospital development in the Newcastle RHB are illustrated. Although some of the Treasury's objections were eventually overcome, the rather rushed preparation of the subsequent Hospital Plan casts doubt upon the status it has been accorded. Chapter 6 presents a detailed analysis and critique of the formulation of this Plan; as an exercise in evidence-based policy it plainly had severe limitations, while the planning capacities of the regional authorities varied considerably. With hindsight, this 'Plan' might better be seen as simply a commitment to an increase in the rate of growth of NHS capital resources.

Periodisation of subsequent events poses the challenge of identifying at what point (if ever) the era of 'planning', inaugurated in 1948, can be said to have ended. The implementation of the NHS reforms from 1991 was one obvious milestone, but how best to divide up the twenty-nine years between 1962 and then? This period was characterised by a gradual loss of faith in planning, which was in evidence before the Conservatives returned to office in 1979. A division into pre- and post-1979 periods thus seemed facile. However, the alternative – of a focus on the 1962–91 period as having some kind of unity – also posed problems. The implication would be that there had *never* been any serious attempt at implementing the Plan; that the era of planning simply ended with the Plan's announcement. Now, given the weak foundations on which the Plan rested, this might appear defensible, and indeed the word 'Plan' was dropped from official pronouncements within four years. However, discussions between Ministry and regions indicate a serious attempt to produce, on the ground, the pattern of services envisioned by the Plan, but a division is made here between events before and after 1973, when the increase in oil prices undermined the growth assumptions on which the Plan had been based. Chapter 7 thus charts the uncertain progress of hospital development from 1962 and it also analyses ongoing debates about the size of hospitals in which professional considerations played a major role, and discusses community resistance to the modernising and rationalising tendencies of the Plan.

Chapter 8 then considers subsequent developments to 1991. There is, first, evidence about the continued difficulties of maintaining the capital programme. Simultaneously there were proposals for more localist forms of development – e.g. the community hospitals movement, and emphases in policy on the retention of physical assets. Other developments are also notable: the expansion of the private medical sector, an increase in charitable fundraising, and reliance on proceeds of land sales all symbolised the way access to care depended to a greater extent on a market allocation of resources. The contention is that while there remained a hospital building programme, whether there was a coherent hospital *policy* is debatable.

Finally, Chapter 9 analyses the impacts on hospital policy of key developments from 1991. First, the implementation difficulties associated with the internal market, and the responses to them (in terms of regulating the market) are analysed. Second, there is consideration of how individual hospitals and communities are responding to the changed external environment, by diversifying their sources of capital, and in some cases by returning hospitals to charitable trusts. Finally, the chapter concludes with a critical assessment of the development and effects of the Private Finance Initiative (PFI) which introduced *de facto* commercial criteria into the process of hospital development.

The concluding chapter reflects on the continuities and discontinuities evident in this discussion of hospital policy. It questions some of the neat periodisations offered in previous work. There is a view advanced by some commentators that the events charted here are simply local manifestations of technical developments (i.e. the changing role of the hospital) and of globalising pressures, which are forcing welfare states down the same inevitable path of market-led reform. In contrast, it is argued that (even in a context of substantial growth in resources) there are risks for the NHS in the rather unreflective drift of policies driven by agnosticism and pragmatism.

The book draws on a range of statistical and documentary sources details of which are given in endnotes. For ease of reference various figures to which reference is made in more than one chapter are presented in an appendix, which thus provides a broad overview of trends in the hospital services nationally and locally. There is also a brief guide to changing administrative structures and to the roles of organisational entities within them.

2 Legacies, donations and municipal priorities

The development of the hospital services prior to 1948

The pattern of hospital provision prior to the NHS is often summed up with reference to two key comments. First, there is Aneurin Bevan's argument, in the Second Reading of the NHS Bill, that the 'caprice of charity' determined the pattern of provision, so that the 'best hospital facilities were available where they were least needed'.[1] Second, there is Abel-Smith's (1964: 405) contention that the distribution of voluntary hospitals depended on the 'donations of the living and the legacies of the dead'. Such ringing phrases have acquired the status of a conventional wisdom, being recycled, as Powell (1997: 30–1) points out, by many commentators. Others have questioned such pessimistic judgements, contending that the voluntary system was thriving prior to 1948. Thus, Seldon (quoted in Green (1996: 37), argues that, but for nationalisation, the voluntary sector would have continued, like a 'galloping horse', to expand hospital services.

In an era during which the institutions of the post-war welfare state have been heavily criticised, some have argued that the pre-1948 period offers potential lessons for policy. The emphasis is on harnessing the perceived flexibility and capacity to innovate of the voluntary sector within a framework in which the state underwrites comprehensive service provision (Ham 1996; Hirst 1994). In addition, the contemporary vogue for 'partnerships' in social policy invites an examination of the impact of those partnerships which operated in the past. As Finlayson (1994) puts it, the inter-war period was a mixed economy of welfare, characterised by a 'moving frontier' between state, market and voluntary provision of services. The precise quantity and quality of services varied from place to place. Resolving problems, whether of duplication or deficiency, required collaboration, either within the private (voluntary) or public (local authority) sectors, or between them.

The aim of this chapter is therefore to examine the extent to which pre-1948 arrangements had produced a comprehensive service in the Northern region of England. This will provide a baseline against which to assess the success of the NHS in rectifying deficiencies. First there is an overview of the scale and character of voluntary and municipal provision. I then consider the strengths and weaknesses of voluntary and municipal provision, in relation to levels of provision and utilisation, financial stability and service quality. Finally, some preliminary proposals for post-war development are discussed.

Voluntary and municipal hospital provision: an historical overview

Prior to 1948, there were two principal forms of hospital provision in Britain: the voluntary and municipal hospitals. The former embodied a long tradition of voluntary service: doctors gave their services on an honorary basis, earning a living from private practice. They largely catered for those unable to afford the services of a private physician but whose income rendered them ineligible for the Poor Law medical service. Over time, however, patient payments, assessed in relation to means, came to play a growing role in hospital finance. In addition many institutions developed contributory schemes, based on weekly contributions from workers, in some cases gathered by deduction from wage packets, with additional contributions from employers.

Voluntary hospitals were established for a number of reasons (Granshaw 1989; Marland 1987; Pickstone 1985) and their distribution thus tended to be idiosyncratic. Municipal hospital provision was based on the somewhat unpromising foundations of the Poor Law medical service, which was available to the impoverished, the elderly and the chronically ill. Given the philosophy of 'less eligibility' which underpinned the 1834 Poor Laws, conditions in such facilities were generally poor and local authority facilities were built cheaply, often on isolated sites (Allen 1979: 10). Poor Law legislation was discretionary and permissive, so there was great variability, but some authorities actively expanded hospital provision to the point where the 1909 Royal Commission on the Poor Law commented that, in some locations, the Poor Law had, *de facto*, become the principal provider of general hospital services. Local authorities also assumed greater responsibilities over time for the treatment of infectious diseases and TB, and for the provision of maternity and child welfare services. But the extent to which local authorities actually exercised their powers varied greatly. This was also true after the passage of the 1929 Local Government Act, the purpose of which was to rationalise public provision and promote greater public–private coordination. Hospital provision had therefore developed according to quite different principles: the *ad hoc* logic of competitive voluntarism and the priorities and financial resources of local authorities.

The contrasts between the two systems are well illustrated in Tables 2.1 and 2.2, which indicate a quite different profile in terms of hospital size and function. Voluntary hospitals had conventionally been identified with the best traditions of medical practice and in particular with high-quality care available in teaching hospitals. However, there was considerable variability; many small institutions lacked resident medical staff and received only occasional visitations from consultants. The growth of specialist units rendered many institutions uneconomic and difficult to staff; this was particularly so with respect to nurses. Some 74 per cent of voluntary hospitals had 100 beds or less, and 33 per cent (345) had no more than thirty beds, while only 2 per cent (19) provided 500 beds or more. Municipal institutions were typically much larger: 55 per cent (230) hospitals had at least 100 beds and seventy-one (17 per cent) over 500 (NPHT 1946). The size of many municipal

Table 2.1 Size distribution of hospitals in England and Wales, 1938 [a]

Number of beds	Voluntary Number	Voluntary Per cent	Municipal Number	Municipal Per cent
	Type of hospital			
30	345	33	96	22
30–100	434	41	99	23
100–500	256	24	159	38
500	19	2	71	17
Total	1,054	100	425	100

Source: Summary Statistics from the Hospital Surveys – held in PRO MH 80/34.

a This is clearly only a sample of hospital accommodation, since at the inception of the NHS over 3,000 hospitals were taken over. However the basis of the sample, and its spatial coverage, were not given. It appears to exclude chronic and isolation hospitals (compare totals with table 2.2)

Table 2.2 Functions of non-psychiatric voluntary and municipal hospitals in England and Wales [a]

Speciality	Voluntary Hospitals	Voluntary Beds	Municipal Hospitals	Municipal Beds	Total[b] Hospitals	Total[b] Beds	Total available beds[c]
			Type of hospital				
General acute	711	60,198	162	69,135	873	129,333	141,721
Special	196	16,105	31	8,543	227	24,648	26,956
Chronic	27	1,730	377	49,199	404	50,929	59,211
TB	66	7,330	134	14,389	200	21,719	27,402
Maternity	54	1,819	98	2,034	152	3,853	4,039
Isolation	3	297	636	42,725	639	43,022	43,665
Totals	1,057	87,479	1,438	186,025	2,495	273,504	302,994

Source: Statistics held in PRO MH 80/34.

a Data refer to 1938 apart from those for total available beds, which are *net* figures for an unspecified date towards the end of the war – see also note 3.
b Since the NHS initially involved state control of over 3,000 hospitals, these figures are evidently incomplete. However, the basis on which they were gathered was not given.
c These figures comprise the total beds available in 1938, *plus* beds provided in EMS (Emergency Medical Service) units, *minus* beds lost through wartime damage. The *net* gain in beds was therefore approximately 30,000. Though the exact date at which these statistics were gathered was not given, from the dates on other papers in this file it seems reasonable to infer that the data refer to late 1944 or early 1945.

hospitals reflected their origins as Poor Law institutions and the obligations imposed on local authorities to treat infectious and chronic diseases. In addition, some municipal authorities recognised the importance of scale and integration, and therefore provided larger institutions than the typical voluntaries. Hollingsworth and Hollingsworth (1985) also identify important differences in the quality of hospital services, with the voluntaries typically spending substantially more than municipal hospitals per bed, reflecting greater capitalisation and better staffing ratios.

The extent to which hospital provision developed depended to a large degree on locally available financial resources. Given the uneven development of the British economy from the nineteenth century, we would expect variability in provision. Mean levels of voluntary bed provision rose nearly threefold between 1871 and 1938, from 0.5 to 1.4 beds per 1,000 population for British counties, but there were variations around this. Typically, high levels of provision were to be found in London and in numerous counties in the south-east and south-west of England. Levels of provision declined in a northerly direction, and were lowest in rural parts of Wales and Scotland. Variability in provision declined over time, as shown by analysis of trends in coefficients of variation (Gorsky *et al.* 1999, Table 2). Such convergence partly reflected the foundation of new hospitals in locations which previously lacked them. Even so, and considering voluntary provision alone, substantial disparities remained. In 1938 six County Boroughs (CBs) had bed:population ratios of greater than 5 voluntary beds/1,000 population, namely Oxford (7.2), Canterbury (7.1), Bath (6.4), Exeter (5.6), Northampton (5.1) and Chester (5.0). Provision in boroughs such as Salford, Rochdale, West Hartlepool and Stockport was characteristically a quarter of this level. Powell's (1992) analysis indicates, however, that the degree of territorial (in)justice in hospital provision did not really lend weight to Bevan's assertions about inequity.

To what extent did municipal provision improve the position? There is some evidence – for example, negative correlations between municipal and voluntary provision (Powell 1992) – which indicates that, for county boroughs at least, municipal provision helped to reduce inequalities in access. Indeed, some local authorities, such as the London County Council (LCC) developed substantial services. Such authorities were the exception, rather than the rule, and commentators associated with the SMA (Socialist Medical Association) cautioned against overgeneralising from conditions in or around London (Stewart 1999: 140). However, the most impoverished local authorities were often unable or reluctant to develop hospital services. Needy areas thus remained underserved (Webster 1982, 1985). Sometimes political will was absent: over three decades after the establishment of the NHS, Kent MPs, who were bemoaning the slow pace of redistribution from London, were reminded that part of the problem was the limited inheritance; the county council had neglected to develop a general hospital service before the war.[2]

The overall picture is thus one of an uneven patchwork of services, variable in quality and quantity and from place to place. The strengths and weaknesses of this system are now illustrated with reference to national statistics and to the experience of the North East of England. This allows a picture to be presented of the challenges to be faced by post-war planning. It also illustrates why questions came to be raised about the extent to which the inter-war public-private mix for health care could deliver an equitable pattern of provision. The focus here is principally upon assessing the state of the region's hospitals on the eve of World War II, which permits consideration of the impact of municipal provision in the decade after the 1929 Local Government Act. Reference is made to earlier periods as appropriate.

Legacies and donations: the strengths and limitations of voluntarism

The region contained hospitals representative of the whole spectrum of the voluntary sector, ranging from the Newcastle Royal Victoria Infirmary (RVI), which was one of the leading provincial teaching hospitals, to tiny cottage and accident hospitals. There was consequently substantial variation in terms of provision, expenditure and activity, quality of services, and financial viability. For reference, Table 2.3 provides various indicators of provision and use within the local authorities which, after 1948, comprised the bulk of the Newcastle RHB.

Levels of provision and utilisation

Possibly the first systematic attempts to compare hospital accommodation across the country were made after World War I, by the Voluntary Hospitals (Onslow) Committee.[3] This showed that in the Northern region per capita bed provision was consistently below the national average. Only three counties had lower bed-to-population ratios than Durham and only nine were below the North Riding's level. Northumberland was close to the national average largely because of the distorting presence of the Newcastle Royal Victoria Infirmary (RVI), but this served a wide area extending well into County Durham.[4]

The Onslow Committee did not present figures for county boroughs (CBs) but Gateshead, West Hartlepool, South Shields and Tynemouth regularly feature in the worst-off CBs in the lists given by Gorsky *et al.* (1999),[5] which cover the period to 1938. However, it was outside the main urban areas that access to hospital care was most problematic. Figure 2.1 shows the size distribution of hospitals with operating theatres in the region, as of 1938, and it can readily be seen that most hospitals were small, containing fifty or fewer beds. Note particularly the limited provision in the western part of County Durham. By 1938 there were only three small cottage hospitals in this area (at Consett, Stanley and Bishop Auckland). The wartime Hospital Surveyors later commented that 'it is remarkable that, in this thickly populated area [their estimate of its population was 288,000] so little provision has been made for the acute sick'.[6] They went on to point out that the lack of access to hospital services must have had a deterrent effect on those in need of treatment since the only alternative was a lengthy journey to Newcastle. In Cumberland, too, Workington and Whitehaven were regarded as underprovided. The Hospital Surveyors regarded West Cumberland as the area where pre-NHS hospital services were the most deficient in England and Wales.[7] Bed:population ratios (Table 2.3) confirm

Table 2.3 Voluntary and municipal hospital provision and activity in the Newcastle RHB area, 1938

| | Voluntary hospitals | | | | | |
	General beds / 1,000 pop.	Total beds / 1,000 pop.	Total inpatients	Total operations	Inpatients per bed	Operations per general bed
Northumberland	0.58	1.77	6,230	4,751	8.50	20.13
Newcastle	2.17	3.20	22,743	19,672	22.06	31.03
Tynemouth	1.02	1.14	1,655	1,898	21.78	27.91
Durham	0.62	0.75	11,699	7,945	17.46	14.39
Darlington	2.32	2.32	3,169	2,031	16.17	11.54
Gateshead	0.38	0.38	978	1,339	21.73	29.76
South Shields	1.33	1.49	2,674	2,421	14.61	16.47
Sunderland	1.64	2.25	9,831	7,548	21.42	25.24
West Hartlepool	0.97	1.11	1,546	1,159	17.98	17.04
North Riding of Yorkshire	0.98	1.57	1,893	1,246	9.33	7.99
Middlesbrough	2.62	2.63	6,892	3,893	17.63	10.64
Cumberland	1.00	1.52	3,341	2,362	10.64	12.05
Carlisle	2.17	3.2	2,851	3,042	14.77	23.22
Westmorland	1.17	4.57	2,038	843	7.03	24.79
			77,540	60,150	15.92	19.35

Table 2.3 (Cont.)

	Municipal hospitals				
	General beds / 1000 pop	Total inpatients	Total operations	Inpatients per bed	Operations per general bed
Northumberland	0.03	558	0	1.41	0.00
Newcastle	2.34	8,588	1,027	7.98	1.51
Tynemouth	3.53	2,480	57	5.59	0.24
Durham	0.21	3,631	194	2.91	1.05
Darlington	0.37	706	0	3.92	0.00
Gateshead	2.41	1,205	626	2.16	2.22
South Shields	2.15	4,207	692	9.31	2.92
Sunderland	1.45	5,912	1,451	6.54	5.48
West Hartlepool	2.98	2,256	537	5.53	2.56
North Riding of Yorkshire	0.02	635	0	2.42	0.00
Middlesbrough	1.62	2,031	406	5.01	1.79
Cumberland	0.02	451	0	3.01	0.00
Carlisle	0.36	1,942	911	14.94	16.26
Westmorland	0.0	112	0	1.22	0.00
		34,714	5,901	5.18	2.47

Source: Ministry of Health/NPHT (1945–46) vols 9, 10.

that, in much of the region, voluntary hospital provision was well below the England and Wales average (1.94 beds/1000 pop.), the exceptions being CBs whose hospitals served much larger hinterlands, and Westmorland, the value for which is inflated by the presence of a specialist hospital.

However, commentators such as Cherry (1980) have repeatedly emphasised the difficulties of delimiting hospital catchments, and argued that comparisons of levels of bed provision between arbitrary administrative areas have little meaning. It is essential, therefore, to assess variations in hospital utilisation. The Hospital Surveys required from each hospital a geographical breakdown of the area of residence of the inpatients treated in 1938 and in what follows I draw on an analysis of this data (reported briefly in Mohan and Gorsky (2001: 61–8) and in more detail in Mohan (2001)). Of the 1,188,095 inpatients treated by voluntary hospitals in 1938, the county or county borough of residence was identified for some 94.2 per cent; the remaining 5.8 per cent were not evenly distributed, but in only a few cases did they exceed 10 per cent of the patients treated in any given administrative unit. For the Northern region the geographical origin of nearly all inpatients seems to have been recorded and this means we have an accurate picture of the main patterns of patient flows in the 1930s.[8]

The data make it possible to calculate a utilisation rate by summing, for each local government area, the numbers treated as inpatients both in that area and in other jurisdictions. The result is a rate for England of twenty-eight inpatients per 1,000 population, but there are considerable variations around this figure.

For county boroughs, utilisation rates varied by a factor of over five. At the bottom, in terms of inpatients per 1,000 population, there are Smethwick (11.3), West Bromwich (11.8), Stoke (16.3), Rotherham (16.5), Salford (17.5) and Carlisle (17.8). Five other CBs had resident utilisation rates of under twenty inpatients per 1,000 population (including Newcastle and Birmingham). Conversely, in eleven CBs utilisation rates exceeded 35/1,000 population. Perhaps surprisingly Tynemouth (58.4) and St Helens (49.2) led the way, followed by Hastings (44.3), Middlesbrough (41.0), Oxford (39.2) and Gloucester (39.1). Also recording rates of over 30/1,000, against an average for CBs of 21.3, were Darlington, Halifax, Southport and Barrow-in-Furness, as well as Bournemouth, Bath, Ipswich, Bristol and Canterbury.

There is no obvious geographical divide evident in these findings and the North East of England alone incorporates almost the full range of utilisation rates. Considering county councils (CCs) (Figure 2.2) there is not quite the same range (from 12.3 (West Suffolk – under-estimated due to missing data) to 39.2 (Rutland)) and the results could be regarded as an artefact of the size threshold required for CB status.[9] There is a somewhat clearer geographical pattern here; of the eleven English CCs where utilisation rates exceeded thirty three, all (except Rutland, and the Holland division of Lincolnshire) are south of the Wash. Note, however, the low utilisation rates for Bedfordshire (14.5) and Middlesex (23.6). Low hospital *provision* here

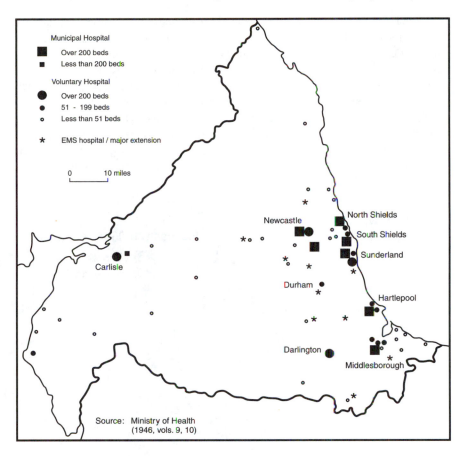

Figure 2.1 Size distribution of hospitals with operating theatres in the Newcastle Region, 1938

reflects the dominance of London, but low *utilisation* must indicate something about difficulties of gaining *access* to services. This is so not merely in a physical sense (travelling difficulties, which would be relevant in some of the low-ranking CCs: West Suffolk, Northumberland, East Riding, Shropshire) but in terms of referral networks.

This point is well-illustrated if we return to the CBs. Low levels of utilisation in Smethwick, West Bromwich and Rotherham might appear at first sight to be related to the presence of hospitals in nearby Birmingham and Sheffield respectively, possibly discouraging the foundation of new institutions and perhaps prioritising requests for admission from the residents of these cities. But that would not explain the surprising success of St Helens and Tynemouth. Despite low levels of local voluntary provision, patients here appear to have had little difficulty in accessing hospital treatment in neighbouring cities. Tynemouth should be contrasted with Gateshead; despite being much closer to the hospital facilities of Newcastle, Gateshead's inhabitants had much less success in gaining access to those facilities. However, availability of beds locally did not guarantee access to them: in the North Eastern region, Newcastle-upon-Tyne had the second-lowest utilisation rate for voluntary hospitals (19/1,000 population), despite the presence of the RVI.

Ideally we would complement this analysis of utilisation data (need which was met) with information on waiting lists (as an approximation for unmet need), but there is no comprehensive data on this prior to the Hospital Surveys. There are occasional *ad hoc* inquiries, such as the reports produced in the 1920s for the Onslow Commission (1925) concerning the adequacy or otherwise of existing hospital accommodation, but these only cover a limited selection of counties.

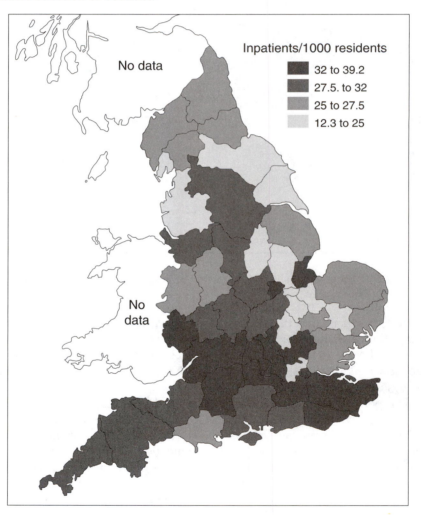

Figure 2.2 Voluntary hospital utilisation rates for English counties, 1938

The report on Northumberland and Durham, for example, referred first to high levels of bed occupancy, exceeding 100 per cent in Newcastle RVI and approaching it (96–97 per cent) in Sunderland RI and Durham County as well as in smaller specialist institutions (Princess Mary Maternity, Newcastle). Waiting lists were also lengthy even allowing for the caveat that cases were only put on the list where there was some chance of admission.[10] On the basis of occupancy levels and waiting lists the report suggested that no hospital could be considered to be underoccupied, and that there was a crying need for additional accommodation.

Increases of up to 50 per cent were required in Durham, for instance. In a reference to supply constraints the report argued that 'the population of the North are not so inclined to seek treatment in voluntary hospitals as those ... further south. ... This may be due to the impossibility of obtaining accommodation'.[11] Equally, reference was made to the difficulty of obtaining the necessary finance to construct new hospitals or extend existing ones. It was therefore believed that, even allowing for the prospect of some assistance from public funds, there was limited likelihood that desirable extensions would be built.

The inquiries undertaken for the Onslow Commission are echoed in various reports of individual hospitals, which referred to Tyneside as being 'gravely underhospitalled'.[12] The adequacy of hospital accommodation was also the subject of comment from local authority health committees.[13] Thus by 1939 Newcastle's Health Committee described the voluntary hospital waiting lists as 'long and pathetic' and stated that the hospitals were dealing 'almost entirely with emergencies'.[14] For more systematic statistics, data from the Hospital Surveys shows that the waiting list in Newcastle was equivalent to 25 per cent of patients treated in the city's voluntaries; for Manchester the corresponding figure was 14 per cent and for Birmingham 10 per cent.[15] Even these figures paled by comparison with Carlisle, where the waiting list was equivalent to 42 per cent of the caseload of the city's voluntary hospitals. The figure for all CBs was 6.8 per cent, so clearly the Newcastle and Carlisle hospitals were under pressure. Given variations between hospitals in the recording and management of waiting lists, it is questionable how much is revealed by these statistics, but for comparison, current NHS waiting lists are roughly equivalent to 8 per cent of the caseload treated in any one year.

Levels of expenditure and financial stability

The resources available to voluntary hospitals depended on the strength of the local economy and so one might expect a degree of variability. Space prevents a detailed exploration of this question here (see Mohan and Gorsky 2001b; Gorsky *et al.*, 2002); a brief comment is made on comparative levels of expenditure before considering the financial position of a sample of hospitals.

The most straightforward way of comparing expenditure levels is to relate them to hospital beds, because relating expenditure to population is subject to the catchment problem mentioned previously. On this indicator, the region clearly emerges as one with comparatively low expenditure.

A list of the bottom ten English boroughs in 1938 includes six (South Shields, Hartlepool, Tynemouth, Darlington, Middlesbrough and Sunderland) of the seven CBs in North East England, the exceptions being Gateshead (only because it had no voluntary general beds) and Newcastle. While in fifteen English CBs expenditure was over £200 per bed, in five of these boroughs the figure was less than two-thirds of that, the maximum being £133 in Darlington. Newcastle (£167/bed) was closer to the national average of £180, perhaps reflecting both the health of the city's economy by 1938 (rearmament had re-employed many munitions and shipyard workers) and the success of the contributory schemes established for the RVI. Only in Carlisle (£184) was expenditure per bed above the national average. Thus the general situation affecting the region was not promising: levels of provision and expenditure per bed were both low, with ramifications for the scope and quality of hospital facilities.

These general comparisons can be fleshed out through an analysis of the experience of individual hospitals, which demonstrates fluctuations in income and expenditure and also the way in which hospitals responded. The following discussion adds some local detail to an analysis of national trends in hospital income and expenditure, surpluses and deficits (Gorsky *et al.* 2002).

We start with the Palmer Memorial Hospital, Jarrow, which, as the Hospital Surveyors accurately observed, 'fell on evil days' when the town's shipyard closed in 1934.[16] Originally established as an accident hospital to serve the town's shipbuilding and related industries, the hospital had always been highly dependent on workers' contributions rather than philanthropy: donations, for example, rarely even approached 10 per cent of ordinary income.[17] It was therefore exposed to the danger that cessation of work at a major local employer could undermine its finances. Its minutes report rising demand for its services in the early years of the century; several local companies sought rights of access for their workers. Despite fluctuations in trade, efforts were made to expand after 1920, with the backing of a loan from the directors of Palmers Shipyard. However, storm clouds were gathering by mid-1923: reductions in fees were negotiated with visiting medical staff; nursing and domestic staff were laid off. There are then discontinuities in surviving records, but by 1927 sales of stocks and shares were being used to reduce the overdraft. By 1934 Palmers Shipyard, the town's principal employer, was no longer operational, and it was recognised that the hospital's financial position would become acute unless there was an 'influx of private patients'. Unsurprisingly, there was not, and in June 1934 the following observation was made by a member of the Governing Body: 'as the hospital was established for the benefit of Palmers workmen, and as Palmers had ceased to exist, *the institution was no longer needed*, and failing the town agreeing to take it over, it should be closed'.[18]

What is novel here is the definition of social need and of obligation: in the absence of the workplace, the hospital's functional role in restoring men to employability no longer existed, and the board member saw no case for continuing to keep it open. The hospital struggled on, treating minimal numbers of patients. The wartime surveyors concluded that 'arrangements for maintaining [the hospital] in an efficient condition by means of voluntary subscriptions do not exist'.[19]

Jarrow has become a byword for economic distress but other institutions suffered as well. The small Lady Eden Cottage Hospital, Bishop Auckland, was the only voluntary institution in South West Durham, and served a densely populated area which experienced some of the worst effects of the depression. However, by 1926 the hospital reported that 'all our reserves are gone'; in 1927, owing to unemployment, the 'miners [had] not been able to send their usual contributions'.[20] The Durham County Hospital, the only hospital of any size in the county for those unable to attend hospitals in Sunderland or Newcastle, consistently ran an overdraft of between £5,000–12,000 throughout the late 1920s; this was at times not far off the hospital's annual income.[21]

Other general hospitals also felt the pinch. Tynemouth Victoria Jubilee Infirmary, for example, relied heavily on workmen's contributions for up to half its income, but these fluctuated substantially. In 1924 this source produced £2,700, out of a total income of £5,948; the corresponding figures for 1926 were £1,739 (£5,726). There was a similar reduction in contributions from £2,532 in 1929 to £1,675 in 1932. In real terms expenditure did not decline substantially but there was no real expansion until the late 1930s. Inpatient numbers, therefore, first levelled off and later declined.[22] The Monkwearmouth and Southwick Hospital, in Sunderland, consistently experienced difficulties in the inter-war years; it only recorded surpluses on ordinary income in 1918, 1919, 1920, 1929 and 1930. By 1933 the hospital was 'quickly coming to the end of its reserves', because (in real terms) income in 1931 and 1932 was some 20 per cent below that recorded in 1930. Despite this the hospital kept its overdraft down by consistently applying extraordinary income to it, and by disposing of stock. Notwithstanding its difficulties, it refused to entertain the possibility of greater collaboration with the nearby Sunderland Royal Infirmary (see Chapter 3).[23]

Even the major general hospitals, such as the Sunderland Infirmary or the Newcastle RVI, were sometimes vulnerable to fluctuations in income from workers' contributions. They did not experience the difficulties of Palmer or Lady Eden – the sheer scale of the workmen's contributory schemes, and the number of workplaces taking part, reduced dependency on single large workplaces. However, the reports of the Sunderland RI revealed substantial fluctuations in income. In 1926, the 'stoppage in the coal trade and industrial depression [had] depleted funds to a greater extent than ever previously'. During 1931, 'one of the most difficult [years] in the annals of the infirmary', £38,501 received from legacies was used for *current* expenditure. By 1932 there were 'practically no realisable free investments', and again in 1933 and 1934 extraordinary income had to be used to meet ordinary expenditure and pay off debt. The Infirmary therefore consistently ran an overdraft, equivalent to between 8 and 16 per cent of the value of its realisable assets, for much of the inter-war period.[24] This was in some respects a risky strategy, since by comparison with some hospitals it had a relatively low asset base. However, it did enable the hospital to expand steadily.

The Newcastle RVI, by contrast, adopted a more parsimonious approach. This institution was the principal voluntary hospital for much of Tyneside, Northumberland and Durham. It is at least plausible that its very scale and importance discouraged attempts to found new institutions in its 'catchment'; certainly it had no problem in attracting subscriptions and workmen's contributions from a wide area. This may be why its income does not appear to have fluctuated to the extent experienced in Sunderland, though its 1926 income was some 10 per cent down on the previous year, reflecting the General Strike.[25] Although the hospital did at times experience deficits on ordinary income, these (and its overdraft) were small in relation to the size of its asset base. A corollary, of course, was that provision did not keep pace with local demand and waiting lists therefore rose (see Gorsky *et al.* 2002, for more details and comparisons with other hospitals). Finally, in Middlesbrough, the main voluntary hospitals both identified the decline in workpeople's contributions as a key cause of financial difficulties in the early 1930s (Mansfield 1991: 27–9 and appendix B2): in real terms income at both the North Riding Infirmary and North Ormesby Hospitals fell by some 20 per cent between 1930 and 1932.

Submissions made by voluntary hospitals to the Commissioner for the Special Areas (see Mohan 1997, and Chapter 3) shed further light on hospitals' perception of their financial position. Of course, they had an interest in exaggerating their difficulties in order to extract grant aid, but their submissions do indicate some limits to reliance on charity. These submissions were requests for assistance with capital projects, revenue subventions having been ruled off the agenda.

Thus, the Newcastle voluntary hospitals, making a joint submission in 1938, emphasised that sources of private charity could not be expected to recover quickly after the depression; firms, 'whose habit of making considerable donations has once been interrupted by the necessity for retrenchment do not readily resume their donations on anything like the scale of previous years'.[26] Other voluntary hospitals referred to the consequences of the closure of major local employers: Tynemouth Victoria Jubilee Infirmary had lost employees' contributions equivalent to 10 per cent of its income for this reason. Durham County Hospital insisted that the stoppage in the coal trade had 'seriously curtailed' its income, and it had not been possible to 'keep up income to meet expenditure ... except by encroaching on the capital fund'.[27] Due partly to declining workpeople's contributions, the Governors of the Sunderland Royal Infirmary had had to resort to overdrafts; although they had considered a contributory scheme or seeking to collect some maintenance charges from patients, they had done neither of these owing to the 'intense depression' affecting the town.[28] Despite these difficulties, some institutions asserted that new capital projects would enhance the attractiveness of their institution, and enable them to raise funds more easily to cover running costs: thus the governors of Durham County Hospital claimed that they had 'every reason to believe that the increase in maintenance costs consequent on completion of [their proposed] alterations can be met',[29] and the Tynemouth Victoria Jubilee Infirmary had 'every hope' of raising funds privately, if a capital grant was forthcoming.[30] But this rather flew in the face of the foregoing evidence about fluctuations in hospital income. The more general issue identified was the impossibility of raising capital sums through charitable appeals; one of the Governors of the Newcastle RVI said that they 'dare not' ask local people to provide the money needed.[31] Allowing for the limitations of evidence which those submitting it were inclined to exaggerate, this material nevertheless seems to demonstrate amply the financial constraints faced by the voluntaries. Yet these circumstances did not always lead hospitals to cooperate, either with each other or with municipal institutions (Chapter 3).

Quality of services

Given the resource constraints identified, the mere existence of hospitals did not mean that a good quality service was available. Hart's (1971) statement of the 'inverse care law' (postulating a negative relationship between provision of services and need) lays as much emphasis on quality as on quantity of service. In the absence of consumerist evaluations the following relies on data on the distribution of qualified medical staff, and on assessments, by the wartime surveyors, of the quality of buildings.

Only the major general hospitals retained resident medical staff and in even fewer were there specialists in residence. The distribution of staff was tied closely to opportunities for private practice, because consultants gave their services free, and voluntarily, relying on their private practice as their source of income. Consequently, access to good-quality medical staff varied considerably between and within regions (Gorsky *et al.* 1999, Table 4). Nationally there were 2.81 medical staff per 10,000 population recorded as practising in voluntary hospitals. In Northumberland, where figures are inflated by the presence of the Newcastle RVI, the figure was 3.79, but elsewhere the region was well below the national average, the relevant figures being 2.28 (Cumberland), 1.63 (Yorkshire (North Riding)), 1.20 (Durham) and 0.61 (Westmorland). For comparison eighteen counties had at least 3.5 medical staff per 10,000 population. Turning to CBs, Middlesbrough, South Shields and Sunderland featured in the bottom twenty boroughs for

England; Gateshead recorded no voluntary hospital medical staff at all in 1929. Only Darlington (2.49) Carlisle (2.97) and Newcastle approached or exceeded the national average for CBs of 2.53/10,000 population. Thus hospitals in areas which offered limited potential for private practice were inevitably disadvantaged; treatment of patients was either carried out by GPs or delayed until a suitably qualified consultant visited a private patient (NPHT 1946). The Hospital Surveyors questioned whether there was sufficient demand in the region to support a large addition to the number of consultants.[32] If access to qualified staff continued to depend on the market for private practice, there was little hope of improving the quality of hospital services other than in large urban centres. Characteristically, many rural cottage hospitals were GP hospitals which rarely, if ever, received consultant visits (e.g. Morpeth, Alnwick, Hexham). In other locations staff divided their time between several institutions – the senior ophthalmic surgeon in the North Riding was 'on the staff of six hospitals, each of which he visits weekly'.[33] Even in some comparatively large hospitals, such as Durham County, 'none of the general beds [were] in the charge of physicians or surgeons who are solely engaged in consulting practice'.[34] Duplication was also evident – the two voluntary hospitals in the Hartlepools both retained honorary consultants in ophthalmology, aural surgery and orthopaedics.[35] In the absence of consultant staff the bulk of hospital treatment was provided by GPs or by local authority medical officers.

The physical plant and sites of hospitals also left much to be desired. Many hospitals, especially nineteenth-century foundations, occupied sites which had been surrounded by subsequent urban development. Buildings were therefore often inconvenient and cramped.[36] Consequently the wartime surveys are littered with comments as to the poor quality of accommodation, the lack of room for expansion, and/or the absence of particular facilities. Several hospitals lacked pathology laboratories or even X-ray departments, giving rise to comments that they were too small for efficient treatment. Even hospitals which were the main source of acute treatment in their locality had deficiencies. The Cumberland Infirmary, Carlisle, comprised a set of buildings which, because of *ad hoc* and sporadic development, formed a 'rambling, rather formless and inconvenient whole'. The only other general hospital in Cumberland, the Whitehaven and West Cumberland Infirmary, was a 'converted castle which forms a very unsatisfactory hospital'.[37] Likewise Middlesbrough was saddled with two general hospitals both of which were in unsatisfactory buildings with very little prospect of reconstruction or expansion *in situ*. The consequence was that in many locations a strategy of 'simply saving existing buildings' was 'often the reverse of economy'.[38] Most hospitals in the region 'did not conform to modern needs'.

The least favourable comments were reserved for outpatient departments which were generally in 'poor, inconvenient and cramped accommodation'.[39] In several cases pre-war plans to upgrade outpatient departments had been put on hold. In respect of support services, X-ray departments were found in most hospitals, but laboratory facilities were often regarded as 'poor' even in important institutions such as Tynemouth Infirmary, the Ingham Infirmary (South Shields), Durham County Hospital and the North Riding Infirmary (Middlesbrough). They were absent from the Darlington Memorial Hospital, the principal general hospital in that area. Many institutions, of course, lacked operating theatres: a 1937 Ministry of Health survey showed that 255 out of 966 (26.4 per cent) voluntary general hospitals lacked an operating theatre; these were characteristically small institutions of a cottage hospital type, with an average size of forty-five beds.[40] Of the sixty-nine voluntary institutions in this category in the study area, however, 33 per cent (twenty-three) did not have an operating theatre; the majority of these were cottage hospitals in Northumberland and Cumberland. In summary, problems arising from the relatively low levels of provision and expenditure in the region were compounded by the poor quality of the facilities available.

Municipal resources and priorities

While local authorities had technically had the power to provide general hospital services for their non-pauper populations since 1875, only three authorities exercised that power before the 1920s. The 1929 Local Government Act is therefore usually taken as the point of departure for accounts of municipal involvement in general hospital provision. This Act allowed for the division of powers between Public Health Committees and the Public Assistance Committees of local authorities. By this division the stigma associated with the Poor Law could be removed, and local authorities could make general hospital services available to all. They were empowered to construct entirely new hospitals but the most common option chosen was the 'appropriation' for general hospital purposes of the former Poor Law infirmaries.

Accounts of the success of municipal effort reach divergent conclusions. Negative accounts emphasise unevenness in provision, suggesting that only in a small number of relatively wealthy areas was much achieved (Abel-Smith 1964: 368–83; Titmuss 1950: 69; Lee 1988). The slow pace of appropriation of Poor Law facilities forms an important plank in criticisms of municipal effort, but Powell (1997: 349) suggests that this may be misleading. Many Poor Law facilities were not worth appropriating and in others the poor quality of the buildings was a major obstacle. Very few Poor Law *hospitals*, as opposed to Public Assistance Institutions, remained unappropriated; Powell contends that when this is considered, the verdict on local authority provision is more favourable. Titmuss (1950: 72) also reminds us that, when local authorities entered the field of hospital provision, 'economy was the watchword'.

Making allowance for these constraints, other verdicts are more positive. Thus, for Pickstone (1985: 6) the inter-war years were the 'high point of municipal medicine'. Likewise, Webster (1988a: 8) suggests that 'where permissive powers were applied to the utmost degree, where rate revenue was buoyant, and where the local Medical Officer of Health was sympathetic with modern developments, the standard of service bore comparison with later counterparts under the NHS' (pp. 5–9). However, he also contends that areas of greatest need were least able to sustain services (Webster 1985), due to financial restrictions and an unsympathetic Ministry.

Municipal provision and utilisation

In quantitative terms, by 1937, ninety-two institutions had been appropriated for general hospital purposes, containing over 50,000 beds, or close to the total beds provided in voluntary general hospitals. But there was considerable variability. Apart from London, only nine county councils had appropriated hospitals; thirty-seven (out of eighty-three) county boroughs (CBs) had done so (PEP 1937: 250). The London County Council (LCC) was justifiably viewed as a pioneering local authority, because of the scale of its activities; it was responsible for over 26,000 hospital beds (Sheldrake 1989; Stewart 1997). In some cases, such as Middlesex, county councils commenced capital programmes which were comparable to those achieved by the much larger Regional Hospital Boards in the early years of the NHS. Other local authorities were said to have 'planned' a comprehensive service (e.g. Surrey, Staffordshire and Essex (PEP, 1937, 255)) but the pace of new development varied considerably. Even where new hospitals were not built, so that net additions to bed numbers were comparatively small, upgrading of Poor Law facilities resulted in substantial increases in the throughput of patients (Powell 1997, Table 1).

As in the voluntary sector there were substantial variations in provision. Municipal provision was substantially greater than that in voluntary hospitals (some 181,000 beds in England and Wales compared to 82,000), and municipal provision accounted for over three-quarters of the available beds in twenty-two CBs and in thirteen CCs. This is potentially misleading, however, because it might indicate the absence of voluntarism as much as the strength of municipal effort. It is also the case that local authorities were required to provide facilities for treatment of infectious diseases and of the chronically sick and a more fruitful comparison is therefore of the respective levels of general hospital beds.

The definitional problems involved are considered by Powell (1997: 350). The data used here – the wartime surveys – rely to some extent on self-definition, but the quality of what some local authorities defined as general hospitals left much to be desired. There were many beds classed as available for general hospital purposes which were provided in long-stay institutions and in which very little hospital treatment (in terms of numbers of operations) was taking place. Acknowledging these difficulties, it is clear that general hospital provision in the public sector was largely carried out by CBs. The data show that CCs rarely provided more than 0.5 general beds per

1,000 population. In the Northern region the figures were even lower; Durham provided 184 beds (0.21/1,000) but even this equated to only 25 per cent of all general hospital provision in the county. Provision in the other counties in the region was minimal. In the county boroughs, municipal beds represented the majority of general hospital provision in Tynemouth (77 per cent of general beds), Gateshead (86 per cent), South Shields (61 per cent) and Newcastle (51 per cent); in Middlesbrough and Sunderland the municipal sector was slightly in the minority; in Darlington and Carlisle it provided less than 15 per cent of general hospital beds. These contrast with numerous boroughs in North West England in which, on Powell's figures (1997, Table 1), the local authority provided over 75 per cent of general beds.

However, we need to provide a fuller picture of the work being carried out in these hospitals. Analysis of patient throughput and of numbers of operations being carried out puts the voluntary sector in a more favourable light. Thus, in the Northern region, the voluntary hospitals carried out over two-thirds of inpatient treatment (77,540 inpatients, compared to 34,714 in municipal hospitals), and over 90 per cent of all operations. Patient throughput, at 15.9 per bed, compared to 5.2 per bed in the municipal sector, indicating that the case mix of patients was clearly very different, with municipal hospitals dealing with many more long-stay patients (table 2.3). It is also the case, as shown below, that the quality of municipal facilities left a great deal to be desired.

For these reasons, caution must be exercised in relation to the following discussion of utilisation rates. Relying on the classification of individual hospitals used in the surveys, voluntary general hospitals treated substantially more inpatients than their municipal counterparts: 950,000, compared to 648,000. If one removes London, the imbalance is greater: 789,000 voluntary against 454,000 inpatients. In terms of the geography of hospital utilisation, it is not possible to separate out with complete accuracy the pattern of general hospital treatment, and so the discussion of municipal utilisation rates incorporates all municipal provision.[41]

Accepting these caveats, there is some evidence which appears to suggest that municipal provision helped in ameliorating variations in utilisation rates. This can be demonstrated statistically in two ways. First, we use the coefficient of variation which divides a measure of dispersion in a set of values (the standard deviation) by the mean. This produces a result which is independent of the actual value of the mean. For the seventy-nine CBs, the coefficient of variation of the voluntary hospital utilisation rates is 0.28 but the CV for the *total* hospital utilisation rate (i.e. voluntary and municipal rate added together) is reduced to 0.22. Second, for the CBs the correlation coefficient between the municipal and voluntary hospital utilisation rates, calculated for those fifty-seven CBs that provided municipal hospitals, is −0.44, which is, statistically, highly significant. The implication is that where access to voluntary hospitals was poor, local authority provision had some effect on improving access to services. In the Northern region the majority of residents of Newcastle and Sunderland who received hospital treatment did so in municipal hospitals and for Middlesbrough and South Shields the balance between use of voluntary and municipal hospitals was roughly even. However, there were also authorities – Gateshead and Tynemouth for example – where municipal treatment took place in antiquated environments not worthy of designation as general hospitals. So while municipal effort did close some gaps in provision, there remained much to be done.

Expenditure and financial constraints

In Lee's (1988) analysis of municipal provision this region is seen as one area where 'low rates of expenditure are matched by indifferent tax effort' (p. 271). Concentrating only on expenditure on general hospital services, as recorded in the Local Taxation Returns, seems to support this verdict. Ranked on a *per capita* basis none of the region's county boroughs featured in the top half of spenders; expenditure ranged from 17 pence per head (Middlesbrough) to 25 pence (Newcastle) but nothing was recorded for Tynemouth, Gateshead, Darlington or Hartlepool and Carlisle's expenditure was minuscule. For comparison expenditure per head in Manchester, Salford, Liverpool and Nottingham was over 50 per cent higher than that recorded in Newcastle. On the face of it the local authorities in this region had not made general hospital provision a priority.

Some, though not all, of this reflected local economic circumstances. Again, there is evidence from the papers of the Commissioners for the Special Areas on this point. Some local authorities were quite emphatic about the financial difficulties confronting them: the Medical Officer of Health for Cumberland reported in 1936 that expansion of health and welfare services depended on receiving assistance from the Commissioner otherwise, 'any substantial rise in County rates, already the fourth highest among English counties, would seriously handicap the prospect of attracting new industries'.[42] Durham CC had proposed a new hospital (at Dryburn, on the outskirts of Durham City), to serve the localities to the west and south-west of Durham City. They had been 'reminded by the Ministry of the very considerable cost of erection and maintenance', and the Ministry had also pointed out, in terms which anticipated the proposals of the post-war settlement policies in Durham to concentrate development in the eastern parts of the county, that 'it was questionable whether Durham was the most suitable centre looking to the trend of industrial development in the County'. The Council had had 'long and serious thoughts as to the heavy cost of this scheme', and had shown 'great hesitation', but had concluded that continuing to maintain the existing hospitals would be less economical. However, Ministry officials believed privately that, given its financial commitments, 'the Council cannot ... afford the cost of Dryburn'.[43] The inadequacies of various infectious disease hospitals, and the deferral of developments because of poverty, were also noted;[44] in Gateshead the local authority reported that most of its proposals for service development had been 'put off for financial reasons', and that in the financial circumstances then existing it would be inadvisable to abandon an existing hospital and replace it, as the Council had proposed, with a new one.[45] In South Shields the financial position of the Borough rendered developments difficult; the Medical Officer of Health's reports did not show the holding up of particular schemes, or delays in the appointment of staff, because of the financial position, but the general tenor of the reports was that the overall level of service was deficient. In Sunderland and Northumberland, desirable planned developments – in maternal and child welfare, and hospital services, respectively – had been postponed because of financial stringency.[46] In submissions to the Commissioner, local authorities repeatedly pointed out the effect on rate poundages if they proceeded with schemes without CSA support; this argument was also deployed to make a case for above-average levels of grant aid. This evidence lends weight to Lee's (1988: 271) emphasis on local prosperity as a determinant of expenditure, though as Chapter 3 shows, local authority performance and commitment were also variable.

Quality of municipal services

Local authorities had inherited a ramshackle collection of Poor Law institutions which could not form the basis of a modern hospital service. In Durham, only the Public Assistance Institutions (PAIs) at Chester-le-Street and Bishop Auckland had 'anything approaching first class hospital accommodation throughout'; the Stockton institution was 'dismal'.[47] Northumberland had inherited 'very unsatisfactory' accommodation, which was 'only fit for ... infirm aged people who are not in need of continuous nursing care'; some of it was not even fit for that purpose.[48] Similar comments could be repeated for many other local authorities in the region. The situation as regards isolation and TB hospitals was in many respects even worse. Large numbers of scattered, small facilities, in old and unsuitable premises, called for substantial rationalisation: there were twenty-eight hospitals for infectious diseases in County Durham, for instance, which the Ministry recommended should be reduced to twelve. Thus Ministry recommendations emphasised the urgency of rationalisation, but (as will be seen) there was less enthusiasm for new construction.

One guide to the quality of local government services is whether local authorities chose (or were able) to develop general hospitals entirely separate from the Poor Law, and whether what were classed as general hospital beds were in institutions with operating theatres. Unpublished Ministry survey data for 1937 indicates, for example, that the proportion of general hospital beds located in Poor Law institutions without operating theatres was 22 per cent. In this area, while Northumberland (15 per cent) was below-average and Cumberland (23 per cent) slightly above it, the figures for North Yorkshire (35 per cent), Durham (47 per cent) and Westmorland (56 per cent) were well above it.[49] This indicates the relative weakness of voluntarism in these areas (because the contribution of Poor Law infirmaries to the bed total was proportionately large) but it also signifies the failure of local authorities to develop municipal services. For comparison, however, there were many rural counties throughout England in which over 60 per cent of ostensibly 'general' hospital beds were provided in Poor Law institutions lacking operating theatres. The wartime surveyors were not always as dismissive of such institutions as one might expect, one reason being that facilities had often been added to them during the war under the EMS (Emergency Medical Service); another may have been a reluctance to condemn available facilities unless they were indisputably beyond redemption. Thus assessments of several municipal institutions, which were subsequently roundly condemned by the NHS, suggested that despite the poor quality of the buildings they were 'not too unsuitable' for accommodating the chronic sick.

Proposals for post-war development

The legacy of the pre-NHS era for this region was thus a poorly developed hospital infrastructure; not only were per capita levels of provision low, but so too were expenditure and hospital utilisation. This supports Hadfield's (1979: 158) view of the region's hospitals as 'underfinanced, underequipped and insufficient'. Evaluations by the Surveyors commented on issues of maldistribution and quality, and identified several key priorities. Cumberland was 'very badly off for hospitals of all kinds' and West Cumberland was 'one place where permission should be given for some of the most urgent work to proceed at once'.[50] Similar comments were made about Durham and Northumberland. The corollary was that patients in these areas were travelling long distances to hospital and there were also substantial waiting lists. The exigencies of the inter-war depression took their toll on voluntary services and inhibited the growth of the municipal alternative. While hospitals did not close, their resources were frequently stretched, and (allowing for the weaknesses of waiting list statistics) there was substantial unmet need, by comparison with other locations. Small wonder, then, that the Hospital Surveyors subsequently observed that 'no inquiry [into the North East] can ignore the fact that this was a distressed region before the war, and this has undoubtedly affected the development of its hospital service'.[51] Not all those hospitals which did exist were available to all; there were various company-owned hospitals (Horden, Ashington, Eston) geared to restoring male employees following accidents, but not playing a wider role.[52] Several facilities were plainly inadequate. For example the miner's lodges of South West Durham had decided, 'quite correctly', not to support the Lady Eden Cottage Hospital (Bishop Auckland), because serious injuries and other accident cases would receive better treatment at the Newcastle RVI – some thirty-five miles away. They had transferred their financial support accordingly,[53] in a sense anticipating the post-1991 purchaser–provider split (see Chapter 9) by over fifty years! Finally, the Surveyors observed that some highly desirable developments had been postponed because of depression, followed by war. This may not add up to voluntary failure – after all, the Newcastle RVI was the largest provincial teaching hospital in England, and had substantial resources – but the limitations of voluntarism were exposed, at least in certain places. Municipal services were also weakly developed; here depression played its part, although Ministry comments (see Chapter 3) suggest strongly that, given political will, local authorities could have achieved more.

How did the Surveyors see the post-war hospital service developing? Their terms of reference precluded consideration of the issue of control and so the emphasis was on managerial issues. Many existing hospitals were obsolete and/or inefficient,[54] and their physical condition had, in several cases, degenerated to the point where they were unsuitable for continued use.[55] Considerable rationalisation and reorganisation of services would also be a necessary corollary of the uncoordinated development of acute hospital services in small or medium-sized units.[56] Hospitals constructed under the EMS[57] had provided an additional 3,719 beds either at entirely new sites (Durham, Hexham) by extensions to existing facilities (Bishop Auckland, Chester-le-Street) or taking over accommodation at mental institutions (Shotley Bridge, Ryhope). However these were, in several cases (Sedgefield, Stannington, Hemlington) located at some distance from major centres of population, and so were not ideal from the point of view of post-war planning. Nevertheless these hospitals represented substantial net additions to general hospital provision in the region.

Making no assumptions about the level of resources likely to be available to the post-war service, the surveyors had to back existing winners. There was unanimity that the region's hospital services should be focused around the RVI in Newcastle-upon-Tyne. Before the war, various proposals had been put forward for a Hospital Centre in the city; several of the smaller specialist units in Newcastle had sought sites within the curtilage of the RVI.[58] The concept of a Hospital Centre was taken up by the Survey; Newcastle was already 'the centre of medicine in the North East ... it should take an even higher place as a medical centre than it has in the past'.[59] Subsequent proposals for the development of this medical complex were, however, to provoke controversial debates in the 1960s.

Second, the Survey made recommendations which, in arguing for district hospitals of 600–800 beds,[60] clearly anticipated the later development of the DGH concept.[61] Two such facilities – the RVI and the General Hospital – would be provided in Newcastle; in Sunderland, Durham and Middlesbrough the district hospital service would be provided by coordination of existing facilities; while in such centres as Carlisle and Darlington one major hospital would be developed.[62] Finally, the Survey recommended the retention of many rural cottage hospitals and the closure of a variety of small, inefficient and/or obsolete units, particularly isolation hospitals.[63]

The Surveyors called for a large capital programme but assumed that a mix of local authority and voluntary services would continue to exist. However, the limits to voluntarism were becoming apparent in cases such as Jarrow. Equally it was recognised that coordination between institutions was not good and that there was a disjunction between the activities of municipal hospitals (responsible, in the main, for patients from their own jurisdictions) and voluntaries (not responsible for designated catchments). This was increasingly perceived as an obstacle to the efficient use of existing facilities (Chapter 3).

Finally the Surveyors acknowledged that because the 'future prospects of industry [were] uncertain … plans for any reorganisation … must not be too rigid'. This was to pose major challenges to hospital planning: were funds to be allocated to correspond to the *existing* distribution of population, or was an attempt to be made to second-guess the *future* distribution? This had been acknowledged in confidential documents such as the Pepler-Macfarlane report (1949), which insisted that social policies in the North East would have to be part of an inevitable process of adjustment of the settlement pattern to the anticipated decline of coalmining. The eastward shift in the centre of gravity of the Durham coalfield had exercised Ministry officials during the 1930s. The likely exhaustion of coal reserves in the west of the county was translated into policy via the controversial settlement concentration policies of Durham County Council (1951). Public sector investment would be concentrated into locations deemed to possess potential for future growth; other settlements would be denied such investment. These policies, and others concerned with the reconstruction of the region's physical infrastructure, raised issues relating to the coordination of hospital investment programmes with other public policy initiatives; these issues feature strongly in subsequent chapters.

3 Regionalism

A positive or negative consensus?

The problems described in the previous chapter were well known but little had been done about them. During the inter-war period there ensued a number of moves towards coordination of hospital provision, in the form of recommendations of Government inquiries, *ad hoc* initiatives within the voluntary sector, and various local developments. The purpose of this chapter is to review the proposals of various reports and some practical steps taken to implement them, the motivations of their proponents, and the criticisms levelled at these proposals. Illustrations from developments in the Newcastle region allow evaluation of their impact.

The key debate to be considered here relates to Fox's (1986) notion of hierarchical regionalism (see Chapter 1). Fox suggests that it was generally agreed that health services would be available at successive levels of speciali-sation, from primary care to specialised forms of treatment obtainable only in teaching hospitals, the apex of the hierarchy. Relationships between hospitals would be established so that patients would be directed to the most appropriate hospital, and so that duplicative development would be avoided. For Fox, there was agreement on such matters on the part of representatives of voluntary and municipal hospitals alike. Consequently the area of disagreement in health policy was confined to questions of administrative detail. Endorsement for Fox's views might be derived from quotations such as the following, which appeared in the 1940 *Hospitals Yearbook*:

> Regionalisation is no more than an obvious and convenient method of dealing with practical problems on a geographical basis ... it follows of necessity in a society that is increasing in size and complexity. Independent local units of the same or a similar kind find themselves obliged ... to combine in defence of their interests or for the promotion of their common purpose.[1]

Regionalism might thus simply be seen as epitomising modernity, ratio-nality and planning: a similar story might have been told of various other initiatives, such as reform of local government (Garside and Hebbert 1989). However, this presupposed that hospitals could agree on their 'interests', or articulate a 'common purpose', neither of which necessarily occurred, and this might raise questions about whether regionalism, as such, could be implemented. Yet Fox (e.g. 1986: 52) implies that, by 1929, 'local authorities, voluntary hospitals and medical interest groups ... had begun to implement the consensus' about hierarchical regionalism, and that the 'governors of voluntary hospitals ... had agreed to coordinate (or pretended to do so) with local authorities'. There are at least two escape clauses here: even minimal cooperation could be viewed as 'beginning' to implement a policy, and agreements as to cooperation might simply amount to the formation of toothless and tokenistic committees, with no practical action. There was obviously an acknowledgement that something better than the existing system was necessary, but this still left room for substantial disagreement. Regionalism signified coordination and rationalisation, but its imprecision allowed it to mean different things to different people. To some, it signified expropriation of voluntary hospitals by the municipal sector, and a degree of state direction; to others, voluntary (if unenforceable) cooperation; for still others, reorganising the activities of individual hospitals in pursuit of a common goal. I therefore seek to highlight the points of difference between the various protagonists in these debates, and to understand the very different perspectives from which they were speaking. I also focus on the extent to which various inter-war proposals extended access to hospital services by making them available in places hitherto lacking them. One might characterise the inter-war and wartime debates as a struggle between two opposing forces: those of rational planning and modernisation, represented largely by local government and the Ministry of Health; and those of individualism, localism and competition, represented by the voluntary sector. Such a dichotomy cannot always be sustained; for instance, some voluntary sector representatives clearly saw the need for a greater degree of planning. But the key themes were (and remain) important elements of health policy debate.

This is particularly so in the context of the emphasis, by the post-1979 governments, on mixed economies of welfare, and on the role of partnerships between public and private sectors in the delivery of welfare services (Chapters 8 and 9). Yet the terms on which partnerships are constructed, and the respective roles, resources and commitment of the partners, have crucial effects on the nature and success of partnership arrangements. It is important therefore to consider the motivations for engaging in partnerships and the incentives and sanctions available, both to potential partners, and to those (such as the government) who wished to encourage partnerships. Appeals to good nature do not appear to have had much success and partners' motivations varied. Articulating a collective interest was difficult.

Moreover, these inter-war debates reveal much about the deep roots of the prevailing orthodoxy favouring the voluntary system, and about the extent to which planning and coordination were (or were not) feasible. State intervention in this sector, as in so many others in the inter-war years (e.g. Ward 1988; Middleton 1996) was heavily constrained by a politico-economic orthodoxy which viewed market failures as problems of a limited and temporary duration, which, consequently, could be solved only by restoring the primacy of market control. Extension of the involvement of the state was therefore conceived as a short-term expedient, not as a new stage in the evolution of welfare policy. Such an orthodoxy imposed quite obvious limits on what were considered legitimate solutions to the difficulties of the hospital system. Hence there was great reluctance even to contemplate greater state involvement beyond informal cooperation. The limits to voluntarist orthodoxy were, however, challenged by the uneven impact of depression, imposing severe stress on the finances of voluntary institutions in the depressed areas, and forcing some policy-makers to contemplate greater intervention.

The chapter briefly reviews some historical background on the question of state intervention in hospital provision. Discussion then concentrates on the emergence of various forms of cooperation (within the voluntary sector and between the voluntary and municipal sectors) and of central government grants to promote coordination.

Historical background

The need for greater coordination and planning of hospital provision was actually recognised as far back as 1870, when the Sanitary Commission advocated the creation of organisations to supervise the trajectory of hospital development. Local authorities were empowered to provide general hospital services in 1875 but hardly any did so. Informed opinion within the voluntary sector held that its greatest defect was maldistribution, leading to calls, in the late nineteenth century, for controls on the location of new hospital development (Millman 1974: 134), not unlike the (much later) 'certificate of need' in the USA. Yet state intervention was resisted even in face of the evidence of maldistribution of services offered by the House of Lords' (1890–2) inquiry which confined itself to a call for informal cooperation (pp. xlvi–xlvii). The large appeal which established the King's Fund[2] in 1897 was essentially an attempt to head off state intervention (Waddington 2000: 191–200) though it is interesting to note that elsewhere, in France and the USA for example, voluntary hospitals had a much more relaxed attitude to receiving payments from the state (T. Smith 1998; Stevens 1999). The minority report of the Royal Commission on the Poor Law (1909) went so far as to advocate a unified medical service provided by counties and county boroughs, but nothing came of this. Labour Party thinking developed along these lines, advocating an extension of the role of local government both in providing services which would be free of the taint of the Poor Law, and in extending preventive services (maternal and child welfare; school health services) (Webster 1988b). Additional pressures for change derived from recognition of the poor health standards of military recruits and post-war pressures for social reform.

These demands led the post-war administration to create a Ministry of Health and then to appoint a Consultative Council on Medical and Allied Services, chaired by Lord Dawson. This produced an interim report in 1920 (the Dawson Report: CCMAS 1920) which, although never formally implemented, forms a useful point of departure for a consideration of inter-war developments.

This report was notable for its recommendations about the integration of primary, secondary and tertiary care, though these had in some respects been anticipated in Labour party documents (Webster 1988b). Dawson saw health centres as forming the foundation of any scheme of reconstruction: here he drew on a pioneering initiative in Gloucestershire, which had attempted to integrate primary and secondary care. Dawson called explicitly for the integration of various forms of health care provision, and emphasised that hospitals ought to be arranged in hierarchies, of successive degrees of specialisation, the better to secure the diffusion of medical technology. Rationalisation was essential because of the rising cost of such technology: 'when a business grows, it grows in earning capacity ... when a hospital grows, it grows in spending capacity' (p. 16). Dawson also criticised the failure of promoters of individual hospital schemes 'to realise that a modern hospital should be part of a more comprehensive organisation'. In order to extend access to treatment, substantial reconstruction would be necessary; as an interim measure, this could be achieved by taking over the Poor Law hospitals although these, 'from their positions or structures, could only be makeshifts' (p. 10). However, the report did not explain how services were going to be extended. The report suggested that 'if a voluntary hospital exists its assistance would be welcomed' (p. 16). It seems to have been assumed that the benefits voluntary hospitals would receive under Dawson's scheme would induce them to cooperate. The assumption appeared to be that by unifying and grouping hospitals together, and by offering doctors access to a greater range of facilities, greater efficiency would result. But there was little information on proposed financial arrangements, nor was it clear how the proposed local health authorities would relate either to existing voluntary hospitals or the established structure of local government. A combination of the vague character of the proposals, and other circumstances (described by Webster 1993: 218–19), meant that the Dawson report was shelved.

In the absence of central initiative, progress towards regionalism can best be traced through a range of reports and initiatives. First, efforts to stimulate greater cooperation within the voluntary sector are reviewed. Second, the post-1929 efforts at public-private partnership, following the Local Government Act are examined. Finally, there is discussion of a little-known initiative, in which central government grants were made available to voluntary and municipal hospitals, on condition that the hospitals agreed to a degree of coordination.

Cooperation within the voluntary sector

Three key reports commented, in the inter-war period, on the need for greater cooperation between the voluntary hospitals and between voluntary and municipal hospitals. These reports were produced by the government-appointed Cave Committee (Ministry of Health 1921) and the ensuing Onslow Commission (Ministry of Health 1925), and by the representative body for the voluntary hospitals, the British Hospitals Association (BHA), which established the Sankey Commission, which reported in 1937.

The financial crisis facing the voluntary hospitals after the war was brought on by rising wages and the costs of treating wartime casualties (Pinker 1966: 149–55). The severity of this situation prompted the establishment of the Cave Committee (1921) which documented inequalities in provision, financial difficulties, lack of coordination, and duplicative and wasteful expenditure. In 'large industrial areas of the North, the expansion of voluntary hospitals had not kept pace with population growth'. There was a 'crying need' for more hospital accommodation, especially in 'the poorer parts of the great cities, in South Wales, and Scotland' (p. 35). There was also 'lack of coordination' and 'much avoidable expenditure', with institutions 'working in isolation or even competition'. Greater efficiency could be obtained if there was a body which had the authority to organise and grade the hospitals in a district and act as a clearing-house for patients and this led to a recommendation that voluntary hospital committees be established in each locality. It was suggested that cooperation could be ensured through conditions attached to grant aid. However, the whole tenor of the report was antithetical to state intervention. Instead, greater cooperation and efficiency within the voluntary hospitals themselves would have the desired effect. Careful delimitation of catchments was essential here (a point also made by the 1925 Onslow Commission). Cooperation could extend to the coordination of appeals for funds and the extension of the embryo contributory schemes. Collections could be made by a central body, and distributed among hospitals on some agreed basis (p. 22). Efficiency could also be promoted through the adoption of a uniform system of accounts. It was thought to be impossible to raise by public subscription the sums necessary to extend hospital accommodation, and so the principal recommendation of Cave was Exchequer support for capital projects. The sum of £1 million was suggested and half of this was agreed by the government.

This grant was to be distributed by the Voluntary Hospitals (Onslow) Commission. The Commission attempted, while acknowledging the difficulties of doing so, to assess the need for additional hospital accommodation, albeit by relying on the recommendations of local voluntary hospital committees, which consisted largely of lists of schemes that were believed to be in the pipeline. What was therefore being evaluated was the vigour, or otherwise, with which the local committees (or their constituent hospitals) had pursued proposals for development in their localities. As a consequence, the proposed additional beds, though welcome, would not have reduced disparities in bed provision very much. Had the proposed developments all proceeded, nine counties (or aggregations thereof) with below-average levels of provision would actually have moved further below the national average; five would have moved from above-average levels of provision to below the national average; and eight local authorities with above-average levels of provision would have moved further above average. Consequently the variability in the bed/population ratio, as measured by the coefficient of variation, would have decreased only marginally, from 0.46 to 0.45.[3] These figures are a demonstration of the limits to relying on the voluntary system to meet social needs; levels of provision were not necessarily rising in localities in greatest need, and spatial inequalities in provision were therefore unlikely to be reduced. However, even on these figures, Onslow's view was that 'when every allowance is made for possible use of beds in Poor Law institutions', there remained an 'ascertained shortage of 10,000 beds, 2,000 of which were [needed] in London'.[4] How were such gaps to be closed? One possibility was to use vacant beds in Poor Law institutions, but this was likely to founder on the 'astonishing differences in the attitude of different areas towards Poor Law hospitals', especially in localities where contributory schemes had been established. Subscribers would regard proposals for cooperation with Poor Law infirmaries as an 'attempt on the part of the voluntary hospitals to escape from an implied bargain'.[5] In any case, voluntary and Poor Law hospital accommodation were by no means of comparable quality. Consequently there was acceptance of the 'broad principle of differentiation' between voluntary and Poor Law hospitals, the former being reserved for 'cases requiring special diagnostic facilities or a high degree of technical skill'. However, this was not to be regarded as a hard and fast rule.

An alternative possibility was to compel local authorities to provide in their own institutions beds for the treatment of cases for which they had statutory responsibility (especially for tuberculosis), but the problem here was that of interfering with the autonomy of local authorities. The statutes under which they could act were permissive, not mandatory. Hence any compulsion by central government was 'in effect an attempt to coerce the ratepayers'. If this was perceived as being associated with the voluntaries, it would 'react in the end to the prejudice of the hospitals themselves' (p. 8).

Thus the scope for a more rational distribution of cases between voluntary and Poor Law institutions was evidently limited. What of the scope for action within the voluntary sector? Some Ministry of Health officials saw the problem as much in terms of utilising existing resources rather than providing additional accommodation.[6] There was spare capacity in many small cottage hospitals, and it was argued that this could relieve pressure on urban general hospitals, if hospitals could somehow be persuaded to delimit spheres of influence. Again, there was reliance on voluntary cooperation; there was no suggestion of directly involving local authorities, or the Ministry of Health. The main recommendation of Onslow was that government assistance, covering up to 50 per cent of the cost of additional beds should be made available. The report also suggested that if resources were limited, they could be targeted on those places in greatest need. It was suggested that any grant aid should be 'accompanied by the clearest possible conditions as to those amendments in organisation which are essential if voluntary hospitals are to live as part of unified health provision'.[7] At a notional cost of £400 per bed, providing 10,000 beds would have entailed government grants totalling some £4 million. The government declined to provide this. However, a steady expansion of hospital provision took place and about 10,800 beds had been added by 1932,[8] though inequalities in provision did not diminish.

Some voluntary hospital representatives clearly favoured greater coordination. Indeed witnesses to the Cave Committee went so far as to suggest that voluntary hospital committees should have powers to shut, or to amalgamate, individual hospitals.[9] Early in 1922 the Secretary of a specialist hospital argued that each hospital 'spins like a star in the charitable firmament, absorbed in shining, and happily oblivious of the radiance of others'.[10] Responding to this, there were proposals for the establishment of a provincial equivalent of the King Edward's Hospital Fund for London, which could counteract the 'spirit of isolation' in which hospitals undertook their work'.[11] In a more outspoken comment, Sir Arthur Stanley, President of the BHA, warned that 'we have ... a large and heterogeneous accumulation of health and hospital services, more or less suited (but not necessarily adequate) to the needs of the population ... inelastic in their organisation, and not fully adjusted to meet the economic status of the several classes requiring their services'.[12] If the necessary 'readjustment, correlation and development' of services were to take place, then the voluntary hospitals would have to give up their isolated existence (p. 96). However, Stanley emphasised a clear line of demarcation between the voluntaries, which were to be specialised consultative centres, and the municipal hospitals, which would receive 'all simple and medical and surgical cases' which were not suitable for treatment at home. This would mean that the voluntaries, 'relieved of all their trivial cases', could concentrate on specialist work.

Despite warnings such as these, little changed within the voluntary sector between the wars, and this was recognised within the sector: Roden Orde, as Director of the Central Bureau of Hospital Information, drafted a memorandum which his Council 'thought rather too strong meat for voluntary stomachs'. It concerned the reasons for establishing a 'Commission ... to enquire what steps should be taken to meet the needs of the present and secure the future of the voluntary hospitals'.[13] In his draft he emphasised the dangers of isolationism and competition: 'today every error … [resulting] from this complete lack of unity is a blow to the voluntary system as a whole'. The hospitals were 'no longer a collection of isolated units'; there were 'questions of a financial character that can only be answered on a broader basis than that of the place in which the hospital is situated'.[14] Identifying a number of themes on which action was necessary above the level of the individual hospital, the BHA proceeded to establish the Voluntary Hospitals (Sankey) Commission, whose 1937 report showed how little had changed since Cave and Onslow.

It acknowledged duplication and inequity; there were some 'redundant hospitals where, perhaps, some generous donor has erected a building and left an endowment at a place already amply served'. The 'thousand separate Exchequers' of the system meant that it was difficult to evaluate its financial stability and viability. It proposed establishing Regional Hospitals Councils; these would have 'no coercive or compulsory powers, but they would be able to correlate hospital work with needs'.[15] They might administer a 'regional fund' – though no indication was given of the source of the money for such a fund. The council would determine the allocation of patients as between hospitals according to need, and would balance the workload of individual hospitals. An explicit hierarchy was proposed ('central', 'district' and 'cottage' hospitals) (pp. 23–5). Moreover, it argued that if the hospitals were able to redistribute their total annual income in accordance with the needs of individual hospitals, by paying into a common pool a percentage of hospital income, their financial position would not be unsatisfactory.[16] If such measures proved inadequate, Sankey suggested that any reluctance to accept state funding should disappear, pointing out that any violation of principle had already taken place (pp. 30–1), as more and more voluntary hospitals were in receipt of local authority funds. In fact, one reason why Sankey was unable to galvanise action beyond that envisaged by Cave and Onslow was precisely that the voluntary hospitals' finances had improved to some degree in the inter-war years, with the growth of contributory schemes and of other forms of support (though not all hospitals, in all places, had benefited to the same extent). This had consequently removed some pressure for collective action. The reception accorded to Sankey was therefore somewhat muted and the BHA did little to put it into practice. And although Sankey did welcome greater collaboration with the state sector, there were strict limits to this; for instance Sankey still proposed that voluntary hospitals would retain a degree of discretion in deciding which patients they would admit. As one Ministry official later pointed out, 'this rather unpromising condition means … that the state hospitals should take what the voluntary hospitals do not want'.[17] It certainly undermined the idea that the voluntary hospitals were acting altruistically. Sankey had emphasised the responsibilities of local authorities to voluntary hospitals rather than the need for reciprocal assistance. It might therefore produce 'organised opposition to municipal effort'.[18]

In practice, the extent of cooperation within the voluntary sector proved to be limited. There was, of course, the King's Fund in London, although it largely concentrated on the promotion of good management through the diffusion of statistics on comparative costs; some control over the trajectory of hospital development was, however, possible because the Fund gave grants to individual hospitals (Prochaska 1992). Discussion of collaboration elsewhere usually focuses on a limited number of well-known initiatives. Joint boards had been established in the Oxfordshire area and in Manchester (Pickstone 1986), while in Scotland an initiative in Aberdeen also involved the local authority hospitals (PEP 1937; Department of Health for Scotland 1936; both of these regarded Aberdeen as very much the exception within Scotland).[19] More detailed descriptions of regionalisation initiatives were given in the 1940 *Hospitals Yearbook*.[20] The schemes reviewed were in Birmingham, Devon/Cornwall, Liverpool, Manchester (see also Pickstone 1986), Oxford and Sheffield. These had grown out of voluntary hospitals and embraced all hospitals, both public and private. There were certainly some successful examples of cooperation, evidenced in discussions about the avoidance of duplication of capital investment, or about referral networks. Pickstone is complimentary about the work of the Manchester Joint Hospital Board (JHB) while other writers praised inter-authority collaboration elsewhere, for example Gloucestershire (PEP 1937: 260).

What was the evidence for cooperation between the voluntaries in the Northern region? There is little evidence of active cooperation, even when economic necessity might have been the midwife of invention. Indeed examples can be given in which institutions were quite openly hostile. In Sunderland, the inter-war period witnessed sporadic discussions about whether the town's largest hospital, the Royal Infirmary (340 beds), should merge with the Monkwearmouth and Southwick Hospital (a 50-bed general hospital in an industrial part of the town). Monkwearmouth consistently refused to entertain such proposals, pressing ahead instead with an appeal for a substantial extension, and declining to discuss the possibility of closer cooperation even when experiencing great financial difficulties in the 1920s.[21] A Ministry of Health survey report commented on the 'senseless rivalry' between the Sunderland voluntaries; a conference, organised under section 13 of the Local Government Act of 1929, had brought together representatives of the town's hospitals, but had 'done little good'.[22] Other survey reports referred to 'competition rather than cooperation' between hospitals in Hartlepool[23] and to the 'maldistribution of beds' between several small general hospitals in Cumberland, which had been 'fostered by local interests'.[24] In Newcastle, there were some small specialist hospitals which declined to cooperate with rationalisation proposals. The Babies' Hospital, for example, indicated to the City's Health Committee that it would prefer to 'preserve its individuality' and that its strategy was to 'make the hospital outstanding', thereby increasing interest in, and attracting financial support for, its work.[25] The Throat, Nose and Ear Hospital was pursuing their own expansion plans in the mid-1930s even though other voluntary hospitals (as well as the municipal hospital) offered treatment in the same areas of specialism.[26] The Princess Mary Maternity Hospital was criticised because it was reluctant to collaborate with other hospitals. The Medical Officer of Health had indicated that he would prefer to see the hospital relocate to a better site, 'preferably in association with the RVI or Newcastle General'.[27] These were not well-resourced hospitals, nor (given their size) were they well-placed to carry out complex treatments and there seemed an obvious case for rationalisation.

In Middlesbrough, too, there was not much by way of collaboration (this discussion draws on Mansfield 1991). The main voluntaries were the North Riding Infirmary (NRI) and the North Ormesby Hospital (NOH), and cooperation between them was initially a negative reaction to the 1929 legislation, because they believed that the Borough Council had taken insufficient steps to consult them. It was a further six years before collaboration was advanced (in the context of the Middlesbrough Hospitals Advisory Joint Committee: see below) and was even then short-lived (Mansfield 1991: 45–54). Initially the prospects seemed favourable and the BHA secretary was called in to advise on the prospects for amalgamation of the two hospitals, which he supported. The proposals were endorsed by the NRI but the NOH, while supportive of coordination, rejected amalgamation, principally because they believed that it would be impossible to raise the funds for a totally new general hospital. However, Mansfield (1991: 60) implies that North Ormesby took a rather 'parochial' attitude, possibly because its finances were in a much healthier state than those of the NRI. Elsewhere in the region the question of collaboration did not arise, since several boroughs only had one general hospital. But the limited examples given do not imply that cooperation within the voluntary sector achieved much. The availability of grants from the Commissioner for the Special Areas subsequently provided incentives for collaboration, but even so, debates about the allocation of grants were notable for evidence of mutual distrust between institutions.

An evaluation of voluntary cooperation would thus suggest a very mixed record. There clearly were examples of good practice, in which hospitals were actively collaborating to avoid duplication and rationalise patient flows. There were other instances of cooperation in terms of fundraising: numerous examples can be found of hospital contributory schemes developing to cover a wide geographical area rather than simply an individual hospital.[28] However, almost by definition reliance on voluntary cooperation had its limitations. The divergent financial fortunes of individual hospitals was one reason why relatively little cooperation took place. And voluntary cooperation could do nothing to address the problems of locations where there were no hospitals in existence; substantial disparities thus remained in access to the voluntaries. Evaluating what voluntary cooperation had accomplished, Ministry of Health officials felt that little of lasting value had been achieved. 'Apart from Gloucestershire', wrote one official, there is very little going on which conforms ... to what [Lord] Dawson [is] always talking about'.[29] The atmosphere among voluntary hospitals was 'one of splendid isolation tempered by financial misgivings'; the main interest of the voluntary hospitals in cooperation lay in what they could obtain from the state, not what they could contribute to a comprehensive service.[30] Subsequently the same author described the weaknesses of several proposals for coordination and planning, and commented that even well-regarded schemes, such as those in Oxford and Manchester, had done little more than 'touch the fringe' of the problem of cooperation.[31]

Municipal development and public–private collaboration

The 1929 Local Government Act empowered local authorities to provide general hospital services. This was an extension of their existing responsibility for the treatment of infectious diseases. However, the Ministry of Health clearly did not envisage the supersession of voluntary by municipal hospitals, because 'the increased burden which would be thrown on the taxpayer by general municipalisation is a thing which we could not contemplate'.[32] Given the financial climate in which local authorities were operating, and a political climate with a presumption against public expenditure, municipal development faced high hurdles. Although the Ministry of Health insisted that needy authorities were not denied assistance, it was suggested that the Ministry had

> necessarily had to exercise great care in sanctioning fresh indebtedness [i.e. capital expenditure financed by loan] in areas with high rates, heavy debts and a doubtful future, but in no case has sanction been refused to a loan for works put forward on urgent grounds of public health.[33]

It may well have been true that no application was actually refused but this presumes that applications were actually put forward, and the Ministry did not always positively encourage local authorities to propose schemes for hospital development.

Not all local authorities responded with enthusiasm to the challenges of the 1929 Act. Quantitative evidence on local authority hospital services, reviewed in Chapter 2, indicates some of the variation, but does not fully capture the vigour – or otherwise – with which authorities had attempted to develop services. A series of Ministry of Health surveys undertaken in the early 1930s provides a comprehensive picture of the initial efforts being made by local authorities to discharge their public health responsibilities. All local authorities were visited by a Ministry inspector; a survey report was made to the Ministry, and there followed correspondence about services which were deemed unsatisfactory. Over one-third of local authorities in

England were viewed as having deficiencies in their services of sufficient magnitude as to require a re-survey: twenty-two (of forty-nine) county councils and twenty-three (of seventy-nine) county boroughs. However, the Ministry's reports tend to emphasise the deficiencies of the local authorities rather than the inadequacy of available resources. Comments on the local authorities selected for re-survey frequently include adjectives such as 'backward', 'reactionary', 'difficult' and 'suspicious'. There are good reasons for scepticism about the Ministry's approach.

First, explanations cast in terms of inadequate resourcing would have had, as their corollary, proposals for additional expenditure, which could hardly be tolerated in the financial climate of the early 1930s. Second, some local authorities were described as reactionary and backward for pursuing precisely those policies encouraged by central government which required economies in public expenditure. Instead of using central government block grants to expand provision, they had deliberately chosen to keep the rates down. It was illogical, in these circumstances, for the Ministry to criticise local authorities, since the Ministry had demanded economies (Bradbury 1990: 308–10). The autonomy available to local authorities in spending the block grant helped them to pursue reactionary policies if they so desired. Third, the Ministry was known to have discouraged some local authorities from pursuing policies which would have involved increased expenditure, usually on the grounds of the uncertain economic future of particular places (Ward 1984, 1988).[34]

Despite these reservations, these Ministry surveys provide a revealing insight into the ways in which local authorities had begun to tackle the challenges of hospital provision. While three of the principal CBs – Newcastle, Sunderland and Middlesbrough – were swift to appropriate Poor Law infirmaries for general hospital purposes, elsewhere progress was hesitant. Some councils were described in the terminology one might expect from colonial officials visiting an outpost of the Empire: 'allowance must be made for the difficulty [the Medical Officer of Health] had in carrying with him a County Council very economical and slow to take up new things'; 'a council economical if not niggardly',[35] 'very dilatory',[36] 'parsimonious ... niggardly ... [the] members seem determined not to spend money although it is obvious that a wide expenditure would be economical'.[37] The most severe strictures were reserved for West Hartlepool and South Shields. The latter had not 'devoted sufficient attention to public health in the past, when it could have afforded to bring its services up to date'. The Council were therefore criticised for practising indiscriminate economy; instead they should 'distinguish between a wholesale course of cutting down expenditure ... and a judicious discrimination between those services which are urgently necessary and other services which, however desirable, are not so urgently necessary'.[38] In West Hartlepool the council had responded very negatively to the first survey report, which had been highly critical. They had 'with few regrets (if not positive satisfaction) deferred all action on grounds of economy'; on receipt of further criticism from Ministry officials the local MP had stepped in and protested to the responsible Minister.[39] The Council had 'been dominated by a few small-minded but influential members whose idea has been to keep down rates at all costs ... so far as West Hartlepool is concerned [the 1929 Act] might never have been passed'. But despite such criticisms there is no evidence that the Ministry penalised backward or irresponsible authorities, as they were empowered to do by the Act: perhaps it was recognised that this would have been counterproductive.

In other circumstances the Ministry saw its role as persuading authorities to make the best use of existing resources. Sometimes this meant urging restraint on Medical Officers of Health. In Cumberland, the 1929 Act 'filled the County Medical Officer of Health with large ideas of hospital development'. On the basis of 'arbitrary and speculative' indices, he had proposed an additional 150 beds, but this 'postulated a generous interpretation of the word "necessitous"', and it 'bore no relation to the former obligations [under the Poor Law] for the hospital treatment of the sick'.[40] The interesting technical point here is that need for services was expressed through existing levels of utilisation. There is no hint that demand might have been suppressed by low levels of provision (despite references to lengthy waiting lists) nor is there discussion of the possibility of latent demand being exposed if new facilities were built. The latter possibility had been hinted at elsewhere; there had been reports in professional journals of 'rising use of hospital accommodation throughout all PAIs since the institutions were transferred'.[41] In Durham, the Ministry attempted to persuade the Medical Officer of Health not to pursue his preferred solution of a new 500-bed general hospital. Aside from the financial consequences (see Chapter 2), the Ministry drew attention to the possibility of better classification of patients, making more appropriate use of available accommodation; moreover, existing hospital utilisation in Poor Law institutions suggested that there was spare capacity.[42] This was accepted by the Council although the result was the retention of a scattered collection of antiquated and inadequate buildings.

Financial constraints and political priorities were thus important, but policy was that active collaboration could close gaps in services if public and private sectors worked together. The 1929 Act required local authorities to consult with representatives of voluntary hospitals, so that a degree of coordination might be achieved. This was honoured as much in the breach as the observance: many authorities did not set up such committees and, where they were established, collaboration was limited.

A Ministry survey of the extent of arrangements for consultation between voluntary hospitals and local authorities showed, in May 1933, that there were fifteen counties, and thirty-one county boroughs, in which meetings between both sides had occurred. It was pointed out, somewhat counter-intuitively, that 'in some of the areas where real cooperation is closest it is most difficult to find evidence'.[43] The Ministry's Annual Report for 1933–4 suggested that in some areas consultation with voluntary hospitals was viewed as a 'somewhat unpleasant statutory duty', to be discharged through a one-off meeting.[44] A view of what cooperation meant in practice is provided by the Ministry surveys. Despite the appearance of Sunderland in the aforementioned list, the survey referred to the lack of cooperation between the general hospitals, both municipal and voluntary.[45] A later resurvey suggested that, despite considerable investment and change in Sunderland's hospital services in the 1930s, the Joint Committee between municipal and voluntary services had met only once. The lack of cooperation was attributed to the 'autocratic and resentful' attitude of the voluntaries,[46] the Monkwearmouth Hospital being criticised for its 'uncompromising' stance. Elsewhere, uncooperative attitudes were found on both sides. Thus in Carlisle the City Medical Officer of Health had been 'frankly antipathetic' to the (voluntary) Cumberland Infirmary, and had sketched a hospital policy with an 'entire and ingenuous disregard for the Infirmary's existence'.[47] However, the governors of the Cumberland Infirmary were castigated, in their turn, for 'choosing ... the prosperity of the Infirmary rather than the service of the city'. The City Council and the Infirmary were thus pursuing separate lines of development. This was unfortunate because, as Carlisle was the *'de facto* medical centre for a large region ... (the) cultivation and strengthening of (its) general hospital resources (was) ... a duty not alone of the city or county, but of regional importance'.[48] The Ministry's post-survey letter to the City Council warned of the risks of 'sporadic developments by individual authorities';[49] however, relations improved later in the decade, possibly spurred by the availability of grant aid from the Commissioner for the Special Areas (see below). In South Shields it was also clear to the wartime surveyors that little cooperation had been achieved.[50]

Cooperation appeared better (or at least more courteous) in Middlesbrough and Newcastle. In Middlesbrough there was established a Hospitals Advisory Joint Committee which sought to encourage greater cooperation. This committee had to deal, as in many locations, with arguments about why voluntary hospitals were not admitting workers despite their regular financial contributions to the voluntaries. Instead, they were forced to seek admission to municipal hospitals and it was claimed that the number of such cases was rising. An agreement was subsequently reached whereby such cases were paid for by the voluntary hospitals which had referred them (Mansfield 1991: 46, 54–5). The Newcastle evidence shows that there were regular exchanges between the public and voluntary sectors. Even before the 1929 Act came into effect, it had been agreed that the RVI should ensure that 25 per cent of its beds were available for residents of Newcastle and a clearing house was set up to allocate patients between hospitals. However, pressure on the RVI meant that it was having to discharge patients swiftly even when their 'home circumstances do not allow of proper attention being given', and it was not always able to guarantee the availability of these beds.[51] These pressures led the city to establish its own general hospital through appropriation, but without developing 'special departments in conflict with existing establishments'. Such links were not formalised for several years, until a Hospitals Advisory Board was established in 1937.[52]

What conclusions can be drawn, then, about public–private partnerships in this region? The verdict can hardly be positive. Both voluntary and municipal providers experienced the effects of depression, but despite this there is little sign of attempts voluntarily to cooperate in the public interest. Arguably a fundamental weakness of this system was that, in relying on partnership, it presumed the existence of partners, but in certain areas these did not exist, in either the public or private sectors. Representatives of the BMA made precisely this point; according to Ministry officials, the BMA

> seemed anxious that as much pressure as possible should be put on the local authorities [to provide further hospital accommodation]. Unfortunately the areas they particularly mentioned, places like Gateshead and Durham, were places where the financial difficulties of the local authorities will render any such provision particularly difficult.[53]

This highlights an important limitation of the public–private mix: it could not guarantee provision of services in locations not already possessing them. The Ministry could warn local authorities of the costs of developments; it could even refuse to approve development proposals although it is clear that it had grave misgivings about so doing.[54] But what it could not do was compel an authority to provide services. There may have been a few examples of good practice and productive collaboration but Fox's verdict – that various agencies had 'begun to implement' a consensus on regionalism – seems somewhat optimistic.

Towards planning: neglected examples of regionalism?

The attempt to rely on voluntary cooperation and on public–private partnerships could not, on the basis of the foregoing, be said to have succeeded. But this did not mean, as a corollary, that proposals would emerge for greater state intervention. This section reviews such proposals that did come forward and attention is also drawn to two little-known initiatives aimed at a greater degree of coordination and planning.

The Cathcart Committee on the Scottish Health Services (Department of Health for Scotland 1936) emphasised the integration of primary and secondary care, and made proposals for the coordination and extension of hospital services. It was concerned to shore up the voluntary system, and it was therefore acknowledged that simply making grants available for capital expenditure (a similar proposal to that of Cave and Onslow) might impose 'a serious burden for future maintenance … (which the hospitals) might not be able to carry' (p. 235). Cathcart, therefore, envisaged that in order to close gaps in the availability of services, a 'definite obligation' should be placed on local authorities to supplement existing facilities, aided by an Exchequer grant of at least 50 per cent of approved capital expenditure. Collaboration would also require more formal partnerships between voluntary hospitals and the Health Department than hitherto. It was proposed that the Department's approval to all planned hospital developments (whether voluntary or municipal) be required, and that the Department be empowered, in the last resort, to veto proposals (p. 241) and to compel combination of (local) authorities for defined purposes. Indeed Cathcart suggested that it should be the duty of the central Department of Health to 'initiate' necessary regional schemes. This is perhaps the most vigorous and positive conception of planning enunciated in any inter-war document; despite its support for voluntarism, it was clear that state intervention was necessary if gaps in the availability of services were to be closed.

However, the official reaction – from Baldwin's Conservative government – studiously avoided support for such recommendations, and the conservative press in Scotland queried the cost implications, the *Scotsman* contending that Cathcart's proposals were 'not far removed' from a state medical service (quoted in MacLachlan 1987: 77). The proposals were also criticised by officials. A Ministry of Health paper on the future development of hospital services regarded Cathcart as 'evading rather than facing' key problems: it was not clear, for example, to whom regional committees would report, nor who would have the final say in their deliberations.[55] For one civil servant charged with evaluating inter-war proposals, Cathcart was 'more promising' than the Sankey Commission, but the 'real arbiter' in planning would be the Department of Health. This degree of centralisation might have been feasible in Scotland, but in England it would be necessary to create regional councils with executive powers. Moreover, the Scottish voluntaries had shown more 'willingness to accept a measure of state control' than had their English counterparts.[56]

The Political and Economic Planning (PEP) *Report on the British Health Services* (1937) argued vigorously that hospital provision was 'essentially regional' and should be approached according to the needs of the region served, without reference to 'arbitrary and extraneous' factors such as local government boundaries and divisions between voluntary and public hospitals. Regionalism would facilitate the elimination of duplication and waste, particularly with respect to the specialist hospitals. PEP also considered at some length the inadequacies of public sector hospitals, arguing that most of the problems of local authority hospitals were problems of the existing local government structure, and consequently could only be resolved through a reorganisation of local government. Civil servants criticised this document for its 'lack of concreteness'.[57] However, the Royal Commission on Tyneside Local Government (1936) made broadly similar recommendations. It pointed to the confused and overlapping network of joint arrangements for delivering health services in industrial Tyneside. In an area the size of Birmingham there were sixteen local authorities with various health responsibilities. The 'inordinate disparity' in the provision and maintenance of services was indefensible, but the various local authorities all had different attitudes towards reform, coloured by the financial ramifications. Owen (1990: 59–103) also points to the political constraints. The most rational solution, an amalgamation of Durham and Northumberland, would have been more obviously regional but was disliked because of the relative size of the counties. Almost any other solution would have enhanced Newcastle at the expense of the counties, and this was not regarded as feasible. The local authorities were simply unable to articulate a shared interest, and the only result was some minor boundary amendments.

The initiatives or proposals described thus far generally relied on goodwill and voluntary cooperation, as well as a vigorous and progressive attitude on the part of local authorities. But they were both likely to run up against harsh economic realities, whether in the form of difficulties of raising private finance, or a limited rate base. Such considerations applied with particular force in locations which either had relatively weak economies to begin with, or which had borne the brunt of inter-war depression. What could be done about such problems of market failure?

In fact, as far back as 1912, a committee of the Scottish Home and Health Department had concluded that 'the private enterprise of doctors was grossly inadequate to meet the medical needs of the Highlands' (Department of Health for Scotland 1936: 22). Consequently, the Highlands and Islands Medical Service was established in 1913, with an annual grant, much of which was allocated to GPs in the remoter areas. Funds were also given to support hospital and specialist services, in conjunction with local authorities; grants from this source prevented closure of the Belford Hospital, Fort William, in 1916 (Kinnaird 1987: 222). The Royal Northern Hospital, Inverness, which experienced 'serious and disquieting' financial difficulties in the early 1920s, also received assistance (Mackenzie 1946: 232–66).

The inadequacies of private enterprise were not, of course, confined to the Highlands and Islands. One of the most visible measures aimed at coordination was through a route which demonstrates how market failures provoked demands for greater state intervention, and which also shows how the problems of health services in particular places led to reappraisals of existing orthodoxy. The Commissioner for the Special Areas (hereafter, the CSA) had been appointed in 1934, with a view to developing schemes which would benefit the economy and residents of the depressed coalfield areas of Tyneside, Durham, South Wales, West Cumberland and Scotland. Given the constraints imposed on him, however, large-scale economic intervention was impossible and therefore much of the CSA's activities focused on social services. The Commissioner asked officials to investigate whether the health services of the 'Special Areas' could be regarded as inferior (or not) to those available elsewhere in the country. Their answers were notable for their evasiveness and for efforts to put the most positive gloss on what they found, but nevertheless deficiencies were identified and the Commissioners were persuaded to make quite substantial grants to health and other social services in the designated areas. What is interesting about the CSA is the extent to which it promoted a vision of cooperation and planned development which would link together both voluntary and municipal hospitals, and it appears to be a largely neglected area of concern in the history of hospital policy. With grant aid in his gift, the Commissioner was able to insist that voluntary hospitals cooperate in the kind of agreements envisaged by the 1929 Local Government Act; further weapons in his armoury were the fact that Ministry of Health approval was required before grants were made, as was the confirmation of the local authority that schemes were consistent with their own plans.

There were lengthy debates about the principle of offering grant aid to hospitals. Initially, it was proposed that assistance would only be available to municipal hospitals, on the grounds that voluntary hospitals had always resisted the controls that would be attached to grant aid. The BHA's conference in May 1935 reaffirmed its traditional opposition to state control.[58] However, according to one official, a 'substantial majority' of the voluntaries were against state assistance on principle, but 'principles are difficult to maintain when poverty is knocking at the door'.[59] While the voluntary hospitals were 'a little nervous of Exchequer grants', in the case of capital grants 'this fear was not well-founded'.[60] Thus resistance to greater state finance was rather less than had been thought likely and, consequently, by late 1935 it was agreed that the commissioner would be empowered to offer grant aid to voluntary hospitals for a proportion (usually between 50–75 per cent) of the capital cost of a scheme (100 per cent grants were approved only exceptionally, the thinking being that such grants would be tantamount to an argument for state control). There was evidence that the voluntary system was reaching its limits, because, in these locations, the task of raising 'large sums by voluntary donations is well-nigh impossible'.[61]

The Commissioner, in concert with the Ministry of Health, took a selective view as to which hospitals should be grant-aided; there was concern at the possibility of being 'inundated' with applications from cottage hospitals.[62] Selectivity in grant aid appeared desirable from the point of view of rationalisation and efficiency, but this also placed the Ministry of Health in a somewhat difficult position: the Ministry was plainly reluctant to discourage any proposals for the expansion of hospital facilities but, conversely, they did not want to support the continued existence of hospitals whose contribution to future health-care provision was likely to be limited. The Commissioner's officials pointed out the Ministry's rather ambivalent attitude: for example, with regard to proposals for an extension at Lady Eden Hospital, Bishop Auckland (whose parlous finances were discussed in Chapter 2), it was suggested that the Ministry '*should tell us whether it wants this hospital to go on or not'.* Given the poverty of the area, a case could possibly have been made for a 100 per cent grant, but as the Ministry had not definitively decided, one way or another, that the hospital was worth supporting, the Commissioner was in a difficult position.[63]

Similarly, with respect to a proposed extension of the Tynemouth Infirmary, the Ministry of Health were alleged to have:

> left the question rather open. *They no doubt have a natural bias towards wishing to see an extension of hospital provision* and if they find a volun-tary hospital apparently prepared to make a substantial extension, provided it gets some assistance, they are reluctant to curtail the plan. The cases in which ... the existing hospital provision is so perfect that an extension ... is superfluous, must be few and far between – both inside and outside the Special Areas'.[64]

In other cases action was more direct. For example the Commissioner had received a request for grant aid for the Palmer Memorial Hospital, Jarrow, which was experiencing grave financial problems (see Chapter 2). Officials doubted whether 'grant was justifiable in the absence of informa-tion as to the hospital's ability to raise part of the capital cost and to meet heavier maintenance charges'. A scheme for Ellison Hall Hospital, in nearby Hebburn, was noted as 'not being proceeded with for lack of funds' and was therefore regarded as 'lapsed'[65] – there does not appear to have been any question of offering a larger grant to ensure that it was developed. Thus, in towns which would have been regarded as among the most depressed places in the Special Areas, questions were raised about the likely financial viability of proposals for hospital development. The inability of the hospitals concerned to raise even a proportion of the capital or maintenance expendi-ture seems to have contributed to a rejection of the schemes, rather than being an argument for greater assistance on social grounds.

The existence of grant aid was also used to promote coordination of hospital development proposals. The best single example of the Commissioner promoting coordination of hospital development was in Newcastle. Although hospital provision was dominated by the Royal Victoria Infirmary (RVI – the teaching hospital) there existed several other, much smaller and specialist, voluntary institutions. The local authority had actively developed its own medical facilities, notably the Newcastle General Hospital. In December 1935 the North Eastern District Commissioner, Mr C. Forbes Adam, wrote that there was 'absolutely no coordination' of the voluntary hospital services. Some younger doctors were interested in a more rationally planned service, but they had 'made no headway against old-fashioned sectionalism', which could lead to waste and delay. Forbes Adam felt, nevertheless, that the Commissioner had the 'opportunity to help in the movement towards coordination'.[66] He himself played an active role in bringing together several voluntary hospital projects, lobbying the hospitals to collaborate on a 'systematised contributory scheme', which would have more prospects of success than 'spasmodic and competitive appeals issued independently'.[67] In recognition of his efforts, the District Commissioner was invited as a principal guest at the launch, in 1940, of a joint appeal for funds by Newcastle's hospitals.[68]

More generally the Commissioner and the Ministry saw in the submission of several disparate proposals for Newcastle's hospital services an opportunity for 'securing cooperation and coordination ... to avoid duplication ... and to effect administrative economies'.[69] The BHA endorsed this[70] and one of the immediate effects was a suggestion that the proposed development of the Throat, Nose and Ear Hospital be accommodated instead on the site of the Royal Victoria Infirmary (RVI).[71] While it was agreed that some form of merger and rationalisation was desirable, however, the plans would require modification if all the beds of the various institutions were to be accommodated on the RVI site. The availability of grant aid helped ensure that the hospitals settled their differences and worked vigorously to arrive at a compromise scheme acceptable to the Commissioner.[72]

This was not the only attempt to coordinate the activities of disparate bodies. In Cumberland aid was granted towards the cost of improvements at Carlisle Infirmary, even though Carlisle was not in the Special Areas. The reasoning was that the County Council, together with Carlisle City Council, were developing a 'unified general hospital system' in which the 'base' hospital was to be the (voluntary) Cumberland Infirmary.[73] Such grants could contribute towards the development of a more rational pattern of service provision, and the hospitals would in any case serve patients from within the Special Areas of West Cumberland. If grants were not given the local authority would have to abandon its scheme for centralisation and various voluntary hospitals would have to patch up unsatisfactory accommodation. Similarly, the Tynemouth Victoria Jubilee Infirmary was refused grant aid to expand their provision for treatment of medical cases, because the local Public Assistance Institution was equipped to deal with them.[74] Several local authorities also found the Commissioner gently twisting their arms. Thus, in respect of schemes proposed in Sunderland, it was suggested that 'the fact that they are all seeking assistance from the Commissioner provides a useful means of persuasion'.[75] In this case the Commissioner appeared prepared to use the stick of withdrawal of offers of assistance rather than the carrot of grant aid: 'if the Council can afford to ignore the facilities offered by voluntary hospitals, we should be justified in concluding that they have withdrawn their request for support'.[76]

The precise impact on hospital development of the Commissioner's activities is difficult to assess with certainty. In terms of the levels of capital investment obtaining in the northern region prior to the 1930s, it seems fair to claim that the CSA made quite a substantial contribution to realising the ambitions of numerous hospitals, both municipal and voluntary.[77] Some expansion in hospital capacity took place but a Ministry of Health survey of bed provision indicated that the three regions which include the Special Areas 'come out badly' on provision of hospital beds (excluding mental hospitals): the average for the country was 7.14 beds/1,000 population, but Westmorland and Cumberland had 5.24, South Wales 5.18 and the North East 6.25.[78] The Ministry thought it was dangerous to suggest that 'completely satisfactory services ... (have been) established';[79] the Commissioner had been 'optimistic' in asserting that public health and sanitary services in the Special Areas had been brought 'up to the general level obtaining in other parts of the country'.[80]

If such equalisation was beyond the powers and resources of the Commissioner, these interventions still have relevance as examples of attempts to achieve a degree of coordination of hospital development. This was not without its costs. One of these was that proposals became tangled up in a web of bureaucracy. Voluntary hospital schemes would have to be discussed by the relevant local authority, the Ministry of Health, the Commissioner, and the Ministry of Labour (and quite possibly the Cabinet Committee on the Special Areas, if disputes arose over levels of grant aid or eligibility). The wonder is that proposals got through at all, and this rather casts doubt on the autonomy, and capacity to innovate, of the Commissioner. On the other hand, there were schemes in which the Commissioner acted as a useful intermediary, and was able to correct mutual misconceptions on the part of voluntary and municipal agencies. The Commissioner, in consort with the Ministry of Health, also took a wider view of the need for hospital services, so that hospital proposals were not considered in isolation, but whether this amounted to a sophisticated concept of regionalism is debatable.

Moreover, if we recall that by relying on voluntary hospitals themselves to submit proposals, to some extent grant aid was given where the voluntary sector was already more active. Thus, despite arguments about whether Newcastle really merited inclusion in the Special Areas, hospitals there were awarded substantial grants, including the wealthy Royal Victoria Infirmary. Strict controls on loans for capital investment meant that those places in greatest need did not necessarily receive assistance. For these reasons the Commissioner's hospital programme did not represent the initiation of 'planning' of hospital services, conceived in the sense of responding to patterns of social need. Nor did it correspond to Fox's notion of regionalism, namely an attempt to devise coordinated hierarchies of health-care facilities. Nothing in the legislation empowered the Commissioners to establish hospitals where they did not already exist or where no local agency had expressed a willingness or ability to provide them. What can be said, however, is that close liaison between the Commissioner and the Ministry of Health did at least ensure that a dose of rationality and coordination was injected into an otherwise largely unplanned system of welfare provision. Constraints on the Commissioners' activities meant, however, that while the first Commissioner was 'persuaded of the advantages of state hospitals',[81] any further intervention was ruled off the agenda.

Concluding comments

While there was broad acceptance of the need for coordination and planning, problems became evident when the mechanisms through which such coordination could be attained were spelt out. Voluntary cooperation had had very little effect, and local authority performance and attitude were variable, even when not constrained by resources. Despite some examples of good practice this mixed economy was characterised in many places by distrust on both sides. The post-1929 consultation process was also asymmetric; voluntary hospitals demanded to be informed about municipal development but were not 'prepared to concede the same right to local authorities' in respect of their own projects.[82] Ministry insiders were well aware of their limited powers. One commented that there were 'practically no dealings with the voluntary hospitals which provided nearly all the acute services'. As for the local authorities, the Ministry was constrained by the 'cumbersome inspection process' which produced 'limited results ... (the) suggestions made in post-inspection letters were out-of-date'.[83] The Ministry might, therefore, have seen its role as an advisory and supervisory one, but it does appear that this role had its limitations.

Despite this, there does not appear to have been proposals for hospital nationalisation. The Cathcart Committee envisaged central grants to local authorities, and advocated greater powers of direction, but Sankey insisted that this would not work south of the border. Even though PEP argued that, eventually, greater public control would have to follow the greater sums of public money being paid to voluntary hospitals, they admitted the difficulties of retaining the good features of voluntary control in a state system, and they argued that moves towards greater state control would take place in a gradualist fashion, as an organic outgrowth of the development of contributory schemes and local authority payments. Left-wing opinion, represented through the Socialist Medical Association and the Labour Party, argued for much greater public provision and control, inspired by the example of the LCC, and Webster (1988a: 190–1) contends that early wartime policy-making was being conducted in response to developments in Labour thinking. On the whole, SMA and Labour proposals envisaged a local government service, though some argued that central finance would be necessary to overcome the variable performance of councils (Stewart 1999: 139–40).

The experience of this period sheds light on the current vogue for public–private partnerships. Cooperation did not necessarily take place even in economically distressed localities, even though it might be thought to be a rational strategy. Hospitals could not be persuaded to sink their differences in the public interest. There was no logic of collective action that could

guarantee socially beneficial results. External circumstances, whether negative as in Middlesbrough, or positive, as in the case of the availability of
CSA grant aid, could occasionally persuade institutions to cooperate, but
this was not so everywhere.

Nor could partnership or cooperation guarantee the availability of
services. Voluntary hospitals with expansion plans could express the hope
that new facilities would enthuse public support and attract payments from
local authorities, but they could not guarantee that this would be the result.
There are parallels, perhaps, with the contemporary purchaser–provider
split, under which provider units must demonstrate purchaser commitment
(i.e. that revenue will be available to fund developments). If financial
commitments could not be given, nor were there bodies able to veto
proposals, at least from the voluntary sector; although the Ministry had
some powers (in the last resort, loan sanctions) with respect to local authorities, it is not clear whether and to what extent they were used.

In these circumstances, there was no mechanism for ensuring that additional services were made available where they were most needed.
Cooperation and partnership depended on the existence of potential partners. The idea that coordinated regional strategies were pursued is therefore
a very optimistic one. The need for rationalisation was agreed but nowhere
in pre-war debates was there an attempt to elaborate just how much hospital
provision was needed and, consequently, what desired levels of capital
investment might be. Nor did any of these reports – Cathcart excepted –
indicate how any additional capital investment might be financed and how it
might be provided in the locations most in need of it. At best (as in the case
of schemes assisted by the CSA) there was *post hoc* coordination rather than
top-down identification of needy places. It is, consequently, difficult to
endorse arguments which imply that regionalism was a settled issue before
World War II. It is better seen as something on which there was a limited
consensus, albeit one which did not extend beyond the lowest common
denominator of agreeing that the extension of hospital provision was desirable. Owen's (1990: 50) verdict, that regionalism in local government was
'inchoate', and that it became 'part and parcel of the conflict it was designed
to resolve', could thus equally apply to health care. Translating vague ideas
about the need for cooperation into practical proposals for extending
services therefore occupied substantial effort during the wartime years.

4   Wartime hospital policy
Attractions and limitations of public–private partnerships

So much has been written about the wartime negotiations on the form of the NHS that further discussion would appear superfluous. However, although the general contours of debates are widely known, a number of technical issues have received rather less attention. The focus here is on the extent to which the various suggestions for post-war policy would, if implemented, have produced the desirable outcome of improved access to services. Although there was some convergence towards 'hierarchical regionalism' (Fox 1986), several important questions remained to be resolved if a comprehensive service were to be provided. These concerned how to extend services to locations from which they were absent, how to rationalise services where there was duplication, how to finance extensions to services, how to respond to variations in efficiency between hospitals, and how to devise an appropriate regional organisation. It will be argued that various wartime proposals all failed to resolve at least one of these problems. This was partly because of the limitations of existing knowledge (e.g. on the comparative costs of hospitals) but, more generally, because officials were operating on the assumption that little change would take place in the existing arrangements. Rather than pushing for ideal solutions, policies therefore became bogged down in a series of unsatisfactory compromises.

The context for these debates is fairly well known. As shown in Chapters 2 and 3, the quantity, quality and financial stability of the hospitals varied greatly from place to place. Changing financial arrangements – notably, the growth of hospital contributory schemes – were inculcating the belief that access to health care was a right. Growing demands for hospital treatment had therefore generated pressures which the voluntary system could not meet, and these were manifested in rising waiting lists and the denial of requests for admission. Although municipal hospitals were beginning to provide a high-quality alternative, the stigma of association with the Poor Law allegedly inhibited use of them (though this clearly was not the case everywhere: the London County Council believed that their hospital service had succeeded in overcoming this problem).[1] Thus, public dissatisfaction with arrangements for health-care delivery was plain enough (Jacobs 1993: 61–2). As early as 1939, a Gallup poll found that 71 per cent of the public advocated making 'hospitals a public service supported by public funds' (quoted in Jacobs 1993: 61). Public opinion gradually crystallised in favour of a comprehensive health service as a key goal of post-war policy. In particular, the public expressed strong opposition to charity, and to arrangements that differentiated patients according to financial means, as well as support for greater government involvement in health care (Webster 1988a: 27–8; Jacobs 1993: 66–70). One Ministry of Health paper suggested in August 1941 that public opinion would not have been satisfied with anything less than a system in which treatment was available to anyone who needed it.[2]

If this was so, and if there was a consensus on the desirability of extending health-care provision, to what extent would the various wartime schemes have achieved this desirable goal? Was nationalisation of the hospitals inevitable, or could the mix of public and private provision have provided a viable basis for the NHS? These questions are not merely of antiquarian relevance. Arguments about the establishment of the NHS were notable for extensive debate about whether some form of public–private partnership could deliver results, or whether greater state intervention might be necessary. A related issue concerns the way a mixed economy of welfare might be managed; there are indications that contractual arrangements, not unlike those eventually adopted in 1991, were considered. Ling's (2000) discussion of partnerships is helpful here. He suggests that partnerships seek to mobilise, for the collective good, the 'values and culture of partner organisations'. A key question here is whether, and to what extent, this realignment of the goals of partners can actually take place. The ethos of the voluntary hospitals was self-evidently rather different to that of the municipal institutions and, as will become evident, there were problems in reconciling the two. Second, Ling argues that, at the turn of the millennium, partnerships reflect a 'genuine shift in the idea of what the appropriate purpose and limits of the state should be'. In the wartime years, on the other hand, it may be that proposals for partnerships were developed to head off the possibility of encroachment by the state on the private realm. These points raise questions about the nature of the (actual and hypothetical or proposed) partnerships of the wartime years. Could these guarantee the desired goal of a comprehensive service? If not, what would that say about the limitations of existing arrangements? The Ministry of Health had always seen itself as an 'advisory, supervisory and subsidising department';[3] could it continue in this role, or would greater intervention be required?

The principal concern of the chapter, then, is with the succession of non-solutions devised in the wartime years. The chapter is divided into two principal sections. The first examines assessments of the deficiencies of pre-war health services, principally those made by civil servants in the wartime years. The second section evaluates various wartime proposals for change. The focus is on the extent to which these could have secured the objective of a comprehensive service, and on whether they could have been politically feasible. The contribution of this chapter lies in refracting the 1940s debates through contemporary lenses, not simply to exhume antecedents of later controversies, but also to reassess whether a mixed economy might have been feasible.

Evaluation of the pre-NHS hospital services

A number of criticisms were advanced of the hospital system as it had evolved prior to 1939. Key criticisms related to the inadequacy and variability of provision, and to the financial position of the voluntaries. Other issues concerned the problem of comparative levels of efficiency, and the 'free-rider' problem, which is inherent in voluntarism. This section reviews – insofar as it can be reconstructed – the evidence available to the Ministry during the war.

By May 1938 the Ministry had identified three key deficiencies of the hospital service: an *overall* shortage of beds; disparities between geographical areas; and the inefficient use of accommodation (for example, 'bed blocking' by chronic cases).[4] The precise extent of the variability and deficiency was not entirely revealed until the Nuffield Surveys (1946), though an undated (but probably 1939) Ministry document points to many areas of the country in which there was a 'known need for additional accommodation for the civilian sick'. However, the source of information on unmet need appears to be the same local authority proposals, the variability of which had been criticised by the Ministry in the post-1929 surveys (Chapter 3). Thus evidence of unmet need in Durham, South Shields and Sunderland appeared to be that the respective local authorities had proposed new developments in the inter-war years.[5] The extent to which these surveys really reflected the position is debatable. For example, boroughs that were at the bottom of the league in terms of provision and utilisation, such as Smethwick, Gateshead, Salford, West Bromwich, Rotherham and Carlisle, did not feature in this document. With the benefit of the subsequent hospital surveys, it is clear that these would have emerged as needy locations. Possibly the data was less-than-comprehensive; perhaps, too, like the earlier report of the Onslow Commission, unmet need was equated with the distribution of proposals for new hospital development. Related to these deficiencies, a further problem was prevention of the ill-balanced development of hospital facilities, but the author felt that merely relying on local authorities and voluntary hospitals could be 'fraught with danger' unless there were sanctions to prevent 'the wrong kind of hospital being built in the wrong place'. Overcoming these problems might well require 'a measure of central direction and control'.[6]

Second, there was the financial position of the hospitals. Here, civil servants were scathing about a system of financing hospitals which relied on hospitals 'being continuously in debt', because overdrafts were 'an asset for the purpose of collecting charitable collections'.[7] The issue of the financial stability of the voluntary hospital system is taken up elsewhere (Gorsky *et al.* 2002). It is certainly true that, in the aggregate, finances had recovered from the difficult years after World War I but this hid a range of local experiences. 'As a whole', reported a 1938 assessment, 'they are solvent but resources are ill-distributed and there are distressed areas',[8] though precisely where (and how 'distressed') these places were was not described. Much attention has been given to London, consistent with the over-emphasis in analysing British health policy on the problems of the capital. The financial difficulties of London's hospitals on the eve of World War II prompted high-level approaches to the Ministry, requesting subvention (Webster 1988a: 22; Honigsbaum 1989: 16–17; Rivett 1986: 221–5). However, the problems were more wide-ranging. Statistics on overall surpluses and deficits conceal a situation in which large surpluses in a small number of institutions could outweigh many small deficits – yet there was no way of pooling funds between hospitals. Moreover, some institutions persistently ran overdrafts which exceeded annual budgets, and many experienced successive deficits during the 1930s (Gorsky *et al.* 2002). Discussion of the voluntary hospitals' finances was limited, however, to a consideration of aggregate surpluses and deficits. There was no discussion of the great variability between hospitals in terms of expenditure per bed or patient throughput. Thus, discussion of surpluses and deficits did not really resolve the questions of whether the hospitals were capable of meeting demand. Looking forwards, it was thought probable that the voluntary hospitals would become completely impoverished after the war; they would have to cope with increased demand from returning military casualties, and considerable capital development would be essential, to make good the bomb damage suffered by many urban hospitals.[9] If this source of hospital care was not to disappear, either the voluntary tradition would have to be revived, or a rather greater degree of state support would be required.

A further issue arose from changes in the funding sources from which the voluntaries drew their income. Traditional elite philanthropy had been supplanted in many locations by hospital contributory schemes, attracting weekly contributions (often organised through workplaces) which gave subscribers entitlements to treatment. These had become the principal source of additional income for many hospitals but the problem was that they had developed very unevenly. In particular they emphasised local attachments to hospitals in fundraising; 'people can be persuaded to support a hospital which they know ... it is far more difficult to get them to subscribe to a hospital 50 or more miles away which they do not know and never see'. The result was that although strong contributory schemes had been built up, the subscribers were in fact helping to pay for patients who did not subscribe, since medical criteria determined admission 'without regard for the locality from which they (i.e. patients) come'.[10] Purely voluntary contributory schemes could never overcome this 'free rider' problem, but as soon as local authorities were charged with providing hospital care, it was argued that ratepayers would 'demand at least an equal right (to hospital treatment) with other ratepayers'. This would then reveal 'the inequity of the present system of mass contributions, concentrated almost entirely in urban areas'.[11] A related problem was that the benefits of contributory schemes were often available in only one particular hospital, so that some sort of reciprocal arrangements were desirable (NPHT 1941). Clearly, then, there were technical obstacles to the extension of contributory schemes on a national basis. Moreover, if such schemes were to cover the whole country, they 'become merely a means of taxing ... a very large section of the community to provide a service which they need and which the prosperous minority do not'. This ran counter to practice in all other health services (NPHT 1941). The very unevenness of voluntary effort, then, posed important challenges for post-war policy.

A final criticism of pre-war arrangements was the variability in performance of the hospitals, as revealed by statistics on comparative costs. Apart from a brief discussion by the Hollingsworths (1985) there is little academic coverage of this but it formed an element in the case for greater state involvement. The Emergency Medical Service (EMS) had been established at the outbreak of hostilities. Substantial payments were made to voluntary hospitals for treatment of wartime casualties; by late 1939 these were already some £40 million. The Ministry would be asked to explain the 'wide variations in published costs' between hospitals and to take responsibility for 'ensuring that these ... are ironed out'. The corollary was a measure of public control,[12] though precisely what that control ought to be was debated.

The diagnosis of the problem could therefore be summarised as follows: inadequacy and maldistribution; financial instability; difficulties of extending voluntary finance nationally; and variations in comparative costs. The remainder of this chapter concentrates on debates about the mechanisms whereby these challenges could be overcome.

The evolution of hospital policy during the war

It is not hard to show that there was agreement on some broad principles of hierarchical organisation of hospital services. There is evidence of convergence on such a view from a range of individuals and organisations. Divergences of opinion emerge concerning the means by which such a desirable state of affairs was to be brought about.

There was a broad agreement that a hierarchical organisation of hospital and specialist services was required. The Nuffield Provincial Hospitals Trust's (NPHT's) Medical and Advisory Council argued both for centralisation, on economic grounds, of the 'more expensive and specialised' methods of investigation and treatment. They envisaged in each region a 'primary' or 'key' hospital, 'connected with a medical school', and proposed that there should be a 'system of interchange' between primary and secondary institutions. The place of smaller institutions of the 'cottage hospital' type was clearly a 'difficult problem', but it was hoped that they would have a future role in low-level surgery and convalescence, subject to appropriate arrangements being made to establish links with specialist institutions, including regular consultant cover.[13] The key hospitals were seen as providing a 'central point' upon which the Ministry of Health and local authorities would rely for the 'raising and maintenance of medical standards at individual hospitals'.[14] An internal Ministry note elaborated on the notion of the 'base hospital' as providing all normal specialist services, including a consultant outpatient department, of *c*. 1,000–1,200 beds. Also envisaged were a series of special centres, offering 'rarer specialities'; the number would depend on population and communications, but the 'unwillingness of patients to go too far from home for treatment' might render it necessary to provide 'more than the theoretical optimum' number of centres.[15] This network would be complemented by a series of specialist units supplying less frequently needed facilities, and the cottage hospital system was worthy of retention in rural areas.[16] The Medical Practitioners Union (MPU), while generally arguing for a prevention-oriented, integrated and less hospital-centred service, nevertheless specified the character of a hospital hierarchy in more detail: at its apex, large general hospitals of a thousand beds or so; then local hospitals, of 50–500 beds, which would have no teaching duties, and would not necessarily be served entirely by a whole-time medical staff. However the MPU did not regard hospitals of under fifty beds as 'economical' or as capable of attracting a nursing staff 'of the type which the health services so urgently require'.[17] There are various Ministry papers which also sketch out these same broad principles, at least one of which was drafted by George Godber, who was involved in the Hospital Surveys and later became Chief Medical Officer.[18] A reading of the Hospital Surveys also makes it clear that these ideas had been absorbed more widely.

Consideration of regionalism was also prompted by the experience of the EMS. Under the Civil Defence Act, 1939, the Ministry of Health's regional organisation of hospital services was set up to discharge the responsibility for treating air raid casualties; by late 1941, an additional 80,000 beds had been made available.[19] These additional resources would be a 'powerful weapon' for any government wishing to extend state control of hospitals, since they would have 'something to offer' local authorities who might otherwise merely defend their own vested interests.[20] The EMS also achieved a degree of regional coordination of services, with the grading of hospitals according to their capacity to deal with cases of greater or lesser complexity. Finally, it introduced uniform conditions of service, greatly improving the pay of junior doctors although somewhat reducing that of consultants (Titmuss 1950; Dunn 1952; Abel-Smith 1964). By dispersing medical staff the EMS also raised awareness of variations in the hospital stock. The EMS scheme was so successful that full state control was seen as desirable in peacetime[21] and it was also thought to have been instrumental in educating those running the voluntary hospitals to accept a coordinated service.[22]

However, though there may have been general agreement on the broad principles of hierarchical organisation, there was little evidence of agreement on how it would be brought about. There were debates about the imprecision attached to quite basic concepts necessary for the delimitation of regions; the powers and resources to be made available to regional bodies, and their relationship to local government and the Ministry of Health; and (ultimately subsuming all of these) the boundary between public and private sectors. These disputes reflected quite fundamental differences over the locus of power and control in any future health service, and about the likely advantages and disadvantages of a public-private mix for health care.

Delimiting regions

If hospital services were to be organised on a regional basis, how large were they to be, and what criteria were to be used for demarcating these divisions? The inter-war period saw extensive debate about the merits of regional administration (Garside and Hebbert 1989) on grounds of efficiency and democracy. The *ad hoc* evolution of local government boundaries had produced a situation in which individual local authorities could not cope with the pressures of suburban expansion or of economic decline. Gilbert (1939: 42; 1948: 182–3) bemoaned the lack of correspondence between existing local government boundaries and what he termed 'natural hospital regions'. However, despite his desire to rationalise these (and other) boundaries, Gilbert devised no practical proposals. There was a tension between devising spatial units which made sense administratively, and delimiting areas which bore some relationship to natural communities, thereby promoting an active, participatory democracy (Daunton 1996: 203–5). The Socialist Medical Association was particularly keen to sweep away 'centuries-old boundaries which bear no relation to changes wrought by the growth of industry'.[23]

There were competing views within the Ministry as to the necessity for and scale of regional organisation. Although some officials favoured a 'general reform of local government on a regional basis', this was unlikely and so regional structures would have to be founded on existing spatial units.[24] Some civil servants thought that the larger local government units would be appropriate. For example, John Wrigley (Principal Assistant Secretary) argued strongly that since 'the great bulk of the population lives in units which contain at least 100,000 people', the existing units would be adequate, at least for the 'primary institutional services'. Where smaller local government units were concerned he felt that it should not be too difficult to produce a 'measure of combination'; this would also be an appropriate way forward for the provision of more specialist services. He did not see that there were strong reasons for interfering with the responsibility of individual local authorities, but was persuaded that regional units were needed, in order to ensure 'some direction of hospital policy ... over a wider area than that of the individual county or county borough'.[25]

As a strong supporter of democratic local government, Wrigley wanted to promote participation rather than provide services 'from above with a mechanically perfect organisation' remote from public involvement. He was therefore prepared to accept a gradual development of services under local authority control, with regional bodies having advisory functions only. He regretted the 1929 Local Government Act, which had separated counties from county boroughs, because 'the most convenient unit of government ... seems to be an urban centre with the county round it'. However, such arrangements were tainted by association with the old Poor Law, and were therefore 'outside practical politics'.[26]

Others in the Ministry, such as John Pater, a principal concerned with hospital policy, put the case for much larger regional units. Regions covering England and Wales had been tentatively sketched out, based on the grouping of hospitals around 'natural medical centres already in existence'. Modernising impulses were clearly on view: it was a 'reasonable course' of action to divide some counties between regions, 'in these days when county boundaries have no real basis but that of custom and when they are irrelevant to the purpose in view, i.e. a properly co-ordinated hospital scheme'.[27] While units of 100–500,000 would attract public interest, larger regional units (populations of 4–5 million) were necessary: 'the advantages of proper organisation of resources outweigh the disadvantages of loss of local patriotism'. Even if the regional authority were somewhat remote, there would be local sub-committees to 'keep interest alive'.[28]

Subsequent papers on policy development show that by August 1941, Ministry opinion was hardening against the possibility that a service could be based on the then existing local government units: 'apart from London and a few of the larger CBs, no county or CB could ever ... form a separate unit'.[29] The NPHT, likewise, suggested that the unit of coordination should be 'regional and not restricted to local authority administrative areas' (NPHT 1941). Both the Ministerial statement on post-war plans, in October 1941, and the War Cabinet Memorandum[30] (statements which are usually taken as definitive sources for the Coalition government's plans) spoke of basing the hospital service on 'areas larger than single counties and CBs'. They were deliberately silent on the question of just how large (or small) the regions would be, and the issue was not resolved (Honigsbaum 1989: 19–29), but it was obvious that the intention was to eliminate some of what officials saw as the 'stupidities' of small local authorities attempting to provide large-scale services, such as Rutland and Canterbury.

The different suggestions for the numbers of regional units are symptomatic of differences of opinion on the most rational way of planning the future service. The BHA, for instance, had around twenty-two regional committees; the NPHT proposed between sixty and seventy Divisions, incorporated into fifteen or sixteen regions; the Coalition Government proposed 30–35 'joint authorities'; the 1944 White Paper suggested a similar number of 'area planning bodies'; and the Labour Government eventually proposed some 16–20 Regional Hospital Boards (RHBs).[31] These signify differences about the locus of power and control. Thus, the 1944 White Paper suggested up to thirty-five joint authorities. If these were sufficiently large – with populations of up to 500,000+ – it was argued that they would obviate the need for a regional tier and would aid integration of services (one of the strong points of the White Paper, which emphasised unification). This suggestion was criticised as timid, because it failed to appreciate that larger units were really necessary for hospital planning, and conciliatory, because it envisaged continuation of the separate development of voluntary and municipal services.[32] More generally the voluntary hospital representatives viewed with horror the possibility that joint authorities might be the dominant players in the system, and held out for a strong regional organisation as a bulwark against state control. Labour envisaged between sixteen and twenty regional authorities, but this was reduced to thirteen (in England) 'in deference to the principle of linking regions with teaching hospitals' (Webster 1988a: 265). However, these arguments about boundary delimitation were symptomatic of more fundamental divisions concerning the purposes of regions, their responsibilities and powers.

Functions and powers of regional authorities

Inter-war proposals for greater coordination of hospital development had had little effect. There might have been broad agreement concerning the desirability of creating hierarchies of services but the mechanisms through which hierarchies might be created were contentious. In examining discussions on these issues I shall emphasise three important themes: the nature of 'partnership', the character of control and planning in the service, and the possible financial arrangements between voluntary hospitals and the public sector.

Early wartime papers in the Ministry drew attention to the limited successes of voluntary cooperation (see also Chapter 3) and pressed the case for greater municipal control. Some extensions of voluntary cooperation (such as pooling of voluntary hospital funds) were dismissed as 'utterly impracticable' and inimical to the traditions of voluntarism, although the possibility of establishing a national fund to aid the voluntary hospitals was considered.[33] On the other hand, any proposal to extend municipal control would only be acceptable to the voluntary hospitals if it had 'the smallest amount of local government and not too much central government'.[34] There was also scepticism about collaborative arrangements developed between local authorities, mainly because the absence of direct democratic pressure removed the most obvious incentive for authorities to improve the quality of services.[35] These general constraints still left much room for argument about precisely what powers and duties were to be made available, and to which agencies.

Most organisational structures proposed during the war therefore envisaged extension of existing collaborative arrangements. There was a need for some 'direction of hospital policy' above the level of existing local government units, but there was vagueness about the extent of this direction. Local authorities would be responsible for guaranteeing the availability of services, their existing power being converted into a duty. They would be under the supervision of a regional body, but such organisations were envisaged as having advisory powers only. This was partly because of limited experience with such bodies, though one civil servant argued that if regional advisory committees worked successfully, a 'regional spirit' could develop. It would then be possible to 'expand the roots of regional advisory committees into a single regional executive organisation'.[36] The evolution of wartime arguments shows that this was a very optimistic view.

The Ministry generally favoured the idea that local authorities would be the key players in developing health services. However, the varying resources, performance and attitudes of local government were such that service development would inevitably be a matter of 'gradual and progressive action over a number of years'. It made little difference whether local authorities were given powers or duties with respect to providing a comprehensive service, since persuasion had generally worked better than coercion. The Minister could not guarantee that local authorities would exercise their powers, but neither could they be compelled to carry out their duties. This certainly implied that there would be difficulties in raising services to the same standard everywhere, and the problem of stimulating 'laggard' authorities was noted, though no definite proposals were made to resolve it.[37]

Local authorities could carry out their statutory responsibilities not only by providing their own hospital facilities but also by making contractual arrangements with voluntary hospitals. It was contemplated that, should a voluntary hospital be unable to carry on financially, the local authority could bail it out or run it as a rate-aided institution. However, nothing could actually guarantee the participation of the voluntary hospitals, and there were lengthy disputes about how this was to be ensured. If local authorities had a duty to secure comprehensive health care, voluntary hospitals would have to choose whether to subject themselves to a regional scheme, or stand outside it.[38] Because of the uncertainty this would cause, it was therefore asked whether it was desirable to impose on voluntary hospitals a duty to cooperate.[39] (Compare the much later 'duty of partnership' introduced in Labour's 1997 NHS Act.) All kinds of difficulties could then follow; it was possible that regional organisation would, in the last resort, entail compelling a local authority to use an existing voluntary hospital, in preference to a municipal one. This was unlikely to be acceptable to local government opinion.[40] Equally, however, the imposition of a duty on local authorities to provide hospital care was seen by some as a potential threat to the survival of voluntary hospitals. Recognising this the NPHT launched a pre-emptive strike, proposing that the most appropriate unit of hospital organisation was regional, not one constrained by municipal boundaries, and arguing for 'advisory and consultative' hospital councils (NPHT 1941). These would be charged with giving effect to the policies of a central hospitals board or council. Because this scheme prioritised voluntary interests, it was vigorously denounced by municipal representatives. The Nuffield proposals spoke of handing supervisory powers in the hospital system to a mixed council (appointed, not elected) of voluntary and municipal representatives. This represented a reactionary and undemocratic attempt to obtain control of 'the people's hospitals'.[41] The result was that the Ministry was forced to announce its own policy.

This took the form of a Commons statement in October 1941 by Ernest Brown, Minister of Health in the Coalition Government. However, this simply made rather vague references to 'co-operation' and 'partnership', and spoke of putting the existing 'informal and unorganised partnerships between hospitals' onto a 'more regular footing'. A duty was to be placed on the larger local authorities to organise a comprehensive service, rather than relying on the permissive powers of the 1929 Act. An expansion of contractual arrangements for service provision was envisaged, channelled through local authorities; it was pointed out that such arrangements already existed in many locations for specialist services.[42] There was no overt reference to regions in the statement, possibly as a conciliatory gesture to local authorities.

Most subsequent wartime proposals endorsed some variant of a mixed economy approach. There were differences of emphasis, for example on the roles of regional tiers of administration, or on the scope for local authority control. Thus, drafts of a Bill prepared during 1943 envisaged that the service would be based on local government, which would secure unification, and that (pending reform of local government) joint boards would be necessary. Compared to the 1941 statement, there was less emphasis on regional organisation. Voluntary hospitals were free to choose whether to play a part in the service; where they did so they were to be remunerated in proportion to their contribution.

The subsequent White Paper (Ministry of Health 1944) stressed the principle of local responsibility combined with 'enough central direction to obtain a coherent and consistent national service'. There was very little mention of regions and the main organisational unit was to be joint bodies (amalgamations of local authorities); these would only have direct responsibility for public hospital services. The voluntaries were assured a role in joint planning and it was guaranteed that local authorities could not gain financial control over them.

Discussions after the White Paper saw the break-up of what had appeared some reasonably promising proposals. In an attempt to reassure the voluntaries there were suggestions for greater hospital and medical representation. There was already a Central Health Services Council, with an inbuilt non-elected medical majority, which had a general advisory function. Then there were to be small, expert regional advisory bodies, charged with overseeing service development at that level. To this there was added a proposed Hospitals Council, which would operate in parallel with the joint authorities (later termed 'Local Health Services Councils') to ensure that, in preparing a plan for a locality's hospital services, medical advice was taken into account. The eventual compromise would have given an equal role in approving plans to both the region and the Minister. Such arrangements, designed as far as possible to insulate the medical profession from elected local government, would have been 'elaborate and cumbersome'; almost any proposal would have to pass through five separate bodies, which was 'intolerably slow'. The proposed regional organisations were a 'fifth wheel to the coach'; there might have been a case for them if hospital provision had remained the preserve of individual local authorities.[43] However, as there were only a few specialist services which would be provided on a supra-district basis, there was the possibility of creating 'vast regional bodies which would find it difficult to do anything except talk'.[44] The role of such bodies was also unclear. There were seemingly endless debates about where power and authority rested. For example, could bodies whose sole function was to act in a planning or advisory capacity successfully secure the implementation of their plans? At best, they could only implement some negative sanctions, such as the withdrawal of grant aid from individual hospitals, but this was 'negative' and 'makes active performance of [a] plan less likely'.[45] Municipal authorities relied on some well-worn objections to joint authorities but were told that it was 'too much to hope' that all councils would willingly accept the plans of an authority that merely had planning powers; there would consequently be no practical way of enforcing a plan.[46] The concern was therefore that the kinds of partnerships envisaged in wartime debates could not have secured the compliance of the partners. In most of the schemes put forward, planning and execution were separated, and inevitably one or another organisation would be 'dissatisfied'; they would have 'ample opportunity' for endless obstruction and delay.[47] In Ling's (2000) terminology there remained much scope for malfeasance.

A related area concerned the contracting mechanisms whereby voluntary hospitals were to be recompensed for their services. The possibility of hospitals providing services on a contractual basis had been mentioned early in the wartime years but the details had not been fleshed out. Even before the war there had been a proposal for a 'national fund out of which grants could be made through regional committees ... in support of voluntary effort'.[48] But part of the difficulty of devising appropriate arrangements was that any state aid to the voluntaries risked discouraging charitable effort. Where that aid was to come from, and how it was to be allocated, became contentious issues. The first proposal, from the NPHT (1941), written at a time when the continued existence of the voluntaries was assumed, anticipated that the diverse mix of income sources from the pre-war period would continue to exist. It subsequently became clear that the scissors effect of the decline in traditional sources of income, combined with the expansion in EMS payments, meant that the financial base of the voluntaries, post-war, would look very different, and this had implications for the way hospitals were to be reimbursed.

Various options for contractual arrangements were considered. If local authorities were responsible for securing the provision of hospital treatment in collaboration with the voluntary hospitals, and if they were responsible for paying the full cost of inpatient treatment (net of any contributions from payments or voluntary sources) then the hospital would have no incentive to keep costs down. Nor was it clear that this system was conducive to the encouragement of continued voluntary support. An alternative was to pool hospital finances on a regional basis with regional bodies being charged with making grants to hospitals according to estimates of expenditure and income as prepared by each local authority and voluntary hospital. [49] It was recognised that such grants should be 'highly selective' and used 'only to support hospitals that are worth preserving'.[50] This idea foreshadowed the 1991 reforms, though a warning was sounded: this system could facilitate planning, as long as accounting arrangements could be devised 'which do not divert patients from hospitals to which they ought to go, merely because there's some financial pull the other way'.[51] The result was a proposal, in the 1944 White Paper, to pay hospitals a 'specified sum for services rendered' based on centrally determined standard payments for different levels of service. In addition there would be direct grants from central funds. The White Paper wanted to avoid 'a mass of financial adjustments between different areas' (Ministry of Health 1944: 15). There was never any intention of a purchasing authority having to make a 'network of separate bargains',[52] as happened after 1991. Contemporary critics would probably regard this as lacking mechanisms to stimulate efficiency, because there was no suggestion that standard charges be used to promote competition.

A shadow cast over all these discussions was the reluctance of the voluntary hospitals to accept a greater degree of public accountability. Payments were to be channelled through local authorities (or combinations thereof), which provoked resistance. As a result the powers of local contracting agencies over the voluntaries were to be restricted. The 1944 White Paper proposed that they would only have limited powers of inspection, and contractual arrangements with hospitals could be terminated only 'by the Minister or with the Minister's consent'.[53]

Although this appeared to insulate voluntary hospitals from control by local authorities, they continued to resist control, proceeding to suggest that all payments should be channelled through the Exchequer. This proposal was born out of paranoia, and rejected with some exasperation by Ministry officials[54] on the grounds that it was 'straining procedure to satisfy prejudice' and 'feasible, but stupid'.[55] The objection was simply to a system in which there would be payments from *individual* local authorities to *individual* hospitals. A verdict on this intransigence was given in Pater's unpublished autobiography. He suggested that what the BHA meant by 'partnership' was a:

> structure which would guarantee the income of the voluntary hospitals and give them a veto in the planning and operation of the services in each locality, while protecting them from any kind of regulation or control by the responsible local authority.[56]

If this was a reasonable view of how things stood in late 1944, one argument would be that the opposing factions had fought themselves to a standstill, failing to develop practical proposals. The voluntary hospitals and the local authorities both fought determinedly to ensure that their interests were given priority, but the result of this stalemate was unwieldy compromises which, had they been put into practice, would not have worked.

Demarcating the boundary between public and private sectors

The foregoing discussions have emphasised the difficulties of devising satisfactory administrative arrangements for making good the wartime pledge to provide a comprehensive health service. Given that these difficulties were widely acknowledged, it is arguably surprising that the possibility of state ownership and control did not feature more strongly in debates.

Though the possibility of state control was discussed in the Ministry early in the wartime years, policy-makers generally circled warily around the subject of nationalisation. Thus, early wartime documents indicate that voluntarism's roots in the national psyche were so deep that a takeover of the hospitals was implausible.[57] There are surprisingly few references in Ministry papers to the necessity or desirability of nationalisation; instead there are arguments about the inevitability and desirability of gradualism[58] with rare dissent. The voluntary system was highly regarded for its capacity to innovate and its flexibility, while its advocates emphasised its localism and capacity for mobilising communities, as well as its role in minimising the need for public expenditure (NPHT 1941). The defenders of voluntarism emphasised that the absence of state interference, the spirit of enterprise and individuality were inherent virtues. Consequently, Sir Farquhar Buzzard (Regius Professor of Medicine at Oxford) argued for a system which would preserve the maximum degree of delegation to individual hospitals.[59] However, other opinion had challenged the view that this competitive *modus operandi* was appropriate. The MPU's 1942 memorandum challenged the argument that the voluntary hospitals contained some 'essence or excellence' that was too valuable to be lost.[60] By 1946 the BHA were being criticised for adhering to the 'negative argument that uniformity does not give the best service'.[61]

The Ministry's approach was non-interventionist – it was an 'advisory, supervisory and subsidising department',[62] whose job was to ensure that services were available, not to provide them. Thus, 'it did not *per se* concern the Ministry' whether provision was made by municipal or voluntary hospitals, and 'apart from a sympathetic interest' the Ministry was not concerned with the survival of the voluntary hospitals as voluntary institutions.[63] There are some relevant parallels between this stance and the fashionable contemporary view of 'reinventing government' (Osborne and Gaebler 1992), in which the role of the state is confined to 'steering, not rowing'.

However, it is questionable whether this role could have ensured a comprehensive service, because the Ministry had no effective powers to secure compliance. The problem of hospital distribution was seen in terms of avoiding competition, duplication and inefficiency, and discussion seems to have emphasised the desirability of rationalisation. Thus, one official raised the possibility of 'suppression' of a voluntary hospital, and it was also suggested that, because of low standards, it might be necessary to 'forbid certain small voluntaries from performing certain operations'.[64] Regulatory mechanisms were limited, though there were some possibilities. Sir Allen Daley, of the LCC, spoke of the need to secure 'sensible investment and avoid duplication'.[65] For local authorities this could be achieved through loan sanctions; Ministry approval was required for loans taken out to finance capital works.[66] No similar mechanism was available to ensure that voluntary hospitals would cooperate with regional plans, and the Ministry did not have the powers to close a hospital down. It was therefore far from clear that the various suggestions proposed during the war could have achieved the desired rationalisation of services. However, it was believed that wasteful development was largely a London problem and was rarely found in the provinces.[67]

A problem which received far less attention was that of expanding services into areas where they did not already exist. The emphasis on voluntary cooperation would not, of itself, call into existence any additional beds.[68] A local government system still faced the problem of ensuring that the laggards would play their part. Two further issues cast a shadow over policy development. First, there was the relationship between voluntary and municipal development. There are repeated wartime references to the likely effect on voluntary support if local authorities were given the lead role in hospital development. The likely consequence would be releasing pent-up demand for hospital services while undermining incentives for financial contributions. Second, the EMS system had provided financial stability for the hospitals, but this meant that the Ministry could no longer continue to operate in a hands-off manner. There was strong evidence of variability in costs between voluntary hospitals, and if state support was to continue, a degree of control was necessary.[69]

Much of the wartime debates therefore originate, to some degree, in voluntary hospitals' objections to the extension of public – and especially local government – control that was thought likely to follow the war. As long as the government insisted on basing the service on local government this deadlock would continue and while one can argue, as Honigsbaum (1989: 171) does, that Ministry intransigence was the problem, the other side of the coin was voluntary resistance to municipalism. The result had been interminable discussions with interest groups producing compromises which were believed to be unworkable. These compromises were necessary because of the lack of political will, in the Coalition government, to disturb existing arrangements.

This was the point that had been reached by 1945. Labour's new Minister for Health, Aneurin Bevan, swiftly prepared proposals for nationalisation. This solution appeared to solve several problems. It would secure unified control and facilitate planning; ensure public control of public expenditure; permit the organisation of hospital services on 'natural' areas unconstrained by local authority boundaries; avoid a separation of hospital planning from the execution of plans; and the medical profession supported it given the alternative of local authority control.[70] Bevan therefore envisaged state control of all hospital services, though the teaching hospitals were to be run by separate organisations. Administration was to be placed in the hands of regional boards, though Bevan hoped that a future local government reorganisation would enable the closer integration of hospital and local government services (see Foot 1973: 263–4). Regional Boards would operate under the 'general direction' of the Minister but 'the aim would be the maximum degree of decentralisation in the administration'. Below the RHBs, day-to-day operation of the service would be entrusted to district committees. Though financed by central government, the service was to be operated in such a way as to ensure a 'free and flexible degree of decentralised control'.[71]

Full state control was advocated because the voluntary hospital system was 'an anachronism'; it had failed to provide a good service and many hospitals were on the point of bankruptcy.[72] Financial support for voluntary hospitals had fallen to such an extent that the state would have to guarantee 70–90 per cent of their income, and contributions on such a scale were inconceivable without an extension of state control. Whether or not it would ever have been acceptable to the medical profession, a local government system could not guarantee the elimination of the existing inequalities, due to the problems inherent in financing a service from the rates; the variations in the extent to which local authorities had developed hospital services were testimony to this. Alternatives to a regional organisation – such as a new, directly elected authority – were administratively complex and remote from public control, and would lead to an 'impossible hotch-potch' of local administrative units.[73] Only through full state control would it be possible to plan the service in such a way as to eliminate inequalities in provision, thereby carrying out the government's pledge to provide a comprehensive national service.[74] In particular, by underwriting hospital finances, the distribution of hospital medical staff was no longer dependent on the prospects for private practice in any given locality.

It is important to note that this proposal did not represent a leap in the dark, because (as Webster's (1998) most recent contribution to the historiography points out) informed opinion outside the Coalition government had consistently argued for nationalisation, as is evident from commentary in *The Economist* about the inadequacies of voluntarism and municipalism. The possibility of nationalisation had been briefly considered by officials as early as 1939, but not pursued: pressure of workload was one reason; a belief that the voluntary hospitals finances would improve post-war was another (Klein 1983: 8–10; Honigsbaum 1989: 18–21). Bevan's proposals were resisted, with the BHA emphasising the traditional virtues of voluntarism and the importance of charitable endeavour in reducing the burden on the state. There were also objections from local government spokesmen. Thus, Herbert Morrison[75] feared damage to the fabric of local government, and was also concerned at the centralisation and rigidity of the proposals.[76] However, Bevan countered such objections on the grounds that a less radical scheme would neither solve the financial and administrative problems of the existing system, nor would it eliminate inequalities in service provision. What was involved, then, was not so much an attack on the functions of local government but rather their 'proper rationalisation'.[77] Whereas previous policy had accepted a degree of 'inequality and inefficiency in order to preserve the political and social advantages of the local government system',[78] in the changed climate the inference was that such inequalities were no longer tolerable.

There was relatively little opposition from the medical profession, reflecting concessions made in negotiations. Thus, consultants were permitted to undertake private practice within NHS hospitals; this helped draw them into the service rather than remaining in full-time private practice. Medical objections were also assuaged by giving teaching hospitals autonomy, and by permitting them to retain their endowment funds for use in medical teaching and research. Not every hospital was nationalised. Hospitals were disclaimed where they did not fit with ministerial plans (e.g. isolation units). But it is not clear how policy towards non-state hospitals was formulated, other than by default. Those institutions that remained outwith the NHS were allowed to retain charitable status. Eventually, this produced taxation anomalies (e.g. emergence of highly capitalised chains of hospitals, or even individual facilities, claiming charitable status: see Chapter 8). Bevan also indicated his willingness to tolerate profit-making nursing homes. To some extent, therefore, elements of the development of hospital services were still partly to be determined by the idiosyncrasies of charity and opportunities for private practice, as is manifest from the distribution of NHS consultant staff. Finally, in terms of Fox's thesis, a tripartite structure for health services was adopted. Under Bevan's scheme, local government – not the NHS – retained responsibility for certain health and welfare services, while primary care was left in the hands of GPs as independent contractors. These compromises posed problems in terms of integrating the various branches of the health service. Arguably some of the Coalition compromises might have achieved this, but at the price of a more inequitable pattern of service provision.

Concluding comments

The organisation and control of the post-war hospital services were contentious issues. It is true that there was agreement on the desirability of something superior to the pre-war state of affairs. Many of the options for policy had been aired as early as 1939, and there was broad agreement that a hierarchical organisation of hospital services was broadly agreed. This is why commentaries on the development of the NHS are prone to the identification of consensus. However, it is an exaggeration to apply this term to hospital policy.

There were extensive disputes about the character of the public–private mix for health care, and about how best to regulate and plan the service. These were not just arguments about technical, administrative detail; the competing (and, eventually, entrenched) positions signified much more fundamental disagreements, which related to the legitimate scope of state intervention and the character of various proposals for planning the post-war service. This is not consensus, and one reason for this was evidently the unwillingness to abandon established positions – even in the face of ample evidence that, in Finlayson's words, the pre-existing systems could not cope (Chapter 2). The vigorous defence of voluntarism, the reluctance of the Coalition government to upset any vested interests, and the Ministry's evident preference for local government produced at best a minimalist consensus, and at worst a stalemate characterised by exasperation and a bunker mentality. When nationalisation was finally proposed, as a way out of this impasse, it provoked far less reaction than other aspects of Labour's proposals for the NHS. Perhaps this was because the various options proposed were just unworkable; perhaps it was simply that the rearguard action of voluntary interests was undermined by the success of the EMS, making a case for greater state intervention and (through payments to hospitals) underwriting them – and simultaneously making a reversion to pre-war arrangements impossible. Though there was resistance it tended to concentrate on the retention of trust fund assets (this was granted only in the case of teaching hospitals) or on ministerial patronage. Some officials in the Ministry also urged caution, but put forward no new alternative.

Interestingly, even though there was recognition that 'in the agency dispensing public funds resided power over the system as a whole' (Webster 1988a: 63), there is little sign of consideration of the possibility that something like the purchaser-provider split might have been developed. There were occasional proposals for contractual arrangements but no suggestion that these would be the subject of local bargaining, nor that contracting for care could have been used to promote competition (and therefore rationalisation). Given the voluntaries' resistance to inspection and regulation it is hard to see how such a system could have been made to work. Preserving the autonomy of the voluntary hospitals could not be reconciled with substantial public payments to them, especially in the light of substantial variations in hospital costs (and it is also doubtful whether there would have been enough understanding of those variations for a purchaser-provider split to have become feasible). Similar comments applied to local authority services: national political commitments could not be reconciled with local priorities and a huge burden would have been placed on the rates, especially in those authorities with limited voluntary provision. At the risk of teleological judgement, voluntarism and municipalism had produced highly variable results before the war, and a whole range of options for a mixed economy had been considered during it. These encountered the problem, identified by Ling (2000) among others, of reconciling the goals of quite different institutions. Bevan had argued in a Cabinet paper that 'the self-contained, independent local hospital is nowadays a complete anachronism'.[79] Integrating the values and culture of such organisations with those of local government would have been a formidable undertaking. On the evidence reviewed here, furthermore, a key problem was to extend access to services rather than promote competition between existing hospitals, and in none of the wartime discussions is there a clear view of how to implement the formidable building programme that would have been necessary. Moreover, the information on comparative costs, on which a quasi-market mechanism might have been based, was simply not available. There were variations in costs, but nobody really knew how to interpret them. It is not obvious, therefore, that there are grounds for lamentations about the failure of the NHS to introduce the purchaser–provider split in 1948. Subsequent critics dismissed the decision to nationalise the hospitals as a mistake, suggesting that most of the NHS's problems can be traced to the decision not to base services on local authorities (Campbell 1987: 177). However, in terms of obtaining the financial resources necessary to develop an egalitarian service, and establishing the planning mechanisms required to distribute hospital services, it is not clear what realistic alternatives were left at the end of the war.

5 'False hopes and frustrations'

The absence of a capital programme, 1948–59

Remedying even the most glaring deficiencies in the hospital stock inherited by the NHS would have required substantial capital investment; considerable further effort would have been required even to ameliorate spatial and sectoral inequalities in hospital provision. However, no concerted attempt was in fact made, during the early post-war years, to do so. Some ten years after the NHS was founded, capital expenditure remained well below estimates of its pre-war level. A legitimate question is therefore why the Ministry of Health was so unsuccessful in obtaining capital funds.

Discussions of hospital policy in the 1950s have generally argued that the Ministry of Health lost out to more powerful Departments in the contest for capital investment. Loss of Cabinet status, a succession of weak Ministers, and the exigencies of post-war reconstruction priorities (notably the imperative to rebuild houses and schools) are usually used in support of such accounts (for example Mullard 1993: 80; Glennerster 1995: 85–6). However, this neglects a number of technical issues relating to the purposes of capital expenditure, which had to be resolved before an expanded hospital programme could be granted. The Ministry had a long struggle to convince the Treasury that benefits would accrue from increased investment. In combination with political reluctance to increase expenditure, the result was a capital programme that was so low, by comparison with housing and education, that it almost appears as an afterthought in the balance sheet. The level of capital investment was arguably dysfunctional, since it effectively debarred construction of new hospitals.

In seeking an explanation for this state of affairs, this chapter focuses on two issues. First, political negotiations between the government, the Ministry and the Treasury are analysed, complementing and elaborating themes discussed by Webster (1988a) and Jones (1992). Second, I develop a more detailed and technical examination of policy on capital investment than has been provided previously, concentrating both on proposed levels of capital investment and the philosophies underlying the use and allocation of capital resources. The Guillebaud Report (1956) is sometimes presented as settling the case for long-term planning and establishing that capital investment would necessarily lead to revenue savings (e.g. Glennerster 1995: 88). I suggest that this is an oversimplification. There is some evidence that the Treasury were well aware of the difficulties imposed by limited capital resources and were willing to consider longer-term allocations, but, working within their terms of reference, they demanded convincing evidence of the likely returns on investment. For some years prior to Guillebaud, therefore, questions were raised about the purposes of new investment and the justification for it. There were discussions about the validity of historical comparisons, the concept of a 'replacement' level of investment, the desirability of standardisation of elements of hospital design and construction, and the relationship between NHS and local authority capital expenditure. Part of the issue here was that the Ministry lacked the technical expertise in hospital planning and design, weakening its ability to make a case. Overlaying these discussions, there were arguments about the relative priority accorded to hospital construction *vis-à-vis* other public programmes.

The structure of the chapter is as follows. First, there is an account of political negotiations concerning the scale of the capital programme. Second, there is a discussion of technical debates about the purposes of increased capital investment, concentrating especially on exchanges between the Ministry of Health and the Treasury. The third main section considers the implications for the allocation of available capital resources, both between regions and within the Newcastle RHB.

Negotiations on the capital programme: the Labour and Conservative governments 1948–59

Considerable attention has been devoted to the Cabinet controversies about rising NHS expenditure under the first post-war Labour government. For some commentators, these illustrate the socialist folly of attempting to build the 'new Jerusalem' before modernising the industrial base (Barnett 1995). Such criticisms are arguably misplaced, as estimates of the cost of the service were pitched at unrealistically low levels (Webster 1988b). It is wildly implausible to suggest that the scale of the NHS capital programme was responsible for an extravagant and unaffordable public burden on the private sector, because, as Tomlinson (1995) observes, the hospital service absorbed only a small proportion of construction resources. The Newcastle RHB pointed out that, under post-war controls of civilian personnel in their area, the number of construction workers allocated to hospitals was one-twentieth of that for factories, and one-eighth of that allocated to schools.[1] Of course, it soon became evident that growing demand would necessitate the allocation of substantial additional resources to the NHS, contradicting the optimistic assertions of the Beveridge Report (1942) that providing a free health service would actually reduce demand, as the population's health improved. NHS finance began to make regular appearances on the Cabinet agenda.

The Labour government was well aware of the impossibility of satisfying unmet need for health care. Estimates were regarded as too low even to maintain existing standards of provision. The government were caught between either avoiding supplementary estimates only by closing down urgently required beds, or implementing charges against all their socialist principles.[2] The Government imposed austere policies, justifying them with respect to severe domestic and international economic constraints, and emphasising the minimal 'margin for readjustments' in public expenditure policy if taxation were to be kept at a reasonable level.[3] The government's credibility and competence were at stake.[4]

Within these rigid constraints, Labour achieved virtually no new capital investment. Tomlinson (1995: 305) suggests that the Ministry seems to have offered little resistance to the tight controls over its investment programme, possibly because the Ministry was also responsible for housing, which was a major competitor for resources. Hence there was an acceptance that the health service would 'have to make do for the time being with existing accommodation'.[5] The Ministry's rather unambitious hope was to restore capital investment to pre-war levels 'as soon as possible'. Vigorous restrictions (both physical and financial) on investment control did not help. Any schemes costing over £10,000 required Treasury scrutiny even though this rarely resulted in modifications. The NHS had been operating barely a year when Treasury officials maintained that 'the NHS was the last place where [the Treasury] ought to weaken such control as it has'.[6] There is a sense here that the lid had to be kept firmly screwed down on a potential Pandora's Box. In addition to financial constraints there were also physical restrictions on the availability of building materials. These meant that new construction was almost non-existent, since it used larger quantities of materials in proportion to cost.[7] In fact shortages of materials meant the very real possibility that even work in progress would actually be stopped.

Following the re-election of the Conservatives in 1951, very little new capital investment was achieved in the early years of the Churchill government (see Jones 1992: 315–16; Bridgen and Lowe 1998). Indeed there were proposals in 1951 for an absolute cut in capital expenditure.[8] The Treasury were committed to limiting investment in the social services to the 'minimum compatible with commitments which have been irrevocably accepted as Government social policy'.[9] The only additional work that was being allowed in the initial years of the service was on mental health facilities, which was felt to represent an identifiable 'new need'. A comparison was made with schools where capital expenditure was permitted when required to accommodate a rising school population, but not to reduce overcrowding. The possibility that some capital investment could be financed out of 'private funds' (e.g. endowments retained by teaching hospitals) was also noted. However, this would have the 'absurd' consequence that a hospital could expand and 'expect the Exchequer to provide funds to run it'.[10]

On the face of it the Ministry appeared to have a strong case for additional investment. The capital programme, initially around £10 million per annum, was well below pre-war levels. Furthermore, bomb damage necessitated a substantial replacement programme, and even within hospitals that remained unscathed, the variable quality of the buildings necessitated replacement or improvement. Moreover, unanticipated demands for hospital construction were being voiced (e.g. from the New Towns). Even pre-war levels of investment were not viewed as extravagant; as an indication of the work thought necessary, one estimate of schemes submitted by local authorities alone in the pre-war years totalled some £65 million at 1938 prices.[11] Even allowing for local authority empire-building, this indicated the scale of the task. The Ministry also argued that at the prevailing rate of investment, it would be at least 150 years before the hospital stock was renewed, demonstrating the 'almost ridiculous inadequacy' of what was being done. The likely relaxation of building controls would give rise to 'odious comparisons' between the health service and what was being done in the private sector.[12]

Iain Macleod (Minister of Health, 1952–5) vigorously argued a case, albeit one based mainly on the political difficulties confronting the Government. The small capital programme actually exacerbated the difficulties faced by RHBs. For example, although revenue-saving investment was thought to be possible, a *specific* allocation for it was necessary, since hospital authorities could not be expected to spend the bulk of their allocations 'on schemes which do not directly affect the medical welfare of patients'. Furthermore, any really large projects would absorb an excessively large share of the capital allocation; the corollary would be almost no visible progress in other areas. Yet there were 'several areas, notably the expanding New Towns, in which it will no longer be possible to make do by adaptation of existing hospitals remote from new population centres'.[13] He repeatedly warned of the undesirable economies that would be forced upon RHBs and the difficulties being experienced in discussions with health authorities. Macleod reluctantly accepted the limited capital programme in light of the general economic situation, though he subsequently warned that reducing capital investment would mean that he could not fulfil 'his responsibilities to the service'.[14]

Later in 1954, Macleod showed that while capital expenditure on housing and education had increased dramatically (by 100 per cent and 43 per cent respectively between 1949–50 and 1952–3), expenditure on hospitals had actually fallen, by 2.3 per cent,[15] rendering the Government vulnerable to Opposition charges of neglecting to invest in the NHS. Churchill recognised the force of this argument, arguing that a 'great campaign should be undertaken to improve this part of our social services'.[16] Following this apparent victory Macleod pressed his case, expressing the hope that the hospital building programme was 'at last on a rising curve towards an annual figure that would be more commensurate with the need'. He envisaged an ultimate figure of £30 million; for comparison the figures agreed for 1956–7 and 1957–8 were £12 million and £17 million respectively. Even with this, Macleod felt it was 'idle to pretend that this adds up to the major crusade for new hospitals' envisaged by

Churchill; the government 'would only be scratching the surface of need'. Nor was it 'practical politics' to use hospital endowment funds to make up some of the deficiencies: if a building scheme is 'demonstrably needed it is difficult for me to insist that part of the cost is met by someone else'.[17] Eventually a programme incorporating £10 million of expenditure on major projects was agreed.[18] As an indication of the political pressures on the Government, shortly after announcing this initiative,[19] Macleod was subject to a marathon session in the Commons, during which he was asked sixty-six questions relating to hospital issues. It was observed that the four-teen New Towns had 'not a hospital between them'.[20]

Although Macleod presented these concessions as an important victory, maintaining the capital programme on a 'rising curve' continued to prove problematic. After the 1955 election, fresh demands were made for restrictions on public investment programmes. These were targeted at local authorities but it was suggested that hospitals could not be exempt. Macleod vigorously resisted this, arguing that the details of the capital programme had been announced and that 'politically we are committed to the hilt'.[21] He publicly thanked the Chancellor for allowing him to keep the 'green light fixed on' the hospital programme.

Yet this was a short-term victory. The Government gave no commitment to implementing the scale of capital investment advocated by the Guillebaud Committee (1956; see below). After the Suez crisis, there were further demands for economies, and advocates of increased expenditure also had to contend with demands from the Government's Social Services Committee, established to review the expansion of the welfare state (see Lowe 1989). This Committee mainly flew a succession of kites about charging for NHS services but it also gave impetus to demands for restraint in capital programmes. There were continued exchanges about the level of investment, which was projected to have reached £22 million by 1959–60, or only three-quarters that envisaged by Guillebaud, just about level in real terms, and less than 1 per cent of gross fixed capital formation.[22] Less than 10 per cent of capital expenditure was going to new hospital construction (Figures A1, A2).

Three points may be made about these restrictions on health capital expenditure. First, cutting social service expenditure was a cheeseparing economy when contrasted with the potential economies in defence, which were not being considered. The obvious political difficulties were captured in a note to Harold Macmillan (Chancellor of the Exchequer) by Henry Brooke (Chief Secretary to the Treasury), drawing attention to the greater potential for economies in defence expenditure than in the welfare state. Second, the contrast between the declining state of the NHS capital stock and the expansion of private-sector housebuilding was all too clear. As Brooke observed, 'it seemed odd to be straining every nerve for higher charges for social services expenditure at the same time that the government was apparently doing nothing effective to check the pressure of housebuilding'.[23] Even within the public sector, Brooke felt that by comparison with the 'lavish' capital expenditure on education, the treatment of hospitals had been 'niggardly'.[24] Finally, it seemed economically irrational to reject the comparatively cheap option of local authority services, which might have the long-term effect of reducing expenditure on expensive hospital treatment and prevent elderly people occupying expensive hospital beds. The Conservatives and the Treasury plainly had some scope for increased capital investment in health care and related services, but chose not to take advantage of it.[25]

In none of these discussions is there a sense of a long-term plan for the hospital service. The first statement of this came from Derek Walker-Smith (Minister of Health, 1957–60), suggesting an attack on the problem of inadequate hospital premises, integrated with plans for prevention and community care. This was followed by discussions in a Treasury-led Long-term Investment Review, in which education, hospitals and housing were in effect competing with one another. Proposals had been advanced for a substantial expansion of capital investment in education – to 'make a reality of the 1944 Education Act' – and Walker-Smith emphasised that if there was to be a long-term programme of investment in schools, he would wish to be in a position simultaneously to announce one for hospitals.[26] However, a decision in favour of education did not imply concession of a similar programme for hospitals.[27] The response of the Ministry had nevertheless been to sketch the basis of a five-year plan, and to persist in pressing the Treasury to accept it. Continuance of existing 'hand to mouth' policies was conducive neither to good planning nor to economy; hospital authorities would be 'too liable to regard [capital] programmes as paper exercises that are not relevant'.[28] The logic of these arguments was broadly accepted by the Treasury but concessions were generally tied to trade-offs in respect of the purposes of investment. As Webster (1994: 59) points out, Walker-Smith's initiative implies that the ancestry of the Hospital Plan goes back before the 1959 election, to an early stage in the tenure of office of Powell's predecessor.

It is difficult to detect a major commitment to hospital expenditure, therefore, until shortly before the 1959 Election. Despite the minuscule size of the NHS capital programme, no serious and consistent attempt was made to expand it. However, there was mounting evidence of dissatisfaction with the failure of the NHS to make a start on what Robin Turton (Minister of Health, 1955–7) called its programme of 'slum clearance'.[29] The contrast with housebuilding could no longer be hidden and this was reflected in growing numbers of debates and questions in Parliament. This might account for why more attention was given to hospital construction from the late 1950s but it does not fully explain why the Ministry was so unsuccessful in obtaining capital prior to that time. For this we need to descend from the level of high politics to the perhaps more mundane and technical level of discussions between the Ministry and the Treasury.

Policy making on the hospital capital programme

Within the macro-political constraints described above, there were debates about the underlying philosophy of public expenditure capital programmes, about the aims to be attained through capital investment, and about the rationality underpinning the allocation of capital funds. I first deal with the attitude adopted by the Treasury to the NHS, before an assessment of technical questions relating to the extent to which capital investment led to revenue savings, the balance between health service and local government capital spending, and the question of standardisation of hospital design and construction.

Treasury attitudes and priorities

Aneurin Bevan chafed at the constraints of post-war austerity. He therefore proposed that the health service be permitted to borrow for capital investment; there was 'no reason why the NHS should be limited to the jog trot of the annual vote'. Borrowing would simply be a continuation of previous local government practice. He linked this to the notion that the NHS could be used as an 'instrument of employment policy'; thus, the capital programme had a wider function as part of Keynesian techniques of demand management.[30]

This submission by Bevan is interesting for two reasons. First, it is very rare, in all the exchanges between the Ministry of Health and the Treasury, that either a Minister or official refers directly to this broader context. Given that the 'post-war consensus' is often identified with Keynesian techniques of economic management, this might appear surprising. Second, it was a proposal which was swiftly rejected by the Treasury. Bevan's analogy with local government did not apply. Local authorities were permitted to borrow because their financial basis was variable, and it was thought unfair to levy the whole cost of capital projects from those ratepayers who happened to be residing in a locality at any given time. Moreover, hospital authorities had no independent source of revenue, so the cost of loan repayment would fall on taxpayers. It was deemed more economical, instead, to finance capital expenditure through taxation.[31] It is interesting to contrast this argument with later proposals, to permit Government departments to escape from the constraints of the vote, in the form of the Private Finance Initiative (Chapter 9).

The question of loan finance was raised again in the deliberations of the Guillebaud Committee, which was established in 1953 to inquire into the rising cost of the NHS. Numerous RHB witnesses argued that loan finance would enable them to undertake works which would produce revenue savings, though others suggested that the net cost of interest payments would exceed revenue savings in the long run, a view endorsed by the Treasury.[32] Other Treasury papers discuss the difficulty of applying quasi-commercial criteria to the NHS. When the hospitals had been nationalised, it had been considered 'out of the question' to value the property taken over, so 'no provision was made for depreciation'.[33] The process was therefore 'very unreal ... no one was in the market to buy hospitals'; any valuations would therefore be 'notional', and costing for depreciation would therefore be a process with, at best, spurious accuracy. Regardless of the difficulties of valuation, the Treasury urged caution in evaluating (actual or potential) capital investments in the NHS. Savings were likely to be whittled away by the 'simultaneous provision of a better service'. While one possible outcome of capital investment was the provision of the same quantity of service at a lower cost, an equally plausible outcome would be a larger quantity of service. The former benefited the Treasury, the latter did not.[34] The former could be dealt with on financial grounds; the latter required a political decision that expansion, or higher quality, was desired.[35]

The relatively low priority accorded to hospital expenditure may also be explained by references in Treasury papers which suggest that health expenditures were viewed essentially as consumption, and not in any wider sense as an investment.[36] This evolved over time into a distinction between those elements of public sector investment which might 'go up with the tide' of national economic prosperity, but no more (category II programmes), and those elements which 'have a substantial industrial or commercial component, and which *directly influence* the expansion of industrial production' (category I programmes). To 'upgrade' from the former to the latter would, in the Treasury's view, encroach upon the private sector.[37] The distinction did not seem entirely watertight. Education was placed in category I, with health in II, which one might justify on the grounds that the former was an investment while the latter was maintenance – if, that is, the purpose of health spending was simply to restore people to functional health, rather than to improve health standards, which would presumably imply 'investment', not just 'maintenance'. We might therefore question the nature of such orthodoxies, and their use as a basis for discriminating between departments. However, capital expenditure on health care was so small – less than 2 per cent of *public* sector fixed capital formation – that regardless of which category it was placed in, it occupied a quite insignificant place.

Given these hawkish views the Treasury took a very restrictive line on health capital investment. Pressing the Ministry to specify in some detail just what the expected results would be seems, on the face of it, perfectly reasonable, but the dismissive tone of many Treasury papers is striking. Thus one Ministry of Health submission was criticised as being 'merely a long-winded way of saying the object is to improve the hospital service. *This is self evident*'.[38] There were continuous discussions between the Treasury and the Ministry concerning not just the scale of the capital programme but also the way the money was spent. Annual capital programmes were regarded as the most straightforward way of ensuring control although ultimately they were abandoned as inimical to long-term planning. There were tight controls over the size of projects which could be embarked upon without Treasury approval. Extensive discussions took place over the value of these controls, and over how they should be exercised. The Treasury was very reluctant to relax its grip; it regarded the Ministry as vulnerable to special pleading. The Ministry was supposed to provide a guiding hand in allocating capital, but 'placed as they are between the Scylla of political pressure and the Charybdis of the medical profession I doubt whether this is, or ever will be, so'.[39] Subsequent comments expressed Treasury scepticism about the possibility of relaxing controls on capital schemes: the Ministry apparently 'did not feel that some of them [the RHBs] were fit to be trusted with so much money',[40] but the Treasury was 'not content to give the Ministry of Health an overall allocation and let them get on with it', because they 'don't trust the health departments and don't think them sufficiently effective'.[41] The result was that over 90 per cent of health capital investment by value, and over 60 per cent of all schemes, were scrutinised by the Treasury,[42] but this rarely resulted in savings, was expensive in terms of the cost of officials' time, and undermined financial responsibility within departments (Lowe 1997: 487). Small wonder health authorities complained of delays in advancing desirable projects. For their part, Ministry officials questioned the value of direct central control of capital projects, arguing that this was the proper role of the RHBs and that to interfere with such decisions would discourage members of health authorities; it also presupposed local knowledge which the Ministry did not possess: 'The Boards were invented in order to ensure that the Minister of Health did not become involved in judging the claims of one district against another', yet several unresolved decisions found their way on to the Minister's desk.[43] Despite the force of these arguments, there was little relaxation of central control. The Treasury's reluctance to permit health authorities greater freedom for manoeuvre, and their general scepticism about increased capital investment, help account for the limited capital investment programme implemented in the early post-war years. This tendency for micro-management, evident through the NHS's history, helped produce an image of the service as monolithic and inflexible, but it is not clear that this was the NHS's fault. Given the minimal resources available, tight central control was inevitable.

Technical debates on capital investment

Even within the limited sums available, the Treasury took a sceptical view and required the Ministry to demonstrate how they would use capital investment to produce a more efficient service. Exchanges between the Ministry and the Treasury were at times theological in character, there being no obvious standard to which the protagonists could appeal. The Treasury sought to close off possibilities that might lead to claims for extra expenditure. Since there were 'considerable differences in standards' within the hospital service, 'we shall be faced with the argument that the highest of these is obviously right'.[44] Any estimates of deferred maintenance would generate a wish list, which could not be published because pressures would develop to obtain more money for the service than the Treasury would be willing to provide.[45] The Guillebaud Committee's (1956) report is often presented as decisive in securing assent for a larger capital programme. Research undertaken for the Guillebaud report (Abel-Smith and Titmuss 1956) showed that, in its historical and comparative context, capital expenditure on the NHS was low. The share of GNP accounted for by the service had actually declined between 1949–50 and 1953–4; likewise, NHS capital investment – expressed as a proportion of gross fixed capital formation – had also fallen. Hospital capital investment for 1952–3 was some 32 per cent of the corresponding figure for 1938–9 (Abel-Smith and Titmuss 1956: 52); the ratio of capital to current expenditure was one-fifth of its pre-war level and one-sixth of that obtaining in the USA; and, at prevailing levels of capital investment, it would take 220 years to replace all existing hospital beds.

The Committee recommended a substantial expansion of hospital capital investment, suggesting that a programme of the order of £30 million per annum would generate important savings in current expenditure (1956: 116). Their analyses had shown that capital investment of £650,000 could generate *annual* savings in current expenditure of £213,000 (Abel-Smith and Titmuss 1956: 136; similar conclusions were reached by the Select Committee on Estimates 1957: xiii). Finally, the Guillebaud Committee argued for a relaxation of some of the constraints under which health authorities had to operate, advocating a raising of the limit (in cash terms) below which capital schemes did *not* require Treasury approval from £30,000 to £100,000 (1956: 85), and proposing notification of capital allocations over three years rather than on an annual basis, to facilitate forward planning (Guillebaud Committee 1956: 120–1).

The Treasury's response was to cast doubt on the validity of this evidence and on the conclusions drawn from it. Many of Guillebaud's arguments were irrelevant since they implied either that there should be a steady trend in hospital capital expenditure, or that it should bear a given relationship to other expenditures on health care. Guillebaud appeared to imply 'a foreseeable diminution in the supply' as hospital buildings 'become obsolete and unusable. From this it is inferred that there is some correct annual rate of replacement ... that the total value of our stock of hospital fixed assets is falling and that we are drawing on our assets and accumulating liabilities.'[46] Weaknesses in Abel-Smith and Titmuss' comparisons served to diminish, but not to eliminate, the inferences drawn; thus, the replacement of capital assets was estimated to take 150 years, not 220! On the question of a replacement rate, the criticism was the difficulties of visualising future needs – 'consider the investment in the 800-odd isolation hospitals'. One corollary, which does not appear to have featured in discussions, was that falling lengths of stay would reduce bed requirements. A further implication, which does not seem to have been developed, was the possibility that the NHS would become less of a curative, hospital-oriented service, though this would arguably have required an even more sophisticated crystal ball. Nevertheless, as the Treasury themselves recognised, in practice budgetary considerations and political priorities determined the level of capital investment. However, this argument was 'to be used with caution',[47] given that public investment in housing and education had far outstripped NHS capital investment.

The conventional view is that the Report made a convincing case for revenue-saving capital investment. Related to this was the argument that standardisation of certain basic elements of hospital design would also effect economies. These were both contested.

Revenue-saving capital investment

The Treasury conceded that failure to replace obsolete assets would be indefensible, but 'clear cut absolute savings [were] not very common'. Improved services generally entailed higher running costs although there were clearly some support services (kitchens, boilers) where money could be saved. Thus the Treasury argued that apart from the 'very narrow field' of revenue-saving replacement, capital investment involved increases in maintenance expenditure, and therefore resisted demands for additional capital.[48] Even if capital expenditure generated savings in current expenditure, it was very difficult to divert such savings to the Exchequer, since they could not be precisely identified.[49] Despite this uncertainty, concessions as to the level of capital investment were usually accompanied by demands for a demonstration of revenue savings. Officials anticipated approving projects which could show annual savings of 15 per cent of revenue costs, and suggested earmarking £3 million per annum for revenue saving investment (thereby doubling it). But it was also suggested that any new developments would have to be 'planned very economically in terms of maintenance costs' and a necessary *quid pro quo* would be economies, or the closure of obsolete facilities.[50]

Officials clearly felt that the Ministry of Health was dragging its feet on revenue savings, expressing frustration with Macleod: '*the Minister has no idea of thinking out ways of making the service more efficient and cheaper*';[51] he was also being 'defeatist' in proceeding as if no substantial economies were to be expected from Guillebaud.[52] While the Treasury were persuaded of the advantages of long-term planning by 1954[53] they linked it unambiguously to revenue savings: 'until Mr Macleod has shown whether he is going to drop the extravagant claims of his Ministry, it would be imprudent to be very forthcoming'[54] on capital investment. Though Ministry officials doubted whether the concept of revenue-saving capital works was 'firmly enough grounded in reality',[55] capital sums were eventually earmarked for revenue-saving works.

Standardisation

Drawing parallels with the experience of other government departments, there were persistent calls for standardisation in hospital design and construction. This arose in the context of Ministry demands for greater devolution of responsibility within the capital programme. All hospital projects costing more than £50,000 had formally to be approved by the Treasury, and this was a constant source of delay. The Treasury indicated willingness to relax these controls if, as a *quid pro quo*, building costs could be reduced, and officials were attracted to the idea of evolving standards for hospital building like those produced for the Ministry of Education.[56] The response of health officials was that hospitals did 'not resemble each other so much as schools' and, perforce, given constraints on capital, 'most building will be adaptations';[57] moreover, there were many more schools than hospitals, facilitating the adoption of standard designs. Progress was slow. Treasury papers commented that the Ministry 'were averse to doing anything effective' and were, indeed, 'half-hearted' about standardisation.[58] Nevertheless, this issue 'was to be pressed most strongly ... there is no hope of advancing [the delegated limit for capital schemes] to £100,000 until there is evidence of progress'. The issue dragged on, without resolution; a 1958 minute was critical of the Ministry's attitude that 'hospitals are so different that the experience of other Departments is irrelevant' and suggested that 'patients' interests would be better served by having a lot of cheapish standardised units rather than fewer custom-built ones'.[59] The Treasury recognised the 'natural concern' of the medical profession and of the health service to 'secure functional perfection', but said that there was a real danger that plans would 'go ahead without regard to economy unless the Government exercise their influence in the formative stages'.[60] Despite eventually establishing its own design unit for hospital building, the Ministry 'did not take' to a 1959 Treasury report which had suggested that it should be 'more proactive' in this matter.[61]

Links to local authority programmes

There are precursors here of much later debates concerning interdependencies between local authority health and welfare services, and hospital provision. The Treasury wondered whether switching investment to the former would ease pressure on the latter. It was, for example, argued that local authority capital expenditure on social care should not be reduced; it should be encouraged, 'for much the same financial reasons as replacing inefficient boilers'.[62] It was therefore argued that the Ministry should think about hospital and local authority investment 'at one and the same time'. The Ministry apparently regarded this as 'quite an unfair question'; they did not regard themselves as 'being under any sort of obligation' to think in those terms.[63] However, it is not clear that this perception of the Ministry was wholly accurate, because the Ministry made a case for a substantial increase in local welfare services in mid-1955 (partly to avoid bed blocking), which was accepted.[64] The Treasury then failed to follow their own lights, rejecting Guillebaud's suggestion of a 50 per cent Exchequer grant towards the current and capital costs of accommodation for the elderly (mainly because it involved new liabilities at a time when the Government was seeking economies elsewhere in the social services).[65] The Ministry subsequently objected to the suspension of loan sanctions for local authority capital expenditure on welfare services, an investment which the Ministry insisted was 'essential for relieving pressure on the NHS'.[66] This comment suggests that, in fact, the Ministry *was* thinking in terms of the parallel development of hospital and community services, and that the obstacle was the narrow financial criteria imposed by the Treasury. Constraints on capital spending, then, occasionally worked against the attainment of desirable improvements in efficiency. Repeated exchanges between Turton and Macmillan during 1956, in which Turton stressed the 'economic absurdity' of restricting the provision of local authority accommodation, failed to alter this position.[67]

Summary

The foregoing does not seem to accord with a view that Guillebaud had authoritatively settled the case. Treasury officials continued to probe the Ministry's justifications for its proposals, and made strenuous efforts to push for standardisation and linkage to local authority proposals. This might be seen as typical Treasury hawkishness and distrust of a Ministry which had acquired a reputation for profligacy. However, it could also reflect a legitimate concern that policy should be evidence based. Although Guillebaud put the issue of investment firmly on the agenda, then, it did not decisively resolve it. Examination of Figure A1 suggests no clear upward break of slope in the trend-line of NHS capital development until the early 1960s. There is an acceleration in 1959, which is just about conformable with the view that Guillebaud had an impact, but it would not appear to be decisive evidence. For all this scepticism in negotiations, Treasury officials acknowledged privately that the hospitals had 'been living on capital ... for 15 years ... the day is coming when really large capital expenditure will be imperative';[68] if not carefully managed, the result would be 'rush, panic and extravagance'.[69] It was eventually agreed that 'Macleod ... is right in stressing the low level of capital expenditure'.[70] There was one last attempt to spike Guillebaud's guns. An internal memorandum wondered if Guillebaud's charges could be undermined by saying that 'other social services ... had had to suffer because of defence', but the writer conceded that 'I doubt if we shall get much change out of this'.[71] Six months later the writer accepted that 'investment in hospitals has been neglected in the past and must be made good in the future'.[72] If such views were sincerely held, there is no evidence that they effected a relaxation in restrictions on NHS capital investment. As indicated above (and in Chapter 6) it was only from late 1958 that the political climate became more favourable to the Ministry.

Formulating and implementing a hospital strategy: national and local policies

Given the constraints on the capital programme, to what extent were the Ministry of Health and the RHBs able to make inroads into the legacy of neglect, and how were decisions taken in respect of development priorities? This is examined using evidence from the Ministry and from the Newcastle RHB. Up to 1952–3, capital allocations reflected population distribution and bed complements, weighted equally. This was modified so that, after holding back sums for centrally financed projects, 95 per cent was allocated in relation to population and the rest in relation to 'particularly grave investment difficulties' (mainly low *per capita* bed provision) in six RHBs.[73] Central finance was necessary as otherwise large projects would have absorbed a substantial proportion of an RHB's capital budget. The allocation of central finance thus provides insight into how the Ministry sought to develop a national strategy.

Because of the scale of resources available, discussion of the relative priority to be given to different locations was 'almost entirely academic', since we 'do not expect to be considering the provision of additional beds in areas where the need for them requires any very fine method of measurement'.[74] This note was accompanied by examples of quite substantial deficiencies, accompanied by the despairing comment that there was 'not the remotest chance of overprovision ...' and no possibility 'of doing away with more than the bare minimum of unsatisfactory premises'.[75] It was 'a waste of time to have any exhaustive scrutiny of regional lists [beyond a few of their highest priorities] since the proportion which there is any hope of starting is so minute'.[76] The problem with this approach was that a list of what individual regions regarded as their highest priorities could, when aggregated, produce results which were difficult to defend. Thus Dr George Godber pointed out that, of a list of schemes produced in this way, 'six are in metropolitan regions, one in the Birmingham region and one in the South West ... there is a great preponderance in the south'.[77] Two years later, of a draft list of major projects to begin in 1958–9, one-third were in the NW Metropolitan RHB ('this will be hard to justify') and seven of twelve major schemes were in London.[78] Godber, for one, sought to adjust the Ministry's priority lists accordingly.

An illustration of the criteria taken into account in formulating policy is provided by the Ministry's annual consideration of major schemes submitted by Boards, taking the schemes for 1956–8 as an example. Although bed deficiencies were important, other factors mentioned included: the state of readiness of projects (to ensure that the funds were not underspent); the regional distribution ('we should presumably try to ensure that each RHB gets a share'); past promises ('some of the schemes have been the subject of pressure on the Department for quite long periods'); and *force majeure* ('projects forced upon us by the termination of our tenure of existing accommodation').[79] One Ministry official described the process of hospital development, no doubt rather tongue-in-cheek, as follows:

> Stage 1: site works followed by stage 2: outpatient and casualty department. Nothing for a year or two until local politics dictate, say, stage 3: twin operating suite and a new acute surgical block, perhaps a new laboratory and mortuary. All these are small beer, say £1/4Mn.[80]

Again, perfectly understandable, given the constraints involved but hardly the most strategic way to plan the programme. If there was an explicit strategy, it was rather vaguely specified, as in a Treasury suggestion that the 'main schemes should be concentrated in New Towns and other rapidly expanding areas rather than improving facilities in places where they already have them ... [this] also makes sense from a Civil Defence viewpoint'.[81]

In developing the hospital service, the Ministry was well aware that the capacities and performance of RHBs, in terms of their assessment of needs and their ability to manage a capital programme, varied greatly. Commenting on a list of proposed major schemes, an official reported that the way in which the Boards carry out their work was 'haphazard and unscientific'. A request for information about their priorities 'caught them in a state of unpreparedness which is hard to believe, when this is just the sort of work we have been expecting them to do for the last seven years'. Sudden switches in priorities, 'blocking the inclusion of schemes ... which are obviously much more urgent', were the order of the day. There was:

> little or no attempt ... to compare the needs of one area with another, ... far too much attention is given to HMCs who are able to organise local pressure groups, and priorities are allotted in accordance with the views and prejudices of individuals rather than on a comprehensive appreciation of comparative needs in the region as a whole.[82]

Similar comments were evident in respect of RHB submissions to the Hospital Plan. The treatment an individual RHB received therefore depended partly on the Ministry's judgement of its competence. Thus one Board was 'backward with planning', while another made 'very slow progress with schemes' so that in both cases 'there is not a great point in giving them too much'; in another region 'we are in great difficulty ... there is great need and practically nothing gets done'.[83]

This unfortunate situation reflected a number of influences. RHBs arguably saw little point in advancing sophisticated plans when they had little chance of effecting them. Both the RHBs, and the Ministry, had to make sure that the available resources were both spent (which meant that places were favoured if their plans were in a suitable state of readiness) and spent roughly evenly (hence a tendency for numerous small schemes rather than a small number of large ones). Inevitably this meant that funds flowed to the well organised and vociferous, leading Macleod to commend that the Ministry would have to 'see that the weaker brethren among the Boards get a reasonable share' of resources.[84]

What were the implications for individual RHBs? The following discussion briefly summarises key themes from the Newcastle RHB; the region, and its constituent Hospital Management Committees (HMCs), are shown in Figure 5.1. The Board persistently emphasised its inadequate legacy and argued that hospital development in the region had proceeded more slowly than in other areas,[85] a situation which was being perpetuated by a capital allocation which, *per capita*, was 23 per cent below the national average. There could be 'no justification' for this in a national hospital service.[86] The deficiencies in the region's services were also occasionally raised in Parliament, with MPs pointing to the region's history of economic depression and contending that there should be a concerted effort to rectify deficiencies.[87] Interestingly, though, by comparison with later periods, it is surprising how infrequently MPs used adjournment debates to complain about the health service (compare the flood of such debates in the 1980s: Mohan 1998).

In practice the Board was unable to do much beyond commencement of a series of small-scale schemes. The RHB's review of its inheritance disclosed a 'serious shortage' of accommodation, though 'some parts of the region had fairly adequate numbers' of hospital beds. However, outpatient, X-ray and pathology departments were either lacking or of very poor quality. The Regional Architect stressed the low standard or unsuitability for hospital purposes of many institutions. Significantly, given the numbers of beds provided in such accommodation (3,700, some 25 per cent of a regional total of 16,000 non-psychiatric beds), he also emphasised the 'regrettably low' quality of accommodation in the EMS hospitals. Nowhere in the region had there been serious efforts at the 'integration' of hospitals, so planning had to start from scratch.[88]

Despite this situation, development was severely constrained by limited capital budgets and restrictions on the availability of materials and labour. The capital allocation available to the RHB – £560,000 per annum initially – was of a similar order to the pre-war level of investment, but this was 'quite inadequate', since virtually no new construction, apart from EMS units, had taken place between 1939 and 1948.[89] Because of the scale of construction required, devising a list of priorities was virtually impossible.[90] Since no major capital development was possible, a considerable amount of minor – and probably 'futile' – capital works would be necessary.[91] Developments

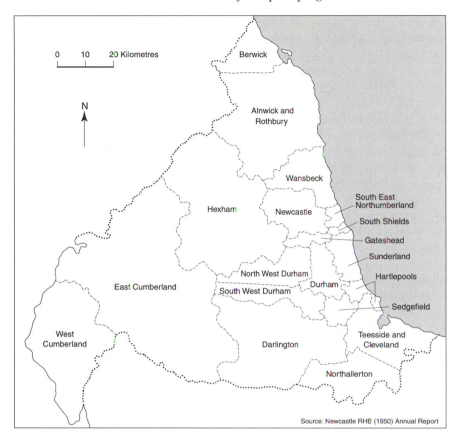

0   10   20 Kilometres

N

Berwick

Alnwick and
Rothbury

Wansbeck

South East
Northumberland

Hexham   Newcastle

South Shields

Gateshead

Sunderland

North West Durham   Durham   Hartlepools

East Cumberland   South West Durham

Sedgefield

West
Cumberland   Darlington   Teesside and
Cleveland

Northallerton

Source: Newcastle RHB (1950) Annual Report

Figure 5.1 The Newcastle RHB and its constituent HMCs

would be geared largely to prolonging the life of the existing capital stock,[92] but this was likely to lead to hospitals becoming 'architectural hotch-potches', as small-scale projects were added as and where possible.[93] As a Chairman of another RHB put it, small-scale works were often undertaken 'more from expedience than priority' (Wells 1951: 45). The Board had little alternative. It had a large number of EMS facilities and would ideally have abandoned them, but concluded that 'from the economic point of view, ... adaptation was preferable to new building'.[94]

How were priorities determined? There are occasional references in the minutes of the RHB and its committees to the needs of particular localities. Thus the Board had established its Special Area Committee to deal with the challenges of Cumberland and Westmorland, partly on the grounds of their remoteness from the rest of the Board's area, partly because of the very limited development of services there, especially in the Cumberland coalfield. In the early years of the NHS this area received a rather higher share of the RHB's capital allocation than its share of the region's beds would indicate.[95] Other localities were less fortunate. For example the Planning Committee was advised, in December 1948, that they should prioritise the Bishop Auckland area, served by the SW Durham HMC: 'there can be few districts with more urgent need for modern hospital facilities for in the main patients are sent to Newcastle'.[96] Several months later it was argued that the Wansbeck HMC, serving several small towns in Northumberland, was 'probably the worst served in the region' in terms of the numbers of beds available. Additional beds were therefore urgently required at the Morpeth Cottage Hospital even though the Board's long-term intention was the provision of a new hospital.[97] The Board were also reminded that they were 'in danger of spending a disproportionate amount of money outside Newcastle', to which the Chairman replied that 'in his anxiety over the needs of other parts of the region his attention had perhaps been distracted from the focal point, but he would try to bear in mind the needs of Newcastle'.[98] Other HMCs drew attention to the poor quality of their hospital stock, the need to complete developments begun before the war, and the desirability of replacing some EMS hospitals. In proposing new hospitals, however, the RHB concentrated on three areas – West Cumberland, eastern County Durham (at the new town of Peterlee), and Bedlington (in the Wansbeck HMC) – which had in common a scattered settlement pattern and a non-existent or minimal inheritance of acute beds. Fourteen major extensions were also proposed, mainly involving increases to the capacity of small general hospitals in several locations.[99]

Having identified these priorities the Board was able to do little about them. *Ad hoc* reductions in capital allocations[100] limited the scope for strategic planning. Thus the RHB's capital allocation for 1951–2 was reduced by 25 per cent shortly before the end of the 1950–1 financial year.[101] This effectively halved the programme, when the effects of rising building costs were taken into account, because Boards were in any event only allowed to spend 85 per cent of their allocations, to reduce the risk of over-spending.[102] These restrictions were regarded as 'calamitous'[103] and they engendered 'considerable irritation' among RHBs and HMCs at their lack of autonomy (Guillebaud Committee 1956: 104). The RHB argued that, in the absence of assurances that funds would be available for proposed schemes, planning was an activity which:

> raises false hopes, engenders a sense of frustration, and degenerates into a theoretical exercise without purpose or justification ... the course of the Board's programme ... has been from crest to trough of successive waves of hope and disappointment.[104]

The Board pressed the Ministry for additional funds, and one result of this was permission to overspend their 1952–3 capital allocation by £82,000,[105] though this had only been possible because other RHBs had underspent.[106] In fact, to avoid overspending on its limited budget, the RHB attempted to slow down the pace of its capital programme by ceasing its practice of 'constantly pressing the contractors to proceed with the work with the utmost expedition'.[107]

There is also evidence that the Board actively considered ways of rationalising the hospital stock. Officials identified twenty-five hospitals to which particular attention was to be given, mainly small specialist and infectious disease hospitals, but also three general hospitals (Dryburn, Durham; Hemlington, near Middlesbrough; Carlisle City General). The conclusion drawn was that what the region principally needed was not a large increase in bed numbers, but rather improvements in the quality of accommodation and support services. The suggestion was also made that it might be sensible to consider closing several hospitals from the point of view of economy and the avoidance of duplication. For example, there were over fifty hospitals in the region where occupancy was under 80 per cent.[108]

Clearly, then, considerable problems were experienced in setting in motion a programme of capital development in the region's hospitals; the results can be illustrated by a consideration of the use of capital resources by the RHB, and by discussing the outcomes of its policies. First, the amount of new construction achieved prior to 1962 was minimal; the proportion of the RHB's capital allocated to this varied between 1.1 per cent and 19.7 per cent, though not until 1957 did this rise above 10 per cent in any one year. Given the limited resources available, investment largely took the form of small-scale projects, though this in turn led to concern that the Board's programme had degenerated into a number of extremely small works.[109] Moreover, there was little scope for replacing the EMS hospitals, for this would have required large investment in view of the size of those hospitals.[110] As an indication of the shortfall in capital investment, RHB and HMC submissions had proposed a total of 1087 capital schemes by late 1955, but only sixty-one of these had a definite place in the programme.[111]

The implications of these developments for the intra-regional pattern of capital investment were twofold. First, only one new hospital commenced building. The provision of a new hospital for West Cumberland had been identified by the Commissioner for the Special Areas and the Ministry as a project of 'national importance', a verdict echoed by the Hospital Surveys (Ministry of Health 1946: vol. 9, 115). But despite the priority attached by the Board to development there, the RHB was advised that the Ministry's central reserve of large projects was being used principally to meet the needs of the mental health services, and the Minister could therefore 'hold out no hope' that authorisation of West Cumberland would be possible.[112] Not until 1955, following a Government announcement of an increase in the proportion of capital resources allocated to large-scale developments,[113] were the RHB able to commence construction of the new West Cumberland Hospital.

The development of West Cumberland was undoubtedly needs-based but the Board was also mindful of the wider context of public policy in the region, which was geared to reconstructing the region's physical infrastructure, the better to attract industrial investment in order to diversify the economic base. An interesting case in point is the shift in the Board's priorities which occurred in the mid-1950s: their initial proposal for a hospital at Peterlee (in an area poorly served by existing hospitals) was supplanted in regional strategy by the claims of Teesside. Peterlee was designated as a New Town in 1948, the idea being to secure a better living environment for the residents of eastern County Durham. This, in turn, would aid retention of the coal-mining workforce and contribute to the maximisation of coal output (Robinson 1978). A hospital would clearly contribute to the social goals of such a development, a site was offered to the RHB, and the Board initially regarded it as a high priority. However, because of the economic imperative to maximise coal output, the NCB had an effective veto on surface development. The site offered was underlain by workable coal and large structures such as hospitals could not be built, but it could be made available for housing. The New Town Development Corporation did not want an 'undeveloped hole' in Peterlee; they were also keen to cooperate with the NCB in minimising constraints on coal extraction. Having released the proposed site for housing, they offered the RHB an alternative, which was accepted.[114] Thus the productionist concerns of the NCB took precedence over the social goals of new town development.

Peterlee consequently slipped down the list of RHB priorities during the 1950s.[115] The town's slow growth may also have contributed to this, not least as the coal industry began to contract, because the prospects for attracting other industries were 'uncertain'.[116] Changing attitudes to the size of general hospitals may also have swayed the RHB against Peterlee and, as the RHB later pointed out, there already existed four hospitals (albeit of poor quality) close to Peterlee.[117] There are contrasts here with the experience of the London overspill new towns, which were prioritised (Welwyn Garden City receiving the first new hospital under the NHS). However these towns were much larger than those in the North East, and they were generally much further from existing centres of hospital provision.[118]

In contrast, by the late 1950s Teesside had become established as the RHB's main priority for new capital investment. Teesside had been identified as a future growth point for industry within the region for some time (see Pepler and Macfarlane 1949: 157–61), and the RHB responded to this. At a meeting of the Planning Committee, it was pointed out that 'the importance of the developments of the Teesside industries ... had been endorsed by the Ministry of Town and Country Planning, the Board of Trade and the Ministry of Labour'. The Teesside HMC therefore argued that 'the proposed developments at Middlesbrough should be undertaken at the earliest date ... major industrial expansion had taken place in respect of chemicals and heavy industries, and extensive additional expansion was planned'.[119]

This matter was stressed at several subsequent meetings of the RHB's Planning Committee, at one of which it was reported that the HMC had actually lobbied the Ministry directly for a new hospital, and had drawn attention to the 'great industrial developments taking place on Teesside' and to the growth of 33,000 in its population.[120] Two direct consequences were, first, that Teesside became regarded as a higher priority than Peterlee, and second, in anticipation of developments on Teesside, the Sedgefield HMC was merged with part of Cleveland HMC, it being recognised that Sedgefield General Hospital would become 'largely redundant' in the event of a new general hospital being built in the north Teesside area.[121] It was recognised that social infrastructures needed to be adjusted, as the pace of industrial development 'was such as to call into question hospital arrangements dating from a period when the development was much less advanced'.[122] It is also notable that, shortly before the Hospital Plan's announcement, the RHB chairman indicated to the Ministry of Health that, of all the projects agreed for the plan, he attached the most importance to the new hospital for North Teesside, even if other schemes were postponed as a result.[123] The implicit prioritisation of an area seen as central to future economic growth is also evident from data about the distribution of capital investments worth over £100,000 carried out in the first fourteen years of the NHS. In this region, they included other significant developments in Cumberland (at Carlisle and Workington), in Newcastle-upon-Tyne, and Middlesbrough. Other important centres of population lagged behind (such as South Shields, Darlington and Sunderland; note, however, that Sunderland had seen major voluntary and municipal developments in the 1930s). Significantly, however, there was very little investment in much of County Durham or in the Northumberland coalfield, a pattern which was to continue. Fox's (1986: 170) statement, that 'almost every hospital was extensively modernised' in this period, therefore requires substantial qualification.

Third, in terms of specific patterns of openings and closures of hospitals, a corollary was that the only *new* hospital to be commenced was the West Cumberland Hospital. New bed provision was confined largely to Cumberland and Teesside. Hospital *closures* were confined largely to a small number of buildings whose physical condition was such that no benefits would accrue from their retention, and to tuberculosis and isolation units. Many of the latter were unsuitable because of their physical condition, while the virtual elimination of tuberculosis was reflected in growing concern at the under-utilisation of several hospitals.[124] However, if little progress could be made on capital investment, the RHB compensated for this by a redistribution of medical personnel and by recruiting additional staff. In comparison with other RHBs, Newcastle was relatively successful in doing so (Webster 1988a: 294-5). By 1957, the RHB felt that the region was well staffed and that its specialist establishment was 80 per cent of what it ought to be.[125] This, in turn, was accompanied by a considerable increase in the efficiency of the service, measured in terms of patient throughput.

Concluding comments

During his tenure at the Ministry, Iain Macleod commented it was 'quite tragic that the result of the introduction of the NHS should be to cripple the capital development of our hospitals'.[126] Conservative critics (e.g. Jewkes and Jewkes 1961) suggest that this was because state intervention stifled voluntary initiative. This is simplistic, because local authority capital investment in the 1930s was substantially higher than that in the voluntary hospitals,[127] but it does raise the question of why the Ministry was so unsuccessful in obtaining capital. Although, the case for capital investment was made with vigour by at least some Ministers, they confronted a Treasury which was convinced, as early as 1949, that the NHS was costly and profligate, and which therefore adopted a sceptical attitude to requests for additional investment. This, plus the low political priority attached to the NHS by the Conservatives, helps account for the absence of a substantial capital programme.

It is not the whole story, however. This view leaves untouched the question of why the Ministry of Health was so unsuccessful (as compared with other Government departments) in obtaining capital for hospitals. The Ministry was unable to convince the Treasury about precisely why they wanted an expansion of investment. My argument here has been that the case made by the Ministry was a statement of the manifest deficiencies in the service, but from the Treasury's point of view, this failed to demonstrate what the benefits of increased capital investment would be. Wary of the possibility of opening a Pandora's Box, the Treasury refused to accept that these deficiencies *per se* warranted substantial investment. The Ministry were repeatedly questioned as to the revenue costs and benefits of investment, the possibility of standardisation, and links with local authority programmes, and efforts were made to tie concessions on the capital programme to developments in these areas. This might be seen purely as a demand for evidence-based policy but it provided the Treasury with scope for resisting any substantial expansion in capital expenditure. The Treasury's determined attempts to refute the Guillebaud Committee's arguments are further evidence of this tendency. What really settled the case for long-term planning was less an acceptance of these arguments than a political realisation that the state of the hospitals, at the end of the first decade of the NHS, was perceived as a disgrace. The technical arguments, which Guillebaud appeared to have settled, continued into the 1960s (see chapters 6, 7).

These 1950s debates are relevant to much broader arguments about welfare provision. They illustrate one response to the problems posed for the allocation of capital investment when services are provided for use, not for exchange. As the Treasury themselves had acknowledged, no one had been in the market to buy hospitals, and political decisions determined capital allocations. These arguments are essentially about seeking to ensure that the public sector was subject to broadly similar disciplines to the private sector. This was an attempt to resolve the contradiction inherent in the welfare state

– the existence of a substantial area of social life which was decommodified, or insulated from market forces. The Treasury's solution has some connections with later initiatives, like the PFI, insofar as it imposed narrow financial criteria on investment in the NHS.

Debates in this period also raise questions about governance, especially the role and capacities of the Ministry. Prior to the war the Ministry had not had direct responsibilities for planning hospital services and its role had been to advise and supervise local authorities. Nationalisation arguably gave the Ministry responsibilities that it was ill-equipped to handle. This was acknowledged by the Treasury; an official referred to the problems of 'an old-fashioned regulatory Department who have suddenly got landed with a senior managerial job' (quoted in Webster 1988a: 239). In common with other departments the Ministry lacked the machinery and capacity to take a long-term strategic view; for example, it was only in the late 1950s that there was serious consideration of technical questions in relation to hospital design and construction. The Ministry was also operating in a context in which autonomy was heavily circumscribed due to controls on capital projects. This meant that governance was top-heavy and bureaucratic.

What was achieved during this period? Fraser (1964) contends that construction prior to the Hospital Plan produced the equivalent of fifty new general hospitals. Some 37,000 beds had been provided. This compares with the ninety new and 134 'substantially remodelled' hospitals envisaged for the ten years of the initial plan. In the Newcastle region the 1,460 new beds in non-psychiatric hospitals provided by 1962 equated to just under 10 per cent of the bed complement,[128] though substantial investments also took place in long-stay hospitals. Development was largely confined to schemes designed to increase throughput in existing hospitals. Both between and within regions there was a dilemma: what was really required was a programme of substantial investment in major schemes, but neither the Ministry nor the RHBs could risk the political consequences of concentrating on them. For example, had the West Cumberland Hospital not been accepted for central financing, it would have absorbed an excessive proportion of the region's capital allocation, virtually precluding developments elsewhere. But having had one new DGH accepted for central financing, the other new hospital projects inevitably slipped further into the future.

A final consequence of the constraints on investment in this period was that the evidence base for future development was limited. The hand-to-mouth method of allocating capital was conducive neither to rational planning or to economy, so that there were few exemplars of good practice.[129] Debates on standardisation, revenue consequences, or bed norms had not been settled. Assessing priorities was therefore approached in an unsystematic manner and the performance of Boards varied considerably (though Newcastle was highly regarded by the Ministry: Chapter 6). This hardly seemed a promising foundation on which to construct a major building programme, and partly because of these weaknesses, which to some degree remained unresolved, the implementation of the subsequent Hospital Plan became a contentious issue which tested the competence of politicians and senior civil servants alike.

6 Explaining and reappraising the 1962 Hospital Plan

The Hospital Plan for England and Wales has generally had a good press. With the parallel plan for Scotland, it remains the most significant declaration by a government of its intention of modernising the acute hospital system. The Plan proposed a national network of large-scale hospitals which would provide, for defined catchment populations, the normal range of acute hospital services. District General Hospitals (DGHs), of a minimum size of 600–800 beds, would serve populations of 100,000–150,000. The logic of the Plan is perhaps best captured by the following: 'the district general hospital offers the most practicable method of placing the full range of hospital facilities at the disposal of patients and *this consideration far outweighs the disadvantages of longer travel* for some patients and their visitors' (Ministry of Health 1962a: 6 – emphasis added).

In spatial terms, this clearly envisaged a considerable concentration of hospital services in the interests of the efficiency of the hospital system as a whole. Thus, while the provision of a system of modern, technologically sophisticated hospitals would involve higher running costs, these increases were to be relatively marginal and, as was explained in the Plan:

> the real increase in running costs ... will be due *rather to a higher standard of service than* to any increase in the number of beds ... opportunities for economy will be created by the concentration of work in fewer centres and the replacement of older buildings by new hospitals which can be more economically maintained and run.
>
> (Ministry of Health 1962a: 13 – emphasis added)

Put another way, efficiency had clearly triumphed over equity in terms of service provision; if longer travel to hospitals was to be accepted, it had to be justified on the grounds that a better hospital service was being provided. The Plan's aim was therefore to provide a more efficient service – in the sense of increasing patient throughput and restraining running costs – or, as one commentator has argued, to introduce 'capitalist rationality' into the NHS (Manson 1979: 42).

The Plan's intentions were to be achieved by increasing capital investment to £200 million in its first quinquennium (1961–2 to 1965–6) and to £300 million in its second quinquennium (1966–7 to 1970–1). The Plan would involve constructing ninety new and 134 remodelled hospitals, 356 other schemes each worth over £100,000, and the closure of 709 non-psychiatric hospitals. The Plan also implied resource redistribution at the inter- and intra-regional scales. Inter-regionally, the Plan sought to redress some of the imbalances in service provision generated by the uncoordinated historical development of the hospital system. This would be achieved by setting 'bed norms' of 3.3 acute beds per 1,000 population.

These proposals undoubtedly represented an advance on the limited achievements of the first thirteen years of the NHS. Perhaps for this reason, the academic reception of the Plan has been largely uncritical, with the exceptions of Manson (1979) and Webster (1994). Yet a number of issues could usefully be explored further. The most basic of these relates to the rationality and coherence of the Plan: did it merit some of the claims made for it as a *planning* exercise? Powell talked of planning the hospital service 'on a scale not possible anywhere else, certainly this side of the iron curtain'[1] while the Permanent Secretary of the Ministry, Bruce Fraser, spoke of a 'new deal' for hospitals when negotiating with the Treasury.[2] Was it, instead, largely – or merely – a symbolic political exercise? There is no doubt that considerable political capital was invested in the Plan: unusually, although it merely involved expanding an established programme, it was launched with a White Paper. It was a large-scale, highly visible and discrete programme, which assumed totemic significance. It therefore became a lodestone of commitment to the welfare state. It was also, of course, a hostage to fortune, in the sense that the implied expenditure commitments rendered it vulnerable to changing circumstances. And the Plan was not without its ironies: it was introduced by a noted free-marketeer, Enoch Powell, whose planning credentials were (to put it mildly) not obvious. In a wider frame of reference, the Conservatives' historical allegiances with localist, community-based and voluntarist welfare initiatives were not entirely superseded by the Plan.

This chapter concentrates on a reappraisal of the origins of the Plan and in this context a consideration of previous work is appropriate. The only extant book on the Plan is Allen (1979; see also 1981). This is based on interviews with several key informants and tends to emphasise the actions of prominent individuals. The Plan was thus seen in terms of the happy coincidence of the arrival at the Ministry of Health of three key individuals: Enoch Powell (Minister of Health), George Godber (Chief Medical Officer) and Bruce Fraser (Permanent Secretary). The credibility of Powell and Fraser (who had both previously been associated with the Treasury) and Godber's 'radical and egalitarian' planning credentials (Timmins 1995: 209; as a former wartime surveyor, he was a long-time advocate of regional organisation and planning)[3] are said to have helped the Ministry overcome the resistance of a sceptical Treasury. Thus, according to Ham (1992: 142), these three individuals 'effectively transformed a vague idea about an expanded building programme into a detailed plan'. But this is not the whole story, since it requires an understanding of the context against which those individuals were operating.

Some of that context is provided by the 'great reappraisal' (Brittan 1969) of government stimulated, it is said, by key reports such as that of the Plowden Committee (1961) on the Management and Control of Public Expenditure. Some writers link the Plan explicitly to a diffusionist model of economic management: according to Rodwin (1984: 151), in the 1960s, 'French-style economic planning spread across the Channel', while Klein (1983: 74) refers to the Plan as the 'child of a marriage between professional aspirations and the new faith in planning'. While Plowden was influential, a key issue here concerns whether the Plan represented a 'properly conceived planning exercise' (to use Webster's (1994: 59) phrase): from an examination of the work that went into the Plan's preparation, substantial questions can be raised about its coherence and rationality. Furthermore (in part following Lowe 1997), I question whether the link with Plowden is any more than a case of prestige by association, and attempt to determine the ways in which the Plowden philosophy influenced hospital development.

A final theme for discussion here is the extent to which the 1962 Plan can be seen as part of a modernisation strategy. Jessop (1992) notes the various connotations of modernity: 'corporate planning, economies of scale, mass production, investment in science and technology, pursuit of standardisation and centralised control, active state sponsorship of Fordist economic growth and a general belief that big was beautiful' (p. 23). In the context of the welfare state Murray (1991) and Mulgan (1991) have noted similar parallels: 'hospitals of the Fordist era were like factories in the Green Belt' (Murray 1991). There are obvious points of conflation here between Fordism and modernism in particular, but the more general point to raise is whether the Hospital Plan shares these general diagnostic criteria. Here I question the extent to which this is so by examining some of the Plan's conceptual underpinnings.

The chapter is divided into three main sections. The first relates the Hospital Plan to the moves towards long-term economic planning, symbolised by the Plowden report. The second details the political negotiations on the scale of the Plan. The third section offers an assessment of key technical issues relating to the Plan's formulation, which leads to a reappraisal of the extent to which the claims made for the Plan can be sustained.

Reorganising the British economy: moves towards long-term planning

Despite the introduction of Keynesianism and the large-scale expansion of the welfare state, economic management in the 1950s entailed little more than marginal adjustments to create the conditions in which the private sector could achieve full employment. However from the mid-1950s a series of balance-of-payments crises, and a growing awareness of the dangers of inflation, prompted a reconsideration of this somewhat 'arm's length' approach (Jessop 1980). Balance of payments deficits occurred in the 1950s and 1960s mainly because government spending overseas, and private overseas investment, were too high (Gamble 1994: 111). The burden of adjustment was placed squarely on the domestic economy.

In this climate the value of public expenditure, and the effectiveness of mechanisms for its control, became subjects for debate. One can detect what might be termed negative efforts to restrain its overall growth. Thus Heclo and Wildavsky (1981: 205–6) refer to the '*ad hoc* and flat rate cuts in public programmes and their effects, namely throwing work out of gear'. The difficulties of managing capital expenditure within such a system produced as many evils as a failure to control overall totals. In particular, stop-go cycles vitiated the use of capital programmes as instruments of demand management and reduced value-for-money (Clarke 1978: 31). From such a perspective, as well as from the point of view of individual departments, there were clear arguments for longer-term planning.

There was also a growing sense of frustration at the failure of indirect manipulation of the economy to promote growth, and envious glances were cast at what were perceived to be successful examples of indicative planning abroad (e.g. in France: Hall 1986; Middlemas 1986). The key political shift, to which the Hospital Plan has been linked, was towards long-term public expenditure programming, associated with the Plowden Report (1961) and the subsequent introduction of the Public Expenditure Survey and Control (PESC) system (see also Brittan 1969: 149–53; Clarke 1978; Ling 1998; Middleton 1996). The Plowden Report clearly saw control of the overall total of public expenditure as its key target, because Treasury scrutiny of the programmes of individual departments was regarded as ineffective. Public expenditure needed to be treated as one subject and not as thousands of isolated decisions. Once physical controls on investment had been abandoned in the early 1950s, there was no effective alternative (Clarke 1978: 17). The purpose of PESC was therefore to devise a more effective system for controlling public expenditure. Under PESC, expenditure was reviewed over a five-year period in the light of the availability of financial resources. The deliberations of the Plowden Committee show, at first, some resistance to long-term planning of hospital capital investment, but then a gradual acceptance of the idea. The Treasury resisted an extended time horizon for NHS capital planning since it limited the scope for adjustment in the economy: 'adjustment of public sector investment [was] a primary weapon to move the economy in one direction or another'.[4] To put this into its context, at the time the NHS capital programme was around £25 million per annum – hardly a sum likely to make much difference to policies of Keynesian demand management – yet the Treasury still felt the NHS 'had not been badly served'. Yet short-term and small-scale programmes had dysfunctional impacts on the capital programme, leading to parsimony in larger projects and extravagance in smaller ones.[5]

During 1960 the Committee came round to accepting a longer-term view, concluding that the present basis for the allocation of capital was 'on much too short a term' and arguing for tentative figures for ten years and 'reasonably firm' ones for five years. (This does not appear in the first version of the subcommittee's draft report (CPE (SC3) 17) but it does in subsequent versions.) Treasury officials accepted the logic of these arguments, but resisted published commitments as to the scale of expenditure on hospital building, which would limit the Treasury's scope for manoeuvre.[6] In some respects there was a contradiction at the heart of these arguments. On the one hand, there was a crying need for longer-term planning in the health service but, on the other hand, the Treasury wanted to encourage only as much detailed planning 'as can be achieved without public commitments'.[7] What the Treasury 'must continue to rule out' was 'implied or actual commitments of resources in the broad old sense'.[8] But it was difficult to see how the Ministry could plan effectively unless it had a clearer view of the likely level of resources that would be made available. In attempting to square this circle, drafts of the Plowden Report refer to capital allocations which 'would have a declining degree of firmness' over time, and which 'could not be binding'.[9] A warning was sounded, however; as the architect of PESC, Sir Richard Clarke, was later to point out, the view was held that in most of the social and environmental services field the 'effective means of moderating the growth of current expenditure is to reduce and postpone the expansion of capital facilities'. This does not sound as if the Treasury was totally convinced that a major expansion of NHS capital investment was imminent or essential, or that they were likely to relinquish such controls as were available to them. Furthermore, as critics have observed (e.g. Ling 1998; Lowe 1997), the aim of Plowden was not merely to force Departments to compete with one another for a share of the cake, it was also to reassert Treasury control at the existing level of public expenditure; in other words, to ensure that, at most, the cake did not increase in size. The pre-eminent concern was therefore not whether public expenditure could be valuable in any sense, but simply to avoid any increase in taxation. As a result the Plowden inquiry did not consider important questions concerning the Treasury's relationship with (and detailed supervision of) departments, and the benefits and costs of collective (as opposed to market) provision of welfare (Lowe 1997: 481–91). The result was that the PESC system was criticised for emphasising the 'softest' expenditure items – in which capital programmes were always likely to be an easy target – rather than 'allocating resources on the basis of a wider economic or social set of priorities' (Ling 1998: 78).

Nevertheless, the climate appeared to be favourable to an expansion of capital investment in the public sector and – given the complaints about political priorities – an expansion of capital investment in the NHS over a long time period. It is clear that there was an upward shift in the hospital capital programme (Figure A1). The increase was not as much as the RHBs wanted, but the Ministry had reservations about the feasibility of excessive expansion because of the unavailability of professional staff and because of the limited spare capacity in the construction industry.[10]

Long-term commitments were assumed in preparation for the Plan, but the difficulties of establishing priorities ten years or more ahead were recognised.[11] Fairly detailed commitments were given in the first quinquennium but thereafter proposals became less precise, and the Treasury, as indicated above, was keen to minimise the extent of published commitments and the detail that was published about the long-term capital programme (i.e. beyond the first decade). One can therefore accept an argument that long-term planning was taken on board, certainly by comparison with the 1950s. One can also discern some shifts in the ways capital expenditure was used – for example, the proportion of capital going to new buildings and to plant replacement increased (Figure A2). This would help avoid futile expenditure on patching up old buildings. At least in these senses there would appear to be evidence that connects developments in policy to Plowden.

But if the Plan was to epitomise the virtues of long-term, strategic thinking, it is less clear what the impact was of the new philosophy on the Ministry. Treasury officials claimed that there was little evidence of strategic planning. First, an expansion of hospital construction obviously involved some choices between, for example, building new hospitals *vis-à-vis* improving existing ones but this was not discussed: 'unless something is worked out on this critical point, talk of a "realistic national plan" sounds to me like a pious hope'.[12] The old chestnut of revenue savings was also glossed over with Powell being criticised for 'pseudoprecision', although the Treasury were willing to accept this if Powell included references 'in the direction of economy, value for money and good management',[13] even though they felt revenue savings had not been demonstrated.

The Ministry's estimates were also a subject for concern. There was no obvious basis for the sums requested. They were certainly not need based (as the Ministry themselves had pointed out)[14] but the Ministry could hardly be blamed for that given constraints on the availability of capital. The Ministry had felt it was more realistic to plan on the amount they thought likely to be available. They had not considered it sensible to 'ask hospital authorities for estimates of their long-term requirements, nor had they devised a long-term plan themselves'. Moreover, their attitude appeared to be that:

> whatever assumptions Boards were asked to plan on, and however tentatively the assumptions were presented to them, the position that would result would be one of virtual commitment and they had little or no responsibility for relating the plans to any conception of long-term national need.[15]

Internal Treasury papers further criticised the Ministry for being unable to produce evidence of any 'master plan'; even the policies of make do and mend should have been informed by a view of:

> what hospitals one will wish to retain on a fairly long-term basis. The Ministry do not see things in that light, and I really think they ought to, instead of proceeding on the more-or-less hand-to-mouth basis which has been their lot (through no fault of their own) until now.[16]

Officials continued to express similar scepticism until shortly before publication of the Plan.[17]

If Plowden was about the long-term planning of the economy, one might have expected more to be made of emerging evidence that the economy was running at close to capacity, which would clearly pose problems for the implementation of the plan. One constraint was the availability of skilled staff such as architects and related professionals.[18] Another was the extent of spare capacity in the building industry; this was mentioned in the submissions of various RHBs. The Chairman of the Bristol teaching hospitals argued, revealingly, that with one exception: 'we have so far failed to attract any firms of national size to our work ... we cannot just rely on the enormous increase in size of our impending programme to put this state of affairs right automatically'.[19]

What is hinted at here is the constraints, within a national economy experiencing growth, likely to attend this kind of expansion of hospital construction; few major firms had much experience and there were emerging capacity constraints within the economy. A 1959 Treasury report on the construction industry observed that, of 100,000 firms, only 150 employed over 500 people, so that there would be relatively few firms capable of carrying out the work.[20] There was evidence that this had been anticipated; in 1960, for instance, the Treasury had argued that emerging pressures on the building industry made it 'out of the question' to accept a more rapid expansion of local authority investment in health and welfare services.[21] The Plowden Committee had also drawn attention to the difficulties of expanding hospital construction on the scale required by the Ministry.[22] The lack of uniformity of hospitals and the limited sums available had meant that the large contractors had taken little interest in the programme, and the Ministry were asked by RHB Chairmen whether more could be done to involve larger firms. Fraser hoped that 'streamlining of planning procedures and mobilisation of larger firms would permit considerable improvement on past performance',[23] but it is not clear what evidence he had to support this. Despite these pressures the Plan was launched regardless, without any obvious attempt to scale back other public sector construction programmes. It might be argued that this was a political decision, but it does cast a shadow over the association between the Plan and the kind of long-term planning symbolised by Plowden.

Thus, it is evident that the case for long-term planning of public expenditure had some influence on debates about capital investment in the NHS. Opposition to longer-term programmes began to melt away; there was a steady upward progression in capital investment; a higher proportion of available funds was spent on new building. Nevertheless, there were definite limits to intervention and planning which meant that the Plan came to be launched in circumstances in which key variables were beyond government control (Peden 2000: 505–6).

Political negotiations on the scale of the hospital plan

Against the background that, at last, a large-scale capital programme might be feasible, the Ministry began to make its case after the 1959 election. The medical profession voiced increased anxiety at the deteriorating condition of the hospitals and compared the lack of action to rectify the situation with the priority accorded to education and housing in post-war reconstruction (e.g. Abel and Lewin 1959: 110). The policy of the BMA – articulated at its annual conference in 1959 – was for an expansion of the hospital building programme to around £750 million, spread over ten years.[24] The Government risked failing to satisfy this key interest group at a time when all major parties had declared their commitments to expansion. Consequently, by the time of the 1959 election, all major political parties had commented on the need for more investment. Key points in discussion were the weight to be attached to the recommendations of Guillebaud and to the election pledges, plus the concept of a 'replacement' level of capital investment.

Most historical accounts of the NHS emphasise the role of the Guillebaud report in making a case for increased capital investment. However, Guillebaud's figures on capital investment featured only marginally in post-1959 negotiations. The Ministry had envisaged a steady expansion to £50 million per annum up to 1965–6, and thereafter they thought that a further £5 million per annum could be added. The Guillebaud figure – of £30 million at 1952 prices – had been arrived at 'with an eye on history and probabilities' and was not drawn from Abel-Smith and Titmuss.[25] Subsequently an official wrote that the Guillebaud figure of £30 million was an 'embarrassment' (presumably because it remained substantially higher than actual capital expenditure on hospitals), but Fraser 'did not attach much importance to the Guillebaud figure'.[26] In comparison to the election pledge Guillebaud was 'the more carefully considered' but its thinking was 'very much out of date'.[27]

The Government's election pledge was clearly more significant, since any shortfall on presumed commitments would be 'asking for trouble'. The Treasury took the view that expansion could not mean more than a doubling of the actual expenditure in the year in which the pledge was made, implying a figure of about £40 million. From the Ministry, Fraser argued for

£45 million for 1964–5 and £50 million for 1965–6, claiming that Ministers could not 'comfortably argue that they are carrying out the pledge if they aim at less than this'.[28] Smaller sums could only be defended if needs had been found to be lower than expected or if, despite the Ministry's best efforts, capacity constraints prevented the money being spent. Despite previously stating that the Guillebaud recommendations were out of date, Fraser could not resist observing that only in the sixth year of the proposed programme would Guillebaud's recommended level of investment be reached. Even these estimates took no account of changes in the bed complement. The need was for 'more beds of some types and less of others, unfortunately the dearer and cheaper types respectively'.

Nonetheless the Treasury expressed their concern that the Ministry was proposing what was in effect a continually rising programme and sought a firm commitment to capping it. However the Ministry believed that to do so would imply that there was a finite amount of work to be done.[29] Even averaging £50 million per annum would leave the NHS 'a long way short of a service whose problems are only those of replacement'.[30] Still the Treasury resisted the implication that the Ministry was seeking increases in the cost of the programme beyond the first ten years (i.e. to something above £75 million per annum). As a result the Ministry undertook 'so to draw the White Paper as to avoid any commitment implying a higher rate after 1970', while emphasising that they did not yet 'see the end of the tunnel, i.e. a levelling off of expenditure'. The figures thus agreed (essentially, steady increases of £5 million per annum on a budget commencing at £25 million) were then confirmed in an exchange between Powell and Henry Brooke (Financial Secretary to the Treasury). Powell thought that the proposals submitted by RHBs had been 'optimistic' but he felt that the Plan was 'the least we could justify as a move towards modernising our hospitals'.[31]

Even these figures had not been won without concessions. Powell had become Minister of Health in July 1960 and within six months achieved a degree of notoriety for increasing NHS charges (thereby raising the proportion of the service's income derived from charges to its highest-ever levels), justifying them as providing the resources to expand the programme.[32] Yet as Willie Hamilton (Fife, West) pointed out, the charges imposed in 1960 amounted to '£66Mn a year, which is more than this programme visualises over the course of ten years'.[33] While such charges did not go as far as some members of the Conservative government had wished – after all, Powell had resigned from the Cabinet over the failure of the Social Services Committee to cut back the welfare state – they were indicative that the Plan in certain respects did not mark a dramatic departure or a shift in public expenditure priorities, being financed by increases in charges, the burden of which fell on the users of the service (Allen, 1979: 61–2; Timmins 1995; Webster 1994). Moreover, Powell was firmly convinced that hospital revenue costs could be reduced and he had agreed with Ministry that growth in the hospital revenue budget would be no more than 2 per cent per annum. This was a tight straitjacket within which to launch an expansion of hospital building. Heffer (1998: 27) contends that it 'was inevitable that some current costs would have to be sacrificed'. However, this glosses over the very real problems that were to be experienced as the NHS sought to modernise its hospitals.

Rationality, modernity and the Plan

There are signs of the genesis of a long-term vision in Ministry papers dating from at least 1958, when Ministry architects visited various RHBs to examine development plans. On the basis of one of these, in the Oxford RHB, it was estimated that a national programme of hospital redevelopment might cost some £600 million.[34] William Tatton-Brown, Chief Architect at the Ministry, drew an analogy between hospital development and town planning: without an overall plan hospitals would simply be located in the 'easiest and cheapest place that becomes available'. The Ministry needed to show that 'haphazard development is even more wasteful than ribbon development and urban sprawl'.[35] Following this, although there were some informal discussions about long-term plans, it was not until 1961 that RHBs and BGs were asked to prepare and submit ten-year development programmes; they were given four months to do this. [36]

The speed of this entailed raised questions about the credibility of the exercise. If the Plan represents the high point of 'modernisation' and 'planning' in the hospital service, it would seem reasonable to subject to scrutiny some of the technical arguments put forward for it. Specific points which are relevant here are the validity of the 'norms' for bed provision used in the Plan and the extent to which the proposals produced could be described, in any sense, as both national and as a 'Plan'.

The Plan arguably represented an apparently consistent attempt to equalise access to services by using standard 'norms' for hospital provision across the country. The first problem here was simply forecasting the population distribution. Some Boards had not obtained any projections of population trends.[37] East Anglia, for instance, was not clear on the effects of London overspill; only the Newcastle region was said to have forward estimates of population;[38] the impact of New Towns produced considerable uncertainty in several regions; in the Liverpool and Manchester submissions there was evidence of some early awareness of the decline of the inner city and the need for more investment in peripheral hospitals. Inevitably a large margin for error had to be allowed for in assessing the likely population distribution some twenty years ahead.

Of rather more importance were the bed/population ratios used as 'norms' for planning purposes. The initial intention of providing 7.0 acute beds per 1,000 population [39] had been invalidated by reductions in lengths of stay, and changing needs (e.g. the decline of TB); it would have been completely unrealistic in the light of the limited resources available for capital development. But what was the desirable level of hospital provision?

Various studies of the relationship between total population and numbers of hospital beds (summarised in Table 6.1) suggested that hospital planning should be based on a somewhat smaller beds/population ratio than had formerly been the case. At least one of them attempted to examine the extent to which the use of beds was justified and found that possibly 25 per cent fewer beds might be feasible (Forsyth and Logan 1960), which indicated a much more rapid throughput of patients in a smaller number of beds (Godber 1958). However, there was such a disparity in these studies that they gave 'very little guidance' beyond a 'rough indication'.[40] These studies were not without their technical weaknesses, such as the lack of consideration of the impacts on revealed demand for services of access to and supply of facilities, a problem which has bedevilled the NHS's attempts to devise an objective measure of need for hospital facilities. They were also, perforce, mainly based on small urban centres with clearly defined hinterlands, located at some distance from other hospital centres. They were consequently not fully representative.

These limitations of existing knowledge were also recognised in the hospital planning conferences organised by the Ministry in 1959 and 1960 in an effort to improve the knowledge base. Nevertheless, bed ratios were viewed as a 'useful tool ... rather like giving a blind man a stick – it may help him even though it won't improve his sight'.[41] By mid-1960, following study visits to the USA (Davies and Lewin 1960), the Ministry was prepared to accept schemes which would not raise the bed/population ratio above three beds per 1,000, though decisions 'must be art as well as science' and would inevitably include a large element of 'by guess and by God'.[42]

Table 6.1 Summary of estimates of 'norms' for acute hospital provision

Estimate produced by:	Recommended norm (beds/1,000 population)	Study area
Ministry of Health Circular RHB(48)1	7.0	Unknown
Nuffield Provincial Hospitals Trust (1945–6)	4.5–6.4	Hospital surveys (various regions)
Llewelyn-Davies (1955)	2.0	Northampton, Norfolk
Barr (1957)	2.0	Reading
Elder (1957)	5.0	Unknown
Forsyth and Logan (1960)	2.56	Barrow
Airth and Newall (1962)	3.6	Teesside

The bed norm finally chosen – 3.3 acute beds/1,000 population – was later criticised for its arbitrary nature (Chapter 7). This imprecision was acknowledged: the norms were 'not … a very sharp tooth', and they were regarded as 'a "touchstone" against which Boards should be asked to justify their proposals'.[43] Notwithstanding these views, the norms suggested by the Ministry were nevertheless used in a somewhat inflexible way. They were to be thought of 'as *maxima* … for the purposes of reducing excesses above them, not supplying deficiencies below them'.[44] One Board was strongly criticised because they had assumed that the bed norms gave them *carte blanche* to plan up to that level.[45] This clearly was not what the Ministry intended, and that particular Board were given 'firm orders' to reduce excesses.[46] Using the norms in this somewhat inflexible way rather contradicts the idea that the Plan was a sophisticated innovation. The norms became a vehicle whereby conformity could be imposed. If the ambitions of the Boards were reined in while the Plan was being prepared, however, this had the advantage of minimising the effect of 'later reductions on financial grounds'.[47]

What of the scientific underpinnings of the idea of a District General Hospital (DGH), the centrepiece of the Plan? Technical developments in hospital planning emphasised the importance of flexibility in design, economies of scale in service provision, and comprehensiveness of service (Abel and Lewin 1959; Godber 1958, 1959; Farrer-Brown 1959) and stressed the importance of integrating the work of the hospitals with the rest of the health service (McKeown 1959; Fry 1959). Concepts such as that of the 'area hospital' (Abel and Lewin 1959: iii) were aired; such facilities were to serve every 'natural area' of population and this concept has clear affinities with the 'base hospital' proposals discussed above (Chapter 4). However, despite the centrality of the DGH to British hospital development, no formal definition appears to exist, many terms used being 'elastic' in their meaning (Harrison and Prentice 1998: 14–15). There were several influences on policy, such as McKeown's (1958) idea of the 'balanced hospital community', providing all forms of care on one site and integrating the hospital with the surrounding community. The implicit assumption was that the DGH would provide better quality care and reduce unit costs. The scope of the DGH followed from the need to provide all the services thought to be required locally; the scale was defined in terms of an appropriate medical staffing structure (Harrison and Prentice 1998: 14–32). However, the arguments about scale and quality could not be substantiated given the state of knowledge at the time, which consisted of various small-scale studies. As Taylor (1960) put it, the conception of optimum hospital size had been arrived at by 'rather imprecise socio-medical studies'. The Ministry did not have the in-house research capabilities that might have provided answers, and in this it was not alone (see Lowe 1997: 488, on the inability of the education and health departments to secure resources for such tasks). The Ministry's architectural department had been pressing for a programme of research into hospital design and construction, but they were rather in a cleft stick: restrictions on capital investment had not justified the large-scale study of building problems, but expansion of the building programme, as we have seen, depended on the Ministry being able to demonstrate the benefits of it.[48] To some extent, therefore, the DGH concept – hospitals of 600–800 beds, serving a population of 100,000–150,000 – was consequently less clear-cut than would appear. As was admitted in late 1960, the concept (promulgated as guidance to health authorities in the form of Hospital Building Note No. 3) was 'inevitably ill-defined' because the Ministry had 'nothing empirical to go on'.[49] The Deputy Secretary in the Ministry, Enid Russell-Smith, was privately more critical: 'we are really making up a policy as we go along ... I really do not think we have been very well-served by the medicos'.[50]

One might also question the concept of the Plan as an attempt to produce an ideal or optimum distribution of hospitals. There was a prag-matic realisation that a *tabula rasa* approach, with all that that implied in terms of the writing off of previous rounds of investment, would never have succeeded. One Board could recognise the attractions of comprehensive renewal but 'could not recommend giving up capital assets of well over £1Mn'.[51] Moreover, the need for visible improvements constrained Boards from putting forward grandiose schemes: 'straight-through planning [was] favoured, but not if it meant no improvement until kingdom come: this would be medically wrong and politically unacceptable'.[52] There were two corollaries of this. There was a 'quite rational process' whereby solutions were conceptualised 'in terms of the present location of hospitals, ... [t]here may also be a tendency to distort the pattern of need to fit the premises available rather than to assess need and then consider how it can be met'.[53] The consequence was that few submissions explored the possibilities of novel solutions to planning problems; many of them failed to grasp poten-tially difficult political nettles. Second, questions of site availability, rough justice, and idiosyncratic preferences informed by rules-of-thumb influenced the choice of schemes and their place in RHBs' plans. The Newcastle RHB admitted, for instance, that it had generally chosen former local authority hospitals for development as general hospitals, mainly for reasons of land availability. While in a sense suboptimal, and thus potentially open to criti-cism, the RHBs were under pressure to produce visible improvements; hence a rather pragmatic approach was adopted.[54]

There were also concerns about the assumptions made in respect of local authority and other health services. Local authorities were responsible for residential care for the elderly and an expansion of such provision was neces-sary if the Plan's targets, of increased hospital throughput, were to be met; many elderly people blocked beds in acute hospitals because they could not be discharged. It was hoped to include a 'general picture of local authority developments which have been included in presenting the Hospital Plan. These ... in their turn, would involve certain assumptions about the amount that could be left to voluntary effort'.[55] This was a prescient observation, since it subsequently became clear that the extent to which local authority service provision had, in fact, been taken into consideration was something which varied greatly, despite Ministerial assertions to the contrary.[56] This issue is discussed at much greater length by Bridgen and Lewis (1999: 51–69): briefly, they argue that the tight revenue envelope, in which the Plan was to be implemented, required circumscribing the scope of the hospital service, by attempting to shift elderly people out of hospital beds and into nursing or residential facilities. However, policy was predicated on assumptions which appeared likely to be (and were in fact) invalidated by an ageing (and more dependent) population. Assumptions were also made about the extent to which local authorities would in practice develop complementary services for the elderly. Greater flexibility in the use of central government grants meant that the Ministry could not guarantee that complementary services for the elderly would be made available. The Plan was consequently an attempt to shift costs from the taxpayer to the ratepayer.[57] As a result of such weaknesses the Plan was a one-dimensional approach to solving the NHS's problems, and officials felt that 'the only part that can be clearly seen is the list of hospital projects'.[58]

The notion that the Plan represented a comprehensive and national blueprint is also suspect. The Plan itself was in effect an aggregation of the individual intentions of RHBs and, to some extent, the HMCs within them, so some variability was inevitable. One reason for this was the different technical abilities and capacities of Boards, some of which submitted 'plans' to which relatively little thought had been given. Russell-Smith thus commented that the building programmes, 'instead of being founded on calculation, reason, logic and mathematical projection ... rest on no ascertained facts whatever', though she also commented on how effectively Powell set about dealing with the variations in the quality of the proposals.[59] Officials were highly critical: one submission was described as 'a list of schemes and their cost, without argument' (E Anglia);[60] of another it was said that 'it is difficult to get a comprehensive picture and one has to discover the "philosophy" in what is said about the various hospitals' (Sheffield)[61] while the SE Metropolitan Board were criticised because 'at the end one will know what the Board wants to do in the next ten years, but will not have much idea of the picture aimed at'. Some more direct criticisms were made of one submission which was a 'depressing document ... put together in a very perfunctory fashion. There is little evidence of a policy and no suggestion of big thinking ... a study of individual hospitals with little view of a wider field'.[61] Thinking back to Fox's (1986) arguments about the hierarchical integration of services, this is not strong evidence to support a claim that regionalism was being implemented. The irony, of course, is that similar comments were made about the Ministry by the Treasury (see above), questioning the Ministry's tendency to think solely in terms of additions to capital.

Moreover, there was a number of *ad hoc* interventions (sometimes quite obvious porkbarrelling) as the Plan was scaled down to the funding levels deemed acceptable to the Government. The programmes submitted by the RHBs had substantially exceeded the funds likely to be made available. Initial bids from the RHBs amounted to over £700 million (Table 6.2) but for comparative purposes Ministry officials seem to have been working to an estimated total expenditure of £1 per annum per head of population over ten years; they compared the cost of submissions with this figure, which would have given a programme worth, in total, some £440 million. As can be seen, some RHBs had put in requests for sums considerably greater than this notional figure – in some cases double it, such as Birmingham. RHBs' programmes were reduced in size by a process of attrition during 1961, in which civil servants pressed Boards to prioritise their most urgent schemes. This process was originally described by Powell, addressing RHB Chairmen, as 'pulling out the concertina' of the Plan.[62] Drafts of the Plan indicate that almost all the original intentions of the Boards were to be achieved but much of this was through the expedient of indicating, in the published Plan, that numerous schemes would have to be started after the completion of the ten-year programme. Comparisons of what Boards requested with what the Plan actually proposed shows that some were cut back substantially, by up to one-third in some cases, while others – notably Liverpool and Newcastle – received more than they had requested initially (in fact, because column C does *not* include figures from the Boards of Governors, but column E does, the changes affecting some Boards are even greater). The effect of Ministry negotiations with Boards was to produce per capita allocations which were generally consistent, with the exceptions of Wessex and Oxford, reflecting anticipated population growth, and Liverpool. The substantial expenditure here was designed to help reduce bed provision from 5.6 beds/1,000 to 3.5, a task which 'came as a shock and was seen as a threat' (Forsyth *et al.* 1970: 21). It also reflected the low quality of Liverpool RHB's inheritance: the region did not have 'a single first class hospital'.[63] There were several frantic months' work involved in the process of scaling down RHB plans, and amendments were being made right up to the last minute. Thus, as the Plan was about to go to press, a note indicated that the Minister felt that the Newcastle RHB should receive additional funds, so as to avoid giving the impression that, by comparison with other regions, it had been 'relatively badly treated'.[64] The gap between the notional £1 per head per annum figure and the publicised commitment of the Plan was some £45 million, and this presumably gave scope for such last-minute adjustments. However the more general point would appear to be that in planning to such politically inspired figures, the government were somewhat undermining claims as to the rationality and equity of the Plan. As a result it is not surprising that one official suggested to a colleague (who was being sent the proofs of the Plan) that 'you may find the most useful sign in the instructions for proof correction is the one for inserting an exclamation mark'.[65]

Table 6.2 RHB submissions to Hospital Plan and actual allocations to RHBs

Board	A Estimated 1971 population	B Cost of RHB's proposed 10-year plan	C Column B Per head p.a.	D Provision in RHB submissions over and above £1 per head over 10 years	E Total capital allocation	F Investment per head of 1975 population[a]
	000s	£000s	£	£000s	£000s	£
Newcastle	3,190	40,335	1.26	8,435	43,000	13.3
Leeds	3,150	48,513	1.54	17,013	41,900	13.1
Sheffield	4,288	67,504	1.57	24,622	63,000	13.3
East Anglia	1,678	33,486	1.99	16,706	22,000	13.3
NW Metropolitan	4,200	62,943	1.49	20,943}		
NE Metropolitan	3,375	55,140	1.63	21,380}	199,700	16.3
SE Metropolitan	3,376	30,954	0.92	- 2,813}		
SW Metropolitan	3,241	60,422	1.86	28,011}		
Oxford	1,831	34,656	1.89	16,342	31,200	16.3
South Western	2,977	51,436	1.73	21,666	42,500	14.2
Birmingham	4,800	98,085	2.04	50,085	75,000	14.5
Manchester	4,497	51,762	1.15	6,792	60,200	13.3
Liverpool	2,332	32,722	1.40	9,402	50,500	21.2
Wessex	1,920	36,882	1.92	17,682	31,700	16.3
England	44,855	704,843	1.60	256,266	660,700	15.0

Sources: MH 88/262; Ministry of Health 1962: 274, 277.

Note: a These figures take account of expenditure to be incurred beyond the first decade of the Plan.

For a Conservative government, the Plan was also somewhat at variance with party ideology, in that it opposed standardisation, centralisation and bureaucracy to localism, decentralisation and voluntary effort. One reason for this was the perceived need to restrain costs. Reflecting Treasury concerns evident in exchanges with the Ministry during the 1950s, the Financial Secretary to the Treasury, Henry Brooke, indicated that standardisation was essential in the interests of economy; there should be 'a pervasive awareness throughout the hospital service that *value for money in this big plan means standard provision at standard cost. I am sure that we are all agreed on this*'.[66] For this reason some commentators have pointed to parallels between developments in the hospital sector and the supposed era of 'Fordism', associated with mass production, standardisation and economies of scale (e.g. Murray 1991; Manson 1979). However, this parallel is too easily and simplistically drawn. Certainly, at the time the Plan was launched, standardisation had not proceeded very far, though the Ministry had begun to use its Hospital Building Notes to secure some consistency of practice, but standardisation and industrialised building of whole hospitals took much longer to become established (chapters 7, 8).

A related issue concerned the political costs of the many hospital closures implied by the Plan. Powell's credentials as a planner were not immediately apparent (see the biographies by Heffer (1998) and Shepherd (1997)) and an obvious problem was the tension between the rationalising imperatives of planning, and the attachments of local communities to 'their' hospitals. Powell attempted to ride both horses simultaneously, on occasions strongly defending the Plan while on others praising the virtues of community support and informal sources of care. Thus, at around the time as he was involved in preparing the Plan, Powell was conducting a series of meetings with voluntary organisations about the role of voluntary effort in the NHS.[67] His defence of the Plan nevertheless emphasised the virtues of modernist rationality; for example, a note from the Welsh Board of Health in 1961 quoted his description of the Plan as 'ruthlessly breaking with habit and tradition where they conflict with reason and common sense',[68] while he regarded the elimination of GP cottage hospitals, with a few exceptions, as a 'touchstone' for a preliminary critique of RHB proposals.[69] This robust approach was not shared by all of the Cabinet; at the Home Affairs Committee, misgivings were expressed about 'indicating in detail the hundreds of hospitals which would probably be closed under the Plan. Many of these hospitals had been maintained in the past by local donations, and attracted a large amount of voluntary effort'.[70] This tension was not satisfactorily resolved before the publication of the Plan and continued to dog the footsteps of Ministers subsequently.

The secrecy and speed surrounding the preparation of the Plan had not helped RHB Chairmen, one of whom stated that he could be 'charged with having misled some of our HMCs to whom I have given no warning that many of the units now slated for closure were to be so treated'.[71]

Demonstrating a sensitivity to this, Powell indicated his willingness to handle the political controversies of hospital closures himself, arguing that one had to be able to manage the minuses as well as the pluses of the programme. He even suggested that he could 'close hospitals symbolically' to demonstrate Ministerial commitment to modernisation and 'capture [the] public imagination'.[72] The apparent lack of flexibility in the proposed pattern of hospitals also exercised RHB Chairmen.[73] At the same time, however, Ministry officials emphasised their disquiet about the apparent slowness with which redundant hospitals were to be closed.[74] The government attempted to soften the blow by emphasising rationality and efficiency in presenting the Plan, using the word 'modern' six times in the first page-and-a-half (Fox 1986: 185), but hospital closures continued to attract criticism from their core supporters (Chapter 7).

A number of criticisms can therefore be levelled against the assumptions, coherence and rationality of the Plan. Some certainly were a function of the state of knowledge at the time, for example with respect to bed norms. Others were perhaps excusable given the speed with which the Plan had been assembled. The weaknesses and criticisms reviewed here suggest that the rhetorical claims made for the Plan were somewhat exaggerated. Weeks before publication, the Plan was described as 'nebulous' and some of its assumptions as 'guff' by Treasury officials.[75]

Concluding comments

Previous interpretations of the Plan have pointed to the influence of key individuals on it, in the context of a wider transformation of the governmental machinery for long-term planning. To what extent are these borne out by the evidence given here?

In terms of giving credit to individuals, the notion of a long-term plan had been put forward by Powell's predecessor, and the arrival of Fraser at the Ministry was perhaps crucial, in terms of overcoming Treasury resistance. However one contemporary witness compliments the way Powell picked up the gauntlet and saw the Plan through; it is also clear that Powell was willing to be associated with difficult political consequences, such as hospital closures.[76] Even Kenneth Robinson, Labour's health spokesman, subsequently gave Powell credit for extracting commitments from the Treasury (Timmins 1995: 210). The irony here, of course, is Powell's association with an initiative of this kind, given his distaste for large-scale bureaucracy. Heffer (1998: 274) records a speech in which Powell argued that 'the great machine … is bound to be cumbrous and unresponsive [and] to abhor variations'. Yet one could argue that the process of cutting RHB submissions down to size was just such a mechanical and bureaucratic exercise, which gave RHBs hardly any scope to argue for variations in planned hospital provision.

Second, as far as Plowden and long-term planning is concerned, the Plan finally marked the acceptance of a long-term programme of capital development for the NHS: there was – eventually – a decisive upward shift in capital expenditure and commitment was given to a long-term programme, though, as pointed out, there was a rearguard action on the scale of it, which constrained what RHBs were able to accomplish. However, the emphasis in this chapter suggests that the Plan rested on somewhat insecure foundations. A number of important questions were unresolved at publication and this clearly remained the case. The Ministry was heavily criticised for the absence of strategic vision and in their turn Ministry officials criticised local agencies. What is evident here is a failure to modernise the technical apparatus of the Ministry and the RHBs, to enable it to deal with the complex tasks inherent in the Plan. Long-term planning had thus only partially percolated into the Ministry and the NHS: there had been efforts to improve the level of expertise but they had not got very far. Whether a more dirigiste state apparatus, with stronger strategic capacities, would have done a better job, is an open (and somewhat counterfactual) question.

Hence there were technical weaknesses in the Plan. Thus Fraser acknowledged that the Ministry was 'proceeding on a mixture of caution and faith and determination', while Russell-Smith observed that 'we are making it up as we go along'.[77] Although no one, surely, would suggest that hospital building should have been delayed until better information was available, this contributes to a revised assessment of the Plan's coherence. It was also an essentially political device: though there was Conservative opposition from people dismayed at the potential loss of their local hospitals, it was also helpful as a symbol of Conservative commitment to the welfare state. But it arguably had further, unanticipated consequences. First, because of its high profile it became a lodestone of commitment to welfare. This meant that hospitals continued to attract a disproportionate share of resources. In effect it defined the nature of hospital care – centralised, remote, professionalised – and precluded alternatives (Manson 1979: 42). Second, perhaps because of the underlying weaknesses and unresolved issues, as well as its long-term nature, it was a candidate for cuts and postponements: its frustration potential was enormous.

It may appear unfair to impose – even if implicitly – a utopian and *post hoc* definition of rationality on the whole exercise, and given the state of existing knowledge, and the short timescale, it could be argued that those involved did the best they could. But if that is the case, it could equally be argued that less grandiose claims ought to have been made for the Plan. In this sense (borrowing Lowe's (1997) verdict on the Plowden Report) the Plan was both a milestone and a millstone: a feather in the government's cap, but one which effectively constrained debate about health policy as the scale of the building programme became a political virility symbol.

There are some interesting comparisons with later initiatives. The 1991 reforms and the Plan had in common a limited evidence base. Both made assertions that greater efficiency would follow from their proposals without strong evidence one way or another. The misgivings of officials in 1962 were echoed, nearly three decades on, by widespread public and professional concern. Although there was some force in these misgivings, at least the Plan's outcomes were largely predictable and visible. That could not be said of the 1991 reforms, which soon led to a destabilisation of the hospital service in some localities, requiring a return to planning. A further point is that to the extent that the Plan was actually implemented, it reduced the scope for competition after 1991, albeit not to the extent originally intended. The other similarity is with Labour's recent NHS Plan, which is really a statement about increasing the rate of growth in resources committed to the NHS, but without strong underlying philosophical foundations. In both cases, the resources were welcome, but there were criticisms of what the policy might mean for the character of the NHS. The good intentions of the Plan were welcomed by Kenneth Robinson, Labour's health spokesman, but Dickson Mabon's characterisation of the Plan's 'combination of pious hopes and unwarranted assertions'[78] proved prophetic in the light of subsequent events.

The submission made by the Newcastle RHB to the Hospital Plan demonstrates well the extent to which a broad regional strategy had been agreed, but it also shows how far the region still had to go in modernising its hospital stock.[79] In the absence of capital allocations large enough to permit substantial new development, the Board had given priority to operating theatres, outpatient and casualty departments, laboratories and x-ray departments. However the most that could be said was that a satisfactory makeshift service was in operation. In no single area was the service 'anything like adequate. Many glaring deficiencies exist'. Even the sums anticipated following the Plan would not eradicate these deficiencies. Thus, the submission to the Plan still spoke of giving 'first priority ... to what is still lacking in so many hospitals – the diagnostic services'. This would pay the highest dividends in achieving a better turnover and greater efficiency, and of course reflected the Board's experience from 1948. Qualitative deficiencies were emphasised repeatedly: 'lower priority has been given to the provision of additional (as distinct from new) beds, because the bed provision is in many cases either adequate or nearly so'. But many existing hospitals would have to continue in their present use 'for the greater part of the next twenty years, before major schemes for their reprovision can be completed'. This would imply a considerably longer timespan than envisaged by the published Plan. It would also necessitate further investment in hospitals which were ultimately to be abandoned. Comments on the Board's preferred order of priorities are generally missing from the submission with the exception of the priority to be given to redeveloping Ashington Hospital, in the 'outstandingly underbedded' Wansbeck HMC, which the Board wished to be treated as a 'continuous exercise'. However, even though Wansbeck HMC was 'underbedded', the Board did not argue the case for including a new hospital in the area in its ten-year programme. Instead it argued that a 'higher priority should be given' to developments in

Newcastle.[80] Otherwise the aim was to spread the incidence of expenditure broadly through the ten-year period. It was assumed that phased projects would be carried out in a way which minimised the intervals between phases. It was also 'assumed throughout that local authorities will have made very substantial improvements' in non-hospital medical and social services, but there was not an attempt to quantify the scale of improvement planned, or required. There were obvious hostages to fortune here. Thirteen years after the foundation of the NHS, the Board was only just beginning to make inroads into its inadequate legacy of hospital services. How far it was able to do so is the subject of the remaining chapters.

7 From 'Plan' to 'Programme', 1962–73

In relation to the history of hospital development in Britain, the Plan could be viewed as marking both the high point of regionalism, centralised development and modernism. It could also be viewed as marking the beginning of the end for all of them. Initially, the period reviewed in this chapter was characterised by considerable faith in state intervention, planning and expertise. Combined in the case of hospital provision, the result would be a network of DGHs which would make high-quality medical services available to all. This optimistic vision came to be tarnished in several ways. The Plan's financial assumptions were partly invalidated by changed economic circumstances, and there were concerns that the associated revenue implications of new hospital development had not been thought through. It was an exercise in modernisation which had to rely for implementation on a construction industry which struggled to cope with the task. The Plan represented an attempt to reform the welfare state through capital investment in labour- and energy-saving technology, and to impose some principles of standardisation on service provision. In this sense the Plan symbolised the triumph of optimism about the capacity of technology to achieve such objectives, but its implementation indicated the limits to such solutions. The top-down nature of the Plan, and the speed of its preparation, almost guaranteed major implementation problems as sites proved unavailable or as local alliances of politicians and professionals threatened major amendments or to derail the plan altogether. As if this were not enough, the period was characterised by growing evidence of dissatisfaction with planning, resulting in opposition to centralised development and resistance to closure of small hospitals.

The general objectives were a redistribution of the capital stock between regions, and substantial rationalisation and concentration of services within them. Table 7.1 shows the variations that existed in availability of acute facilities in 1960 and indicates that a degree of convergence in bed:population ratios was anticipated by 1975. Considerable variation in development was envisaged, both to rationalise the existing capital stock (e.g. in the Liverpool RHB) and provide for the influxes of population anticipated in certain areas (e.g. in the Oxford and Wessex RHBs). The Newcastle RHB was slightly

over-provided with beds relative to many regions, and the anticipated investment in it was comparable with most other RHBs. The main planning
problems identified *within* the region concerned not so much an overall *deficiency* in bed numbers but rather that hospitals were inconveniently located
and composed of old or unsuitable buildings. Looking at the age distribution
of hospital accommodation within the region over half the hospitals dated
from the nineteenth century and these were to be replaced with a small
number of DGHs providing a full range of specialist services (Ministry of
Health 1962a: 17). Most of the smaller facilities would ultimately close, thus
increasing the average size of hospitals within the RHB from 107.2 beds to
156.6 beds (Table 7.2); likewise, forty-six of the seventy-two hospitals built
before 1900 were ultimately to be closed.

The reception of the Plan, inside and outside Parliament, highlighted
themes which were to recur. As well as perhaps predictable Opposition criticisms of the government for doing too little too late, the Plan was also
criticised for having been scaled down in the first place. The regional submissions implied a programme worth around £800 million over ten years,
compared to £500 million as announced, and even that was not a firm
commitment. Parliamentary critics also reminded the House that the Plan
was effectively being financed out of the receipts from raised prescription
charges. While the Plan was welcome news in many areas, a London MP
anticipated some 1980s debates, expressing concerns that 'some of our
teaching hospitals might be displaced from world leadership', and saying

Table 7.1 Actual/intended distribution of acute beds by region

RHB	Acute beds		Beds/1,000 population	
	Available in 1960	Proposed (1975)	Available in 1960	Proposed (1975)
Newcastle	11,475	10,770	3.8	3.4
Leeds	11,836	10,860	3.8	3.4
Sheffield	13,501	14,160	3.1	3.0
East Anglia	4,581	4,960	3.0	2.9
Metropolitan RHBs	58,529	53,340	4.2	3.6
Wessex	5,926	6,450	3.6	3.3
Oxford	5,336	6,410	3.3	3.3
South Western	10,627	9,930	3.7	3.3
Birmingham	15,671	16,130	3.3	3.1
Manchester	15,908	15,580	3.6	3.4
Liverpool	12,388	8,590	5.6	3.5
Wales	11,623	9,310	4.5	3.5
England and Wales	179,456	168,550[a]	3.9	3.4

Source: Ministry of Health 1962a: 274, 277.

a This figure includes 2,055 beds in London's Teaching Hospitals used by patients from
outside the Metropolitan regions; these beds were not included in the regional figures.

Table 7.2 Size distribution of hospitals in Newcastle RHB

Size (no. of beds)	At 31.12.60	Proposals for 1975	Long-term proposals[a]
<50	79	36	8
51–100	28	23	6
101–250	33	16	12
251–500	16	12	9
501–1,000	4	8	11
>1,000	–	3	3
Total	160	98	49

Source: Ministry of Health (1962a).

a These are strictly accurate only for the lower size ranges; in the two largest classes the precise   figures for the distribution of beds between hospitals were not always given.

that 'if some hospitals are not treated more equally than others, we shall not get the pace-setters we ought to have'.[1]

Medical critics raised two other points. One pointed out that the Plan's proposals had 'started as braver and more ambitious projects' and had already been watered down; 'few people realise how little this will achieve'.[2] Various doctors working in small cottage hospitals argued against the 'enormity of this ruthless plan', which was removing local hospitals by edict of a 'central planning committee'.[3] A BMJ editorial continued this theme, suggesting that 'anything tailor-made in Savile Row [where the Ministry was then located] will not necessarily be a good fit for the men on the spot in the hospital regions'.[4]

A more fundamental point was raised regarding the technical basis of the Plan, because the studies of 'need' for hospital care on which it had relied were regarded as unsystematic (Chapter 6). Labour's Health spokesman, Kenneth Robinson, duly attacked the limited scientific basis of the Plan:

> The Minister sticks in his thumb and pulls out a figure marked 3.3 [beds per 1,000 population] and that is to be taken as the normal requirement for acute beds. The present figure is 3.9 – very much larger. It may well be that the need for acute beds can be met by a much smaller figure but *surely such a vital figure, on which the whole ten-year programme is based, should be the result of something more than guesswork?*[5]

Other criticisms were raised concerning the accuracy of the norms used for planning geriatric and maternity services, the lack of integration with local authority services, and the speed with which the whole exercise had been carried out. *The Times* also questioned the central 'paradox' of the Plan – the assertion that capital investment would assist in the containment of revenue expenditure: Powell might be unable to have his cake and eat it.[6]

These technical weaknesses and unresolved questions perhaps made it harder to defend the Plan against retrenchment.

A discussion of the Plan's implementation is used here to illuminate several themes. These include: the rationality and coherence of this exercise in 'planning'; the extent to which it did indeed signify a victory for the virtues of modernism and of Fordist principles of organisation; the constraints on state intervention which influenced both the resources available for, and the on-the-ground implementation of, the Plan; and the extent to which subsequent representations of this era, as one of lumbering, hierarchical bureaucracy, are valid.

Four key issues are considered in this chapter. First, there is consideration of the impacts of national public expenditure policy decisions on the implementation of the Plan, including the tight revenue 'straitjacket' agreed by Powell. Second, developments in policy on hospital size, construction and location are noted. Third, the bulk of the chapter is taken up with examination of the development of a hospital strategy within the Newcastle RHB. This is followed by a discussion of the social consequences of implementing a hospital policy which came to place greater emphasis on spatial concentration of acute hospital services.

Public expenditure policies and the building programme

Two interrelated issues are considered: the scale of the capital resources committed to hospital building, and the question of the likely revenue consequences of hospital investment.

Progress with the building programme

Because of capacity constraints in the economy, the real-terms cost of hospital building soon began to rise steadily; this was linked to the small number of contractors bidding for hospital work and the 'relatively "easy" climate from the point of view of the contractor'.[7] By December 1962 the Treasury was resisting proposals for an expansion of the programme; grant 'substantial increases ... [would] be embarrassing *vis-à-vis* other departments'.[8] Kenneth Robinson claimed that the government's statements, that expenditure was nevertheless rising, were 'misleading to the point of dishonesty'. He pointed out that the NHS capital programme compared unfavourably with the road programme, which was experiencing double the rate of growth of hospital investment.[9] He believed that the Ministry had 'no idea' what it cost to build a hospital, and contended that a realistic Plan would cost 'very nearly double' the original sums announced. Significantly Anthony Barber, the Health Minister, did not refute these figures, instead confining himself to rhetorical questions about what Labour would spend.[10] Revisions to the Plan in 1963 and 1964 (Ministry of Health 1963, 1964) avoided mentioning in detail the implications of rising costs for deferments of schemes, but it was becoming evident that some projects scheduled for the ten-year programme were unlikely to be completed within fifteen years. These revisions were also much less specific, omitting references to detailed schemes in the second and third quinquennia of the Plan. Yet the process of investment was raising expectations as the existence of new hospitals led to dissatisfaction with the second-rate.[11]

Labour returned to office in 1964, having made manifesto commitments to double the amount spent on new hospital building; this was notwithstanding a comment, attributed to Jim Callaghan (as Shadow Chancellor), that the Conservatives' building programme 'could not be exceeded by any party with a degree of responsibility'.[12] The relationship between public expenditure and the growth of the economy had become an issue of concern within six weeks of the return of Labour to power. The Conservatives had announced substantial increases in public expenditure programmes, which Labour could not reduce drastically for fear of losing electoral support; on the other hand the government could not restore foreign confidence in the pound without such cuts (Crossman 1976: vol. I, 80, 82–4; Brittan 1969: 171–6). Initial attempts by Robinson, the new Minister of Health, to obtain additional resources were therefore rebuffed, despite clear warnings from RHB Chairmen that the Plan's aims were now 'completely unrealistic',[13] as well as growing dissatisfaction from the medical profession.[14] Robinson subsequently argued, to Cabinet, that the original Plan had been seen, by the public and the hospital authorities, as a 'plan for the erection of specific named hospital projects'. These were now threatened by rising costs and if more resources were not committed, the 'impression created will be one of deliberate cuts and "stop-go"' and this could not be blamed on the Conservatives. On the other hand, the Chief Secretary to the Treasury argued, *ad hoc* expansion of individual programmes would 'cast doubt on the efficacy of the Government's forward planning ... [the] consequences of overloading the economy were far more serious than the political embarrassment of appearing to delay hospital projects'. This view was endorsed by Cabinet;[15] Labour's credibility and competence in economic management were at stake. In subsequent internal discussions with officials, Robinson emphasised that the published version of the revisions ought not to be made easily comparable with the 1962 Plan, and it was agreed that the information released would be deliberately non-specific so as to avoid being held to commitments.[16] He later explained to the Prime Minister that 'I believe my proposals, unlike the original plan, to be realistic'. While involving broadly the same number of new hospitals as the 1962 Plan, rather fewer reconstructions were envisaged.[17] The published revision – entitled, not without significance, the 'Hospital Building Programme' – claimed that its initial aims had been over-optimistic and that many of the proposals were 'inadequately defined and imprecisely costed' (which was hardly surprising given the speed with which the Plan had been assembled); consequently it was necessary to 'bring greater realism to hospital planning' and 'get the best possible value for the resources provided' (Ministry of Health 1966: 1, 10). Stricter financial control was an explicit aim: the programme of developments was stated in terms of available finance rather than as a list of approved physical development schemes. Hence adjustments to the estimated cost of schemes would have to be made within the total sum approved for hospital development, and Boards would not be able to allow for the effect of delays on their programmes.[18] Thus, if a major development project was delayed, for whatever reason, the capital programme for subsequent years would not be expanded to allow for this. The overall effect of the 1966 revision was a slight slackening in the rate of growth of NHS capital expenditure (Figure A1).

The building programme was spared in the 1966 round of public expenditure cuts. It also survived the 1967 devaluation crisis, thanks to a Prime Ministerial undertaking, given in a television broadcast, though prescription charges were reintroduced as part of the *quid pro quo* for the latter decision. Nevertheless this did not prevent the BMA repeatedly criticising the government for failing to modernise the hospital infrastructure. The 1964 Annual Representative Meeting (*ARM*) pointed out that when they had accepted the recommendations of Abel and Lewin's (1959) report on hospital building, they 'had not intended that they should come into effect long after the representatives were dead'.[19] There were similar comments at the 1965 and 1966 *ARMs*; far from being feasible in ten years, the plan could nowhere be completed 'in the working lifetime of any doctor now in hospital service'.[20] It was suggested that other countries (Sweden, Israel) were devoting ten times as much of fixed capital formation to hospital development, figures later challenged by the Ministry (Sweden's hospital building programme, comparatively, was merely double that of the UK).[21] The 1966 *ARM* deplored the 'continued failure' to implement the Plan.[22] A particularly memorable and outspoken attack came from a prominent North-Eastern doctor, Henry Miller, a neurologist and Dean of Medicine at Newcastle University. He contrasted the 'extraordinary sense of priorities' that tolerated the 'public squalor' of London's teaching hospitals, in a 'city rendered almost unrecognisable by an orgy of commercial building'. He went on to deplore the 'outlay of astronomical sums' on defence commitments from 'Berlin to Borneo'. In his own region, one district would have to 'put up with its present antediluvian facilities until 1997' (Miller 1967: 11) – a comment which actually proved optimistic. The continued economic difficulties faced by the government kept major public expenditure programmes on the Cabinet agenda, as the government sought to raise the level of productive investment and restore competitiveness. The trade-off between hospital and prescription charges and the capital programme was once again a major issue. Kenneth Robinson had been succeeded by Richard Crossman, who became Secretary of State for Social Services upon the formation of the DHSS in 1968. Crossman's Diaries record a protracted and heated argument during 1969 concerning proposed cuts of some £39 million in DHSS expenditure. Reflecting concern about rising NHS expenditure, the

Chancellor (Roy Jenkins) expressed his 'disappointment that we [i.e. DHSS ministers] couldn't make any positive proposals for squeezing hospital revenue'. Crossman responded that revenue savings from 'closing down the little hospitals' were outweighed by the 'enormous expense' of running the new ones. Jenkins consequently called for a halt in new hospital construction. Crossman resisted, arguing that Jenkins' demands would require a twelve-month halt in new starts, which would be politically unacceptable: a six-month moratorium would be 'seriously damaging and would produce all sorts of anomalies', while a three-month delay was just about manageable.

There were two key issues in subsequent discussions. First, as the government had introduced prescription charges in order to protect hospital construction, any cuts or postponements 'would put us in an appalling fix' (Crossman 1976: vol. III, 556), since the scars of the 1951 Cabinet resignations over prescription charges had hardly healed. Second, a public announcement of the cuts or postponements would be essential, because the government would have to absolve RHBs from blame. Having agreed that the political costs of even a six-month delay could not be contemplated the issue amounted to a gap of £4 million, between what Jenkins wanted (£9 million; a three-month delay) and what Crossman believed could be saved in the absence of a public announcement. Crossman felt that:

> *It was absolutely demented* to be squabbling about £4 million from the Ministry out of a £17,000 million total. We had already had prescription charges and teeth and spectacles, and now the Chancellor wanted an announcement that we were cutting the hospital building programme as well, just for the sake of £4 million. (Crossman 1976: vol. III, 600)

Although the Cabinet eventually sided with Crossman, he clearly regarded this as a pyrrhic victory, because the Cabinet 'had all known that electorally the Chancellor couldn't cut the hospital building programme'. Hospital building expanded under Labour, then, but they never achieved the acceleration of the rate of growth in investment that had been promised in their manifesto (Figure A1). On taking office at the DHSS following the 1970 election, Keith Joseph sought an expansion of hospital building (Webster 1996: 383). The Heath government subsequently adopted an expansionary programme, ensuring that hospital capital expenditure continued to grow until brought to a sudden halt in late 1973, with expenditure cuts imposed in response to the hike in oil prices. However, this does not mean that all building work proceeded as planned because it became clear in this period that, for a variety of reasons, health authorities experienced difficulties in containing costs. Notwithstanding this expansion, by 1973 the NHS's share of fixed capital formation was still barely 2 per cent of the total for Great Britain as a whole; the proportion of new building was higher, at 3 per cent. Although NHS capital expenditure at constant prices was four times as great as in 1962, the NHS was still only slowly renewing its asset base. Assuming a sixty-year lifetime for hospital buildings, a figure endorsed in a 1967 paper,[23] around 1.66 per cent of hospital capacity would need replacing each year. Bed numbers are an imperfect index, but are used here to provide a broad-brush comparison. Not until 1967 did the number of new beds provided equate to 1 per cent of the total in a single year, and the figure only passed 1.66 per cent in 1971–2.[24]

Revenue consequences of capital investment

The exchange between Crossman and Jenkins underlines the persistent debate about the relationship between capital and revenue expenditure. Powell had publicly argued that substantial revenue savings would accrue from capital investment. He had, of course, agreed with the Treasury that revenue growth in the hospital service would be held at 2 per cent per annum. However, it was not entirely clear that the requisite savings could be made in practice. This can be exemplified with reference to some HMCs from the Newcastle region.

In the South East Northumberland HMC, for instance, the closure of five small hospitals would, on their 1961 budgets, have generated savings of £169,000, or 21 per cent of the HMC's revenue budget. However, the RHB proposed a new ninety-bed maternity unit to improve on and expand the closed services, a new A and E department and a fifty-bed orthopaedic unit, and a new outpatient unit. It was also intended to see major redevelopment of the main general hospital in the HMC. The likely revenue implications can be estimated from the RHB's summary of hospital accounts. Assuming levels of occupancy, inpatient costs, and lengths of stay at around the regional average, it can be estimated that the cost of the new maternity unit and outpatient department alone would have wiped out the revenue savings.[25] The casualty unit and outpatient department, and any other developments, would have had to have been resourced out of 2 per cent revenue growth. Another example, from Newcastle, casts further doubt on the validity of the assumptions made. The HMC's proposals entailed closure of six peripheral hospitals which would have saved approximately 10 per cent of the revenue budget, but a number of new schemes were proposed, including doubling the size of one general hospital from 320 to 650 beds, and how this was to be reconciled with Powell's revenue straitjacket – indeed whether it *could* be – was not at all clear.

These revenue constraints (see Webster 1996: 89–91) soon had visible effects on the hospital stock. A typical response by HMCs was that maintenance expenditure was being 'bled white', but the NHS would pay 'compound interest' for this, because deferred expenditure would cost 'far more at the ultimate reckoning'.[26] The Ministry therefore, risked 'very silly spending' on unsatisfactory accommodation, and pressed for some relaxation of revenue constraints, without success.[27] The Treasury response was its usual condemnation of the Ministry's failure to resolve the relationship between capital and revenue. As in the 1950s this issue rumbled on, without resolution. The Treasury suggested that the Department needed to stop claiming that the building programme carried an 'inescapable' increase in running costs. An official castigated the Ministry for failing to 'get a grip' on the relationship between hospital openings and rationalisation, and 'the sums which *can be expected to be made available*' for revenue costs.[28] The political commitment to the building programme was therefore circumscribed by prior assumptions about revenue. Among other things this led to pressures to accelerate hospital closures. But the attitude nevertheless appears to have been a reluctance to endorse the increased expenditure resulting from the improved quality or increased quantity of service permitted by new hospitals.

Policy on hospital size, design and location

In parallel with – and indeed partly stimulated by – debates about the capital investment programme, this period saw innovations in policy. These involved a reconsideration of the nature of the DGH concept, proposals for greater standardisation in hospital design and construction, and initial formulations of the community hospital concept.

The notion of a DGH was not contested in either the 1962 Plan or in subsequent revisions and so a professional definition of the nature and organisation of health care was accepted, almost by default. A subcommittee of the Central Health Services Council was charged with reviewing the DGH concept. Its report (CHSC 1969 – more generally known as the Bonham-Carter Report, after the Chair of the Committee) concentrated on the more economical and efficient use of medical manpower and reaping the benefits of scale economies in hospital construction. The report argued that DGHs 'should be planned around teams of not less than two consultants in each speciality, with all their inpatients at the DGH' (CHSC 1969). This partly reflected concern as to the future number of consultants likely to be available for the hospital service; the report had assumed that there were unlikely to be large increases in the number of such personnel and therefore their efficient use was imperative.

The report caused considerable concern. Concentration of hospital facilities into units of 1,200–1,800 beds followed logically from the report's contention that at least two consultants in each speciality should be available, but the social implications of such developments caused some alarm. The report had support within medical circles,[29] but the response of the DHSS and of the RHBs was less than enthusiastic. The implications for accessibility, and for the management of the capital programme, both attracted attention. There is some evidence that, while the Committee was deliberating, the Ministry sought to persuade it of the error of its ways, without success. The Committee concluded that smaller DGHs could not sustain the required level of expertise. One official saw this as a victory for

McKeown's (1958) idea of a 'balanced hospital community': McKeown, he said, had 'carried all before him' in the Committee discussions.[30] But there were still concerns that a capital programme made up of large projects lacked flexibility, which was necessary to cope with changes in economic circumstances or in attitudes to patient care. One official put it bluntly:

> We have already made a frightening investment in our own infallibility in the teaching hospital programme (... saddling the country ... with physical appurtenances to medical education ...) and if the same mega-lomania informs the DGH programme we could end up looking pretty ridiculous in the eyes of our successors.[31]

It was 'practically and politically impossible' to spend large sums on a limited number of projects while other places had to wait for many years. Patients might eventually become accustomed to lengthier journeys but it was not possible to hasten the process. Official views also echoed the need for flexibility in managing the capital programme and expressed reservations about the impacts on access.[32] Consequently, the Secretary of State's intro-duction to the report argued for flexibility, speaking of the needs of patients requiring long-term care and of the future role of peripheral hospitals (CHSC 1969: iv; see also Crossman 1972). Within the Newcastle RHB, the response was that developments in Newcastle, Sunderland and Teesside could be planned on the assumption that only two DGHs would now be necessary in each centre, rather than three as previously proposed. The populations of other HMCs (Gateshead, Darlington, SE Northumberland, South Shields, Hartlepool and North Teesside) were large enough to permit the planning of hospitals to serve around 200,000 people. There remained the problem of the smaller HMCs. Both the Cumbrian HMCs would require DGHs because of their remoteness, but Wansbeck, Durham and the periph-eral HMCs would have to rely heavily upon adjacent areas. Thus acute hospital services for Wansbeck would be provided from the DGH to be developed in SE Northumberland HMC. Finally, while it had never been the RHB's intention to provide full-scale general hospitals in the Alnwick and Berwick HMCs, their proposals for 'peripheral' hospitals in Northallerton and Hexham caused some concern.[33] The effects of the Bonham-Carter Report on planning were therefore felt most severely in the peripheral HMCs; the consequences in urban areas were rather less serious.[34]

While Bonham-Carter 'undoubtedly influenced in an upward direction the size of hospitals planned at the time' (DHSS 1979: 11), its recommenda-tions were never formally adopted by the DHSS. Indeed, by late 1969 there were indications of greater emphasis on retention of physical assets. The building of 'new "glass palace" hospitals was no longer all-important' and the DHSS were thinking of scaling down the size of DGHs and of retaining more hospitals to provide longer-term care.[35] Later pronouncements on hospital policy favoured a maximum size range of 1,100 beds, a conclusion supported by a DHSS study which claimed that a size range of 540–900 beds was one in which hospitals functioned most efficiently (DHSS 1972).

A second important issue, in the context of debates about long-term changes in the character of the welfare state, was the question of standardisation. This had been a fixation of the Treasury (and the Public Accounts Committee) since the 1950s, and in granting resources for the Plan, the Financial Secretary had emphasised standard provision at standard cost (see p. 127). Aside from cost saving these demands reflected difficulties with the construction industry, which was characterised by large numbers of small firms, many of which were not capable of the large-scale and complex work required. In some locations there were few, if any, firms with the right capabilities. This meant little competition because there were so few firms interested in or capable of tendering. Contractor bankruptcies could cause major disruption (e.g. completion of the North Tees General Hospital was held up in the late stages of construction). RHB witnesses to the 1970 Estimates Committee inquiry suggested that the construction industry was not known for its 'highly organised management factor' and Boards therefore had to make allowances for the 'generally inefficient' way of doing things.[36]

It was therefore believed that without substantial gains in productivity, 'the [construction] industry would not be able to meet the country's building needs'.[37] But little could be done to reorganise the industry; the indicative planning of the 1960s 'had little effect' on construction (Smyth 1985: 172). To the extent that the state could do anything about this, it was via reorganising the demands placed on the construction industry, via attempts at standardisation and at streamlining the processes involved in commissioning construction.

Standardisation and industrialised building were seen as one way of reducing pressure of demand on the industry in a context of labour scarcity.[38] The BMA's Central Consultants and Specialists Committee had endorsed standardisation in 1964, though it was suggested that this acceptance reflected desperation at the Ministry's failure to invest.[39] Standardisation was pursued through central guidance: the Ministry's Hospital Building Notes, technical memoranda and the like, as well as the procedures used to process individual submissions (CAPRICODE – the capital projects code) (Vann-Wye 1992: 171). These initiatives logically pointed towards standardisation of the design and construction of whole hospitals, and the use of industrialised construction methods. One unsuccessful pilot was the 'Best Buy' design, a minimum-specification hospital which attempted to maximise hospital throughput, and which did not allocate beds to particular specialities. The aim was to maximise the use of hospital space by providing a central core (theatres, treatment rooms, ITU, maternity unit) surrounded by wards, with support services all being provided off-site. The assumption was that bed requirements could be reduced substantially if appropriate support was available from community care, local authorities and GPs. These were heroic assumptions, which were duly criticised for altering 'the distribution of capital costs'; the promised local authority services failed to materialise in one of the demonstration projects;[40] two pilots were built but not widely replicated. Vann-Wye (1992: 165) argues that 'Best Buy' was not centrally imposed, but became a standard by default. It was followed by the 'Harness' design, projecting hospitals of 600–1,000 beds, using standard designs for departments based on work by individual regions, and 'harnessing' them together via a framework of communications and engineering works. It posited rather more generous standards than previous Hospital Building Notes, and consequently expenditure cutbacks limited its impact, but it evolved into the successful 'Nucleus' design (Chapter 8). It cannot be said, then, that the aim of 'standard provision at standard cost' had even begun to be achieved in this period, and while the principle had been accepted by the BMA, there was still evidence of resistance to it.[41]

The final issue considered here is the commissioning of capital developments. This is where the NHS has been heavily criticised over many years for failing to manage the capital programme effectively. The National Economic Development Office (NEDO 1969) and the Commons Select Committee on Estimates (1970) both examined this issue. NEDO (1969: appendix 2) demonstrated substantial variations in the time taken to progress from approval in principle for capital development, to the start of construction, ranging from thirty to 114 months. In some extreme cases even agreeing on content and sketching designs was taking up to six years (NEDO 1969: para. 2.11). There were many examples of changes to the scope and cost of large capital schemes, causing delays which members of the Estimates Committee found 'pretty shattering'.[42] A good illustration is the North Tees General Hospital, on which the exchanges between RHB and Ministry over design, content and cost took from early 1961 until 1965.[43] For some commentators, such delays symbolise the inflexible and bureaucratic character of hospital planning. For the NEDO, the solution was a rationalisation of the process by which the NHS commissioned capital developments. Not all the RHBs would be responsible for enough work to gain the necessary experience, and so their main recommendation was the creation of specialised hospital development organisations, covering two or more RHBs; the volume of work for which they would be responsible would mean that they would swiftly develop expertise (NEDO 1969: para. 5.2). These might coincide with economic planning regions. The recommendation was not adopted, but the 1974 reorganisation partly solved this problem by bringing teaching hospitals within the ambit of RHAs, thereby increasing the capital programmes for which RHAs were responsible. Various other recommendations were made which were designed to speed up various stages of the building process.

The issue here really concerns where the sources of delay were to be found. Ideas about medical practice were changing, and expectations were rising: RHBs and Boards of Governors did not want to be left behind and they had to attempt to meet the professional aspirations of medical staff. The Ministry appeared restrictive – using its design guidance in an attempt to enforce conformity – but given the Treasury's emphasis on standardisation, it is debatable whether there was an alternative. And shortages of labour (e.g. architects and other design professionals), difficulties in the construction industry, and an inflationary climate all played their part. Certainly some procedures could have been improved – e.g. reducing scope for variations in the later stages of contracts – but this period arguably demonstrates the constraints on planning; the extent to which the state could control any of the foregoing influences was debatable. Nevertheless these problems with the building programme contributed to a broader sense of disillusionment with top-down, centralised planning.

Issues of strategy and policy in the Newcastle RHB

Even though the resources available to the RHB grew steadily, their capital budget did not exceed £3 million per annum until 1963 and so they initially relied for large-scale developments on schemes which were financed centrally by the Ministry. The RHB had benefited substantially from such schemes in the 1950s and it is indicative of the priority attached to the new North Teesside General Hospital (Chapter 5) that the central financing of this development was announced in October 1963. The Ministry's attention then turned to other regions, posing difficulties for the RHB because they were anxious to progress phase II of the redevelopment of Ashington Hospital, in the under-provided Wansbeck HMC. They had engaged in preliminary planning in the belief – encouraged by the Ministry – that this scheme, which could not easily be accommodated in their capital programme, would be centrally financed. When the Ministry agreed to fund North Teesside but not Ashington phase II, it was an embarrassment for the Board, as they were 'deeply committed publicly' to both projects. Further exchanges with the Ministry proved largely fruitless; the Ministry could not guarantee any central finance for Ashington in the two financial years in which most expenditure would be undertaken, leaving over £500,000 to be found from within the RHB's allocation in 1965/6 and 1966/7. Failure to accept this project, as the RHB observed, would mean an actual reduction in the sums to be spent in those years. The Ministry's view was that this simply reflected other RHBs 'catching up' with Newcastle in obtaining central finance.[44]

The Ashington case is illustrative of the difficult balancing act faced by RHBs, a situation exacerbated by rising building costs. Constrained from above by tight limits on the programme, the Ministry took a great deal of time to scrutinise schemes, but the result was that the Ministry were perceived by the RHB as 'indecisive and hesitant' in reaching major decisions.[45] In the early years of the programme, Ministry control was exercised on total expenditure, which meant a steady procession of slight delays in start dates of schemes. There was therefore a temptation to artificially restrict the cost of schemes in order to keep as many in the programme as possible, but the Ministry viewed this as the 'antithesis of sensible financial planning'.[46] Seen from the RHB's point of view, of course, this was a rational response; it was important to the RHB to be seen to be doing something in as many locations as possible even if they were then criticised from above.[47] There was an evident tension in the Board's activities. There were difficulties (due to increases in the content and cost of schemes in the programme) in bringing major schemes on-stream, and so the development of new hospitals proceeded slowly. In turn, this aggravated the problem of existing hospitals having to continue in inadequate premises, and hence there was a need to spend money to maintain existing hospitals;[48] in some cases these were hospitals which the Board would have preferred to close.[49] The Ministry would clearly have preferred the Board to plan 'on the basis of real priority of need',[50] but this implied concentrated effort on a small number of HMCs, which would have exposed the RHB to criticisms from all the others.

Capital expenditure rose rapidly for the first two years of the Plan, but its growth then slackened slightly in the term of office of the Labour government; after increasing again in the early 1970s, the 1973 cuts represented the first setback to the expansion of hospital building. This period also witnessed an overall expansion in the proportion of NHS resources used for capital expenditure, while the proportion of capital devoted to new hospital construction also rose steadily (Figure A2), though the corresponding proportion in the Newcastle RHB was rather lower throughout this period, indicating that the RHB was redeveloping existing hospitals, rather than concentrating on a few major new projects.

The impact of such policies can be assessed from evidence submitted to the major inquiry into the building programme by the Select Committee on Estimates. Restraint of and uncertainty about capital allocations was regarded as disadvantageous in terms of temporary provisions, changes of use of facilities, the small size of building contracts, long gaps between successive phases of building at individual hospitals, and the need for continued expenditure on maintenance.[51] An indication of the implications of such problems can be seen in Figure 7.1. This gives the RHB's tentative programme of major capital developments and shows that (given certain assumptions about the capital resources likely to be available to the RHB) it was hoped to complete the DGH programme for the region by the end of the century. Even this target – which was considerably more optimistic than those of some RHBs[52] – ultimately looked unrealistic when later delays in building schemes were allowed for. To take two examples, the commissioning of the Freeman Road Hospital, Newcastle, was seriously delayed by successive financial crises in the late 1970s, while construction of phase 1 of the new hospital for South East Northumberland (at Rake Lane, North Shields) did not commence until late 1980 – almost three years after the date indicated here. Space prevents a full charting of the delays to and rescheduling in the capital programme, but the potential for frustration was all too evident. For example, after the announcement of the Plan, several schemes were advanced during 1963, only to be postponed to later dates than originally envisaged barely a year later. Furthermore, because of the complexities of some of the larger projects, it was not possible to postpone the Plan *en bloc*; rather, individual schemes might find themselves postponed still further, or alternatively brought forward, simply because of the exigencies of minimising unspent funds in any one year. The HMCs which suffered in all this seem to have been those where there were constraints on and arguments about the most appropriate location of services; schemes could not take a definite place in the programme until these were resolved. Hence the RHB were unable to commit themselves on the dates at which it might be possible to provide new facilities in some of the relatively deprived HMCs within the region, for instance, Sunderland and South East Northumberland. It was clear that the latter would, by the mid 1970s, 'resemble the metaphorical "sore thumb"'.[53]

It is nevertheless clear that – intra-regionally – capital development was uneven. The most favoured area in this period was Teesside, reflecting substantial expenditure on the new North Tees General Hospital. By contrast, in the peripheral rural HMCs (Alnwick and Rothbury, Berwick, South West Durham), investment was limited to minor schemes at the relatively small hospitals in these HMCs, since the RHB did not intend to provide full DGH facilities in such areas. Analysis of data on hospital

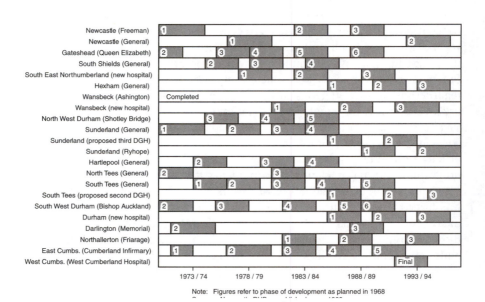

Figure 7.1 Newcastle RHB's programme of DGH development: progress as of 1968

Source: Newcastle RHB, unpublished paper 1968

Note: Figures refer to phase of development as planned in 1968

investment at constant prices clarifies these issues.[54] Over the first twenty-five years of the NHS, the most favoured areas, receiving over twice the regional average *per capita* investment, were West Cumberland and North Teesside, reflecting new hospital construction. Most other HMCs were within about 10 per cent of the regional average, indicating a reasonable degree of equity. However, several HMCs had received 70 per cent or less of the regional average level of funding: Gateshead (70 per cent), Hartlepool (63 per cent), South Teesside (61 per cent), Sunderland (48 per cent) and SE Northumberland (45 per cent). While Sunderland had received important investments in the 1930s (Mohan 1997) that could not be said of SE Northumberland, nor of Gateshead or Hartlepool, and SW Durham, one of the worst-off HMCs, had benefited only to a limited degree from new investment (83 per cent of the regional average). The largest elements of expenditure to 1973 went to Newcastle, which received one-sixth of the RHB's capital expenditure, 45 per cent above the regional average; this is actually an underestimate of expenditure in Newcastle.[55] One would not, of course, expect each HMC to receive an entirely proportionate share, but such disparities clearly persisted over a long time period.

There is evidence of Ministry concern about the RHB's emphasis on Newcastle. This was noted in early 1963: there was 'more emphasis on improving hospitals in the "central" part of the region' (principally Tyneside and Teesside). While this was to the 'detriment' of peripheral areas, the Board considered that improvements 'at the centre' had a higher priority.[56] By early 1965, the RHB had agreed to the development of Newcastle's hospitals taking place in two 'large and costly' stages, necessitating an increase in Newcastle's capital allocation from £3.3 million to £8.8 million.[57] An immediate consequence was delays in capital projects elsewhere which were identified as being for 'budgetary' rather than 'planning' considerations. One Ministry official questioned whether hospitals in Newcastle should get 'such a lion's share',[58] which was equivalent to 25 per cent of the RHB's programme.[59] Although the RHB's policy was ostensibly designed 'more or less to do something for each group' it was felt that 'Newcastle is always more equal than the others'. A Ministry official felt that too much had been spent on Newcastle in the past, and this underlined the view that the RHB was proposing to spend too much money on Newcastle in the future. He was 'horrified' to learn that over £2.5 million had already been spent on Newcastle General Hospital (a rather ramshackle collection of former local authority hospital buildings) in what were 'patchwork additions' when a new hospital was really required.[60] The 1966 revision of the Plan gave priority to the three major industrial estuaries (Teesside, Wearside and Tyneside), in conformity with other efforts to pursue a policy of spatially selective investment. However, the corollary was that other schemes in the region, lacking the high profile of these localities, slipped down the pecking order.

In fact, the development of hospital services in the region was threatened by the persistent dispute over how best to develop the hospital services of

Newcastle-upon-Tyne. This dispute engaged not just the RHB, the HMC and the Board of Governors; other public agencies became embroiled in it (Newcastle City Council, the University, and, tangentially, the Northern Economic Planning Council); prominent politicians and medics expressed their views forcefully; and ultimately the argument was resolved only with the personal intervention of Richard Crossman. The saga is recounted briefly here to illustrate how the social goals of hospital policy became subordinate to a variety of professional and political criteria.

The concept of a major hospital complex in Newcastle dates at least to the Hospital Surveyors. Efforts to coordinate the city's hospital services date from the 1930s (Chapter 3) and a short-lived 'Hospital Centre Committee' had in the wartime years attempted to coordinate the activities of the city's voluntary hospitals.[61] The Hospital Plan envisaged three general hospitals in the city, including a new DGH in the eastern suburbs, but problems with the proposed site (mining subsidence, and the Council's preference for maintaining a kind of 'Green Belt' around it to check suburban expansion) led to delays and these created an opportunity for a powerful alliance to emerge, consisting of consultants, local politicians, the Board of Governors and the University. This group favoured a central hospital complex, uniting the teaching hospital (the Royal Victoria Infirmary – RVI), the former municipal hospital (Newcastle General) and a new hospital, to be accommodated on land between the RVI and the General. Unusually, seventy consultants had, in 1966, publicly petitioned the Ministry to intervene along these lines. The supporters of this proposal included prominent regional politicians such as T. Dan Smith[62] who was a passionate advocate of improving the region's infrastructure, and of boosting Newcastle's image as an important urban centre. A well-connected figure in the Labour Party, Smith lobbied at the highest levels for his scheme: Richard Crossman described a meeting with 'Smith ... the big boss of the North East ... full of his concept that the hospitals must help in the export trade and must provide a base for Newcastle's industry' (Crossman 1976: 589). Newcastle was seen as a regional capital with a modern environment to match (Burns 1967) and the City Council had by 1967 swung behind proposals for a scheme of centralised development. The medical lobby weighed in; Henry Miller (see p. 137), from 1968 Vice-Chancellor of the University, argued that their proposals would offer 'potentially the finest medical centre in Europe, with three closely-integrated hospitals'.[63]

This dispute ran for nearly seven years and only the outlines can be given here.[64] The RHB's argument was that a suitable site for a third DGH had been found when the City Council made available land at Freeman Road, on the north-eastern fringe of the city. To postpone Freeman Road implied substantial delays (plans for the hospital could not simply be transferred to an alternative site *en bloc*), with consequential effects on regional strategy: it would not be easy to spend the capital sums released by the delays while, once construction eventually commenced, other schemes would have to be postponed. Either way, the RHB would be put in an embarrassing position. Moreover, the RHB claimed that hospital development in Newcastle was lagging behind that elsewhere in the region.[65] As some £3 million had been spent at the General since 1948, and as capital expenditure in the Newcastle HMC had been above the regional average, this claim was not entirely water-tight. It was also at variance with the Ministry's view, that Newcastle had benefited disproportionately from capital allocations (see above). The RHB also contended that the Freeman Road site was important on social (accessi-bility) grounds, since the hospital's catchment would extend into Northumberland (and, though not mentioned explicitly, the Board was aware that SE Northumberland HMC had received a very small share of RHB capital allocations since 1948). Finally, centralised development would entail further delays, because of the complexities of *in situ* redevelopment of two hospitals.

Opposition to the RHB focused on the advantages for medical practice, research and education of an integrated complex, achieving economies of scale in specialist departments as well as ancillary services, and avoiding duplication. The contemporaneous Royal Commission on Medical Edu-cation (1968) (Chairman: Lord Todd) lent weight to a case for a teaching hospital complex, under one authority, while the deliberations of the Bonham-Carter Committee implied greater concentration. Accordingly, medical opinion in Newcastle was said to be united in 'preferring a central development and in regarding Freeman Road as a disastrous and uneco-nomic anachronism'. A central complex would not produce an 'impersonal medical mammoth, but three interlinked hospitals, virtually adjacent, permitting integration of specialist services, ... and furnishing an undergrad-uate and postgraduate teaching potential that will be unsurpassed in Europe'. By contrast, Freeman Road would be a 'truncated' hospital because, in an effort to secure medical support, the RHB were prepared to relocate certain specialist services to the central site. A further key point was that, under the RHB's proposals, Newcastle General was to contract to 450 beds, of which some 370 would be in geriatric medicine, and some of its facilities, such as its cardiothoracic unit, were to transfer to the new hospital, which was 'especially indefensible' as they would be isolated from other cognate specialities.[66] This generated substantial resistance from doctors at the General, who could not be persuaded that it was sensible to run down their hospital while reproviding some of its facilities on a new site three miles away.

Many of these arguments were conceded by the RHB but they were focused firmly on the need to avoid delays because of the political costs of so doing. The problem with the centralised medical complex was partly a social one: accessibility would be improved if Freeman Road were built (although the issue did not feature strongly in the RHB's case, the local MP pushed it strongly); conversely plans for a central medical complex were described by Crossman as a 'case of elephantiasis' (1976: vol. III, 589).

Furthermore, a Private Member's Bill would have been necessary for the acquisition of the central site, as part of it was owned by the Freemen of the City. Even without this complication an independent architectural assessment indicated delays of at least four years. Since that was universally felt to be excessive, the Freeman Road proposals were eventually agreed.

What is interesting about this case is the way professional considerations, allied to political ambitions, combined to cause a substantial hiatus in hospital development. Pursuing a somewhat utopian vision of a future teaching hospital, the proponents inadvertently held up the development of Newcastle's hospital services. The question of the social implications of the proposed developments scarcely featured at all. Part of the reason surely lies in the autonomous status given to teaching hospitals in the 1948 compromise. They were charged with advancing medical education and research and, in conjunction with the University, mounted a case based on the efficient organisation of clinical science and education, the benefits of which were claimed to be self-evident. Opposition on the part of the RHB was simply dismissed by Miller, the Vice Chancellor, as an example of 'administrative inflexibility' by an organisation which was solely concerned with 'budgetary expediency'. Where Miller referred to Freeman Road at all he was concerned with its 'usefulness as an instrument of medical education'.[67] This signals the principal concerns of those involved with the medical school, and is in certain respects a contrast to inter-war experience, in which some teaching hospitals played an important role in integrating voluntary and municipal provision (see, for example, Sturdy and Cooter 1998; Pickstone 1985). In essence, those favouring centralisation presumed an identity between their interests and those of the public who would use the hospitals. These arguments had a certain rationality and consistency, albeit one which discounted considerations of accessibility, but they were trumped by the political impossibility of rescheduling the capital programme.

The question of the relationship between spatial and social policy also arose in the context of new town development. The various new towns in the region – particularly Peterlee and Washington – were seen as symbolic of the new modern infrastructure that the region required for economic success. The Development Corporations, charged with ensuring the success of the new towns, voiced claims for capital investment. Peterlee's case had been the subject of discussion in the 1950s (Chapter 5); however, given the definition of a DGH enshrined in the Plan, it was evident that it could not be considered seriously as a location for a general hospital.

Washington was a different proposition because of its larger target population (80,000) and its location in between hospitals in Sunderland and Gateshead. It became a planning issue because of the possibility that, in the absence of a local hospital, Washington's population might gravitate towards Gateshead. The latter would be an embarrassment to the RHB as it would greatly overload the capacity of Gateshead HMC's hospitals. Hence the RHB provisionally agreed to provide a hospital at Washington.[68]

However, this development could not be accommodated within the RHB's ten-year programme, and for the Development Corporation, this posed the problem of 'sterilising' some 30–40 acres of land.[69] If Washington developed as planned there would be considerable pressure to release this land, so they sought assurances from the RHB, which were not forthcoming. The future population of Washington was uncertain, as it would depend on voluntary migration, and so having initially favoured hospital development in Washington, the RHB then felt justified in waiting until they had a clearer view of the town's likely growth.[70] However, with the emphasis on spatial concentration in the Bonham-Carter report it was clear that Washington could not constitute a viable site for DGH development, and the issue slipped quietly off the table, resurfacing from time to time as the continued existence of the Development Corporation provided an institutional voice. What these examples do show is the difficulty of coordinating the intentions of state agencies, in circumstances in which external constraints limited the scope for manoeuvre of both the RHB and the NTDC. Similar difficulties were evident elsewhere (House of Commons 1970; Aldridge 1979). The scale of the hospital programme meant that RHBs could not afford to risk the opprobrium of constructing new hospitals in advance of full demand – a problem which, in the wider context of the new towns, meant that provision of social and welfare facilities always lagged behind population growth.

Rationalising the hospital stock: social and political challenges

Announcement of the Plan immediately generated substantial criticism, not just from those distressed at the prospect of losing cherished hospitals, but also from defenders of cottage hospitals, though the latter's motivations were sometimes coloured by an opposition to any variant of 'planning':

> the ideological centralization proposed in the Hospital Plan is about as realistic as would be a plan to scrap all the ships in the fleet except the aircraft carriers, and about as moral as would be a plan to close all the parish churches on the grounds that the work done in them could be more efficiently organised in cathedrals.[71]

Strong reactions were forthcoming from around the country. Representations continued to be made in the early 1960s, notably from backbench MPs, about the perceived threat to treasured local facilities. For example, the Conservative Research Department regarded hospital closures as 'quite the most difficult issue' with which they had to deal.[72] Civil servants could dismiss community protests as sentimental attachments to institutions dating from 'the horse and buggy age' in which 'modern treatment cannot be given'[73] but Ministers were more constrained in what they could say. It was nevertheless acknowledged that a vigorous closure policy would have to be pursued if the aims of the Plan were to be achieved, particularly if revenue expenditure were to be held within the agreed limit of 2 per cent growth. Powell felt that establishing the pattern of DGHs took precedence, and that if there was to be consultation with community interests, it would be on matters of minor detail. However, by late 1963 the Ministry was taking a more open and conciliatory approach on closure proposals, in order to allay suspicions that RHBs were acting in a 'hole-and-corner way' on closures.[74]

In common with other RHBs the Board had kept a watching brief over hospital occupancy, identifying institutions where occupancy appeared particularly low, and investigating the underlying reasons. It is clear, from a reading of papers recording such investigations, that the Board had good reasons for wishing to dispose of a number of facilities. These were often (though not exclusively) buildings inherited from local authorities, which provided accommodation for geriatric patients or for those with infectious diseases. In a number of cases occupancy was as low as 60 per cent or less, while several hospitals contained small specialist units, which really required relocation into DGHs. Staffing difficulties were also an important factor contributing to low occupancy, especially in rural areas. On the face of it, there appeared good grounds for a vigorous programme of closures.

The reality was rather different. The Plan proposed closure of some 700 hospitals in ten years but such a net reduction in hospital numbers was not achieved until the early 1980s.[75] Progress of closures was uneven, reaching a peak of thirty-nine (in England) in 1968. The Plan had proposed the closure of forty-one hospitals in the Newcastle RHB by 1975, but only fourteen closures had been effected by 1973. Thus, by 1973, the Board had been able to achieve only limited rationalisation, having closed a total of twenty-six hospitals since 1948 – largely isolation or chronic units, or single-speciality facilities, containing small numbers of beds and often housed in poor-quality buildings (Figure A4). Nationally, trends in the numbers of non-psychiatric hospitals indicate a slow decline in this period, which accelerated only *c.* 1969, as more new buildings were commissioned (Figure A3). One reason for slow progress was delays in important capital schemes; another was the problem RHBs had in obtaining agreement to closure proposals. The DHSS hoped that opposition to closures would cease once the public accepted that a spatial concentration of facilities was in everyone's best interests, due to the superior service that would be provided.[76] In practice, considerable resistance developed to hospital closures. Under the terms of the 1946 NHS Act, the Minister of Health was obliged to ensure that hospital buildings were, as far as possible, used for the purposes for which they had been employed immediately prior to the setting up of the NHS, and the arrangements for consultation on closures or changes of use emphasised this Ministerial obligation.[77] However, a different emphasis emerged in policy from 1968; reflecting concerns that anticipated revenue savings had not been achieved, RHBs were 'actively encourage(d) to promote closures and change of use of uneconomic units as an essential measure to facilitate the provision of a planned service'.[78] Yet even this, which explicitly promised Ministerial support for closure proposals, proved of limited practical value. Ministers did not follow Powell's lead on closures. Crossman indicates on more than one occasion the view that more could be done to preserve physical assets (1976: vol. III, 608, 639). He emphasised the need for much greater attention to public relations aspects of closures, proposing new procedures in which RHBs liaised much more closely with local authorities, and suggesting that approval would only be given to closures after all possibilities had been considered for alternative health and welfare uses of hospital buildings.[79] However, the Treasury interpreted this revised guidance as indicating that Crossman was unwilling to pursue a closure programme with the necessary vigour; it was argued that if the political difficulties were so great, perhaps RHBs should be encouraged to retain hospitals and scale down DGH programmes.[80] Given what appears as a less-than-firm Ministerial approach, it is not surprising to find that some RHBs were perceived, by the Ministry, as being somewhat dilatory in their approach to hospital closures. One Board had been 'repeatedly advised' that their capital programme 'must be accompanied by planned closures of existing unsatisfactory hospitals'; 'unless they resolutely close beds and hospitals ... they will face an intolerable revenue burden'.[81] Simply running down old hospitals once the new facilities were in place was not going to generate the required revenue savings.

The social consequences of hospital closures were felt most acutely in rural areas. As was observed in Parliament, it was an 'unhappy coincidence' that the Plan was announced 'at the moment when the Minister of Transport is busy dismantling rural transport services by both rail and road'.[82] The interesting point here is that the decisions to concentrate hospital provision *and* to rationalise the transport network had been taken with the same objective in mind: the more efficient long-term management of public expenditure. Yet between them they exacerbated the problems of accessibility to services (and, in practice, the greenfield or peripheral locations on which new hospitals were built sometimes made such problems worse).

The implied accessibility problems were causing concern shortly after the Plan's announcement. Thus the Newcastle RHB reassured various local institutions that their aim was not an excessive centralisation; rather, small units would be retained in some local centres (Alston, Penrith, Alnwick, Rothbury) and additional facilities would be provided in places not already possessing them (e.g. Millom, Kirkby Stephen).[83] On the grounds of economies of scale, the Board were unwilling to consider a scattering of acute hospital facilities, but local hospitals would be retained for the reception and treatment of 'social cases'.[84] However, following the publication of the Bonham-Carter Report, there developed considerable local opposition to the RHB's proposals, particularly in the case of Northallerton which could not support a DGH along the lines indicated in the Report. Consequently the RHB envisaged running down the existing Friarage

Hospital in Northallerton, according it the status of a 'peripheral' hospital.[85] This generated a fierce protest, orchestrated by several local authorities and voluntary agencies, and articulated in local newspapers. One consequence of protests against the concentration of services were proposals to provide community hospitals to serve rural areas (see Chapter 8).

Concluding comments

This period undeniably saw a steady expansion of hospital capital expenditure, and RHBs began to make inroads into the challenging task of renewing the hospital stock. The expanded programme allowed greater numbers of large schemes which were crucial in attacking problems of obsolescence. The effects began to be visible; by 1970, BMA representatives admitted to the Select Committee on Estimates that their attitude had changed from 'despair' to 'cautious optimism that their sons will work in modern hospitals'.[86] On the other hand, many inadequate buildings remained in use: as an indication, in 1965 nineteen hospitals in the Newcastle RHB still consisted wholly or partially of temporary wartime accommodation, built (in twelve cases) of wood, corrugated iron, or even tin.[87] The expansion of investment enabled new hospital development, or substantial reconstruction of existing hospitals, in several HMCs, though others lagged behind. It also became possible to spend larger sums on individual schemes. Moreover, the RHB's minutes do show a Board determined to maximise the use made of capital funds; there was a constant process of rescheduling of schemes to ensure that, as far as possible, available monies were spent.

This era has been characterised disparagingly as one in which a 'command-and-control' bureaucracy moved with sloth-like speed to produce a set of half-built, cumbersome and inflexible hospitals which the nation could not afford. Norms-based planning is the villain of the piece here (e.g. Mallender 2000). However, given the scale of the task faced by the NHS, and the need to prioritise given limited resources, it must be acknowledged that despite its inflexibilities the Plan was at least a starting point; bed norms, however arbitrary, gave a basis for determination of priorities. It was also the case during this period that attempts were made more systematically to steer revenue and capital resources towards areas of greater need greater weight being given to a demographic structure and to projections of regional growth and decline, though as in the 1950s, the absence of comprehensive data about the condition of the hospital stock hindered redistribution. However the extent of interregional redistribution was constrained by a policy decision to ensure that there were no actual reductions in capital allocations, thereby provoking 'less disappointment, and therefore less criticism'.[88] The evidence from this period also shows flexible responses to changing needs. Thus, reviews of the RHB's capital programme took account of differential and selective population change as well as attempting to make allowances for the needs of new towns and for rural areas. There may be an argument that there could have been more flexibility, but consider the counterfactual case: what would have happened if the RHB had arbitrarily altered its order of priorities? The Board was implementing a set of development proposals within a constrained budget, which meant that shuffling the order of schemes, once they were under way, was almost impossible. This may have given an appearance of inflexibility, but the problems arose from the need constantly to refer development proposals up to the Ministry and the Treasury. RHBs had little scope to depart from agreed plans without authorisation, and this caused much frustration among senior RHB officers.[89] In short, flawed though the Plan was, what we see in this region at least is an attempt to maximise the resources available to the region and ensure that (allowing for the inevitable 'lumpiness' of large investments) efforts were made to respond to changing circumstances.

In other respects one might raise questions about the credibility of this exercise in planning. There is evidence of both skill shortages and capacity constraints: could a more interventionist state planning apparatus have had the capacities to steer resources in the desired direction? The pressures on the construction industry were known but proposals to do something about this focused firmly on the demand side, indicative of the limits to state intervention. It is also clear that the extent to which there was parallel investment in local authority services for the elderly varied considerably, yet this was essential if bed blocking was to be avoided. Publication of local authority health and welfare plans revealed substantial variations: Gateshead proposed thirty-five residential places per 1,000 over-65s whereas Northumberland envisaged 15.5.[90] Bridgen (2001: 518–22) shows that hospital geriatric provision remained static, as hospital authorities adhered to the 1962 norms. Because complementary community care did not expand consistently, and because of the growth in the elderly population, the 'bed blocking' remained. Insofar as the Plan might be represented as an exercise in the integration of health and welfare services, this is not strong evidence.

In addition, the central presumption of the Plan was that efficiency would be increased as hospital services were rationalised on fewer sites. There were three interrelated problems here. First, though not publicly acknowledged in the Plan's presentation, the candidates for closure generated the smallest revenue savings. The revenue consequences of new developments were substantial but the NHS was constrained within a tight financial straitjacket. Second, arising in part from delays in providing new facilities, the benefits of the Plan were not obvious to the affected communities. In fact, for many communities, the Plan appeared to threaten the removal of cherished facilities, with only vague promises of new provision. Resistance to closures therefore was vociferous and vigorous. Third, the planning apparatus was not set up to process closures quickly. Although management circulars encouraged a firmer policy, RHBs were criticised for indecision while, in their turn, they criticised Ministers for failing to back them. Clearly, not all Ministers shared Powell's willingness to explain to communities why their hospital should close. But the unfortunate result was that even hospitals where the case for closure was self-evident clung to life for far longer than envisaged.

What of planning as the embodiment of modernist virtues of scale economies and standardisation? There are those who see hospitals of this era as reflecting broader trends in the organisation of production. Such standardisation could be perceived as an attempt to regulate the labour process within hospitals, in much the same way as was attempted in factories, by paying attention to the efficient use of space, but there is not strong evidence of this even in the face of rising capital and revenue costs. However, hospitals were largely designed on an *ad hoc*, one-off basis and the process of standardisation had little impact in this period. This may reflect on the capacities of the administrative machine, which simply had not had the opportunity to put experimental designs into practice given limited capital resources. The question of the efficacy of standardisation was not really settled properly, however, because there were changes of policy in fairly rapid succession and before pilot projects had been properly evaluated.[91] So those looking for superficial parallels with Fordism in the welfare state will not find them here. Instead they will find a tortuous process of experimentation which did not produce much in the way of useful results.

There was also an emergent critique of standardisation, drawing on a distrust of authority and expertise. Kemp's (1964) critique of the blind 'bed worship' of hospital planners is an early example, as is Hunter's (1963) argument that DGHs would only make more pronounced the 'superficial and mechanistic' basis of the NHS. Those defending the cottage hospitals argued in like vein, against hospitals as a 'mechanical repair service'.[92] The eventual acceptance by the BMA of standardisation indicated their desperation to see new hospitals built, but there is ample evidence of professional interests shaping the development of new hospitals. The strength of resistance to standardisation gave subsequent policy-makers something to build on, in terms of advocating a more localist line in policy; as shown in the next chapter, however, they arguably did so in a negative sense.

The process of planning thus faced considerable obstacles. Even if funding for the capital development programme expanded, rising costs and revenue constraints limited its direct impact. Planning agencies existed in a relationship of resource dependence (on subsidiary bodies and on the private sector) and also required cooperation with other public bodies to achieve their goals. The exercise of power was not, therefore, a straightforwardly hierarchical process. Hospital Boards continued to pursue their strategy, however, and it would be unfair to characterise this period as one of government failure; it is clear that there were substantial improvements in hospital provision, even though the blueprint of the Plan may not have been implemented quite as intended. Before we reach verdicts of government failure, it is also necessary to acknowledge the external constraints on the modernisation programmes pursued in this period, Lowe and Rollings 2000: 117). However, as politicians became aware of the risks of nailing their colours too closely to the Plan's mast, the word 'planning' disappeared from their vocabulary. Hence the period is aptly characterised as one in which a 'Plan' simply became a building programme.

8 A programme without a policy?
Hospital developments 1973–91

The 1973 cuts in public expenditure seemed an obvious point at which to break the narrative of hospital policy developments. Subsequently, however, there seemed to be no obvious point at which to break this chronology until 1991. Within that eighteen-year period, it can broadly be argued that, once Labour adopted monetarism, continuities existed in attitudes to economic policy between Labour and the Conservatives, and these had ramifications for the management of the welfare state, albeit with some differences of emphasis. The difficulties of managing the hospital building programme were common to both governments but there were differences in terms of the emphasis placed on voluntary effort and commercial criteria in the capital programme.

The socio-economic backcloth to this chapter is a period in which there were substantial challenges to the Keynesian welfare state. Historians have questioned the existence of a stable consensus regarding the welfare state, but there is general agreement that both governing parties regarded the NHS as a core element of welfare provision. However, the period under consideration was marked by a constant search for new ways of managing health care (involving major reorganisations), new incentive structures (for managers and hospitals), and new sources of resources. There are certain continuities in approach between the Labour and Conservative governments – at least in terms of the adoption of monetarist economic policies, though there were also substantive differences, certainly as the Thatcher era wore on.

The immediate causes of the perceived 'crisis' of the welfare state were economic. A combination of high and accelerating inflation, and the onset of recession, partly induced by substantial increases in the price of oil, simultaneously increased the need for public expenditure (associated with unemployment) and limited the government's scope for raising revenues. In turn, greater government borrowing became necessary, which in its turn eroded the value of sterling as confidence evaporated. However, these were really short-term economic shocks – albeit ones with very real consequences (in the form of cuts in the capital programme) for hospital development. There were much more fundamental challenges to the welfare state, however. First, there was mounting dissatisfaction with the 'British disease': a combination of endemic stagflation, and the persistent failure of governments to increase economic growth. This was partly a result of changed external circumstances. The internationalisation of production and finance limited the scope for Keynesian economic management and thus contributed to a crisis of legitimacy, as governments were seen to be unable to deliver full employment. These circumstances offered fertile ground for a monetarist critique of public expenditure, adopted by Labour after the IMF crisis of 1976, and (with greater vigour) by the Conservatives after 1979.

More generally, there was an emerging sense of a crisis of legitimacy, symbolised by high levels of industrial militancy, and reinforced by perceptions of rising crime and a terrorist threat. This was associated with apocalyptic statements that Britain had become 'ungovernable' (Lowe 1993: 302), and that there was governmental 'overload'.

In this climate, reviews of the institutions and practices of the welfare state became possible. Moreover, there was growing dissatisfaction with the way welfare was delivered: professional, centralised bureaucracies came under attack from all points of the political compass. From the right, such services were attacked as inflexible and hierarchical, and as organisations which limited the freedom of individuals and communities. Coercion through taxation became a watchword: the obvious response was to expand scope for market forces. However, there were also criticisms from the left, that centralisation and professionalisation had gone too far, and that state welfare services were alienating and unresponsive. Critics such as Illich (1973) argued that high technology health care could in some circumstances be positively harmful. In the period in question such views did not lead to a wholehearted challenge to the dominance of hospital-based health care. However, along with the influence of commentators such as Schumacher (1975), these ideas provided an intellectual justification for proposals for smaller-scale organisation, and for greater pluralism in welfare provision (Johnson 1987).

Three broad strands can be discerned in the acute hospital sector in this period. First, there was a continued effort to maintain a substantial building programme, accompanied by efforts to redistribute resources within the NHS. Managing the capital programme became difficult in the austere economic climate, while redistribution became politicised as limited revenue growth focused attention on apparent over-provision of hospital capacity in certain locations. The result was a greater emphasis on standardisation and low-cost solutions in hospital development. Second, there was a revived localism. In part this can be seen as a response to the centralising tendencies of the Hospital Plan; in part, also, it was an attempt by communities to retain cherished local facilities. But this localism was also encouraged by the state, certainly after 1979. Third, discussion of market criteria featured to a growing extent in debates on the distribution of hospital facilities. In part reflecting criticisms from the private hospital sector, there were arguments about whether, and how, the NHS's capital assets ought to be valued and paid for, while NHS estates were treated in a *de facto* commercial manner following the 1983 Davies Report; as a result, proceeds of property disposals played a growing part in the NHS capital development programme. Questions of commercialisation, competition and regulation surfaced again as a result of the expansion of private health care.

The period was also one of ideological ferment, in which possible alternative ways of financing and running hospital services were hawked around the policy marketplace. Although one might see some of these initiatives as forerunners of the innovations rolled-out nationally in the 1991 reforms, a more circumspect view would be that they created a climate in which it became possible to question the value of 'public' solutions to problems of hospital capital development. The chapter first discusses the management of the NHS capital investment programme, emphasising the attempts to maintain the scale of investment in hospitals but also looking at efforts to manage the stock more efficiently and supplement public funds. There is then an examination of the changing character of policy on hospital size and design. The effects of these developments in the Northern region are exemplified. Finally, consideration is given to efforts to diversify sources of capital for hospital provision, in the form of charitable and commercial provision of services.

Managing the capital programme: a 'crisis of crisis management'?

The early 1970s are often now perceived as a turning-point in terms of economic management, and as a period in which managing public expenditure became an increasingly problematic process. This is well illustrated by debates about the hospital programme.

The commitments of the Hospital Plan were always likely to be vulnerable in such an expenditure climate. Barbara Castle's diaries describe some of the political difficulties to which this could lead. Castle, as Secretary of State for Social Services (1974–6) recorded a Cabinet discussion, in April 1975, of budget proposals initially designed to reduce public expenditure by some £900 million. However, the Chancellor subsequently sought agreement for further cuts to bring the total savings up to £1,000 million. Castle (emphases added) reports that there ensued:

> a chorus of complaints ... *that Ministers were never given the chance of discussing priorities or overall economic strategy.* Instead we were faced with ad hoc demands from the chancellor from time to time, pleading sudden crisis or necessity. In particular, I pleaded that we should look ahead to 1979 and decide what objectives we would wish to have achieved by then and which we were prepared to sacrifice. *How could I get my health authorities to plan the NHS properly when the capital allocations were abruptly changed?*
>
> (Castle 1980: 359–60 – emphases added)

A consequence was that, at the beginning of the 1975–6 financial year, health authorities had not actually known what their capital allocations were to be.

This throws into sharp relief the difficulties of sustaining a planned development of the hospital service, given such restrictive – and unpredictable – constraints. As Castle (1980: 546) went on to say, 'although demography, the condition of the capital stock, and the under-investment in the service' all constituted good grounds for investment, 'this finessing is wasted when the public expenditure chips are down. It is only political muscle that counts'. Later entries find her arguing that:

> Further transfers from capital would merely create a *frightening deterioration in our capital stock for the next decade* when we already had a far worse legacy of out-of-date hospitals than we had of houses or schools, *thanks to long years of neglect of the NHS. The cuts the Treasury were demanding would mean something like a moratorium on new hospital starts.*
>
> (Castle 1980: 593 – emphases added)

However, faced with growing economic crises in the mid-1970s, the Labour government saw little alternative, although an effort was made to restore some of the December 1973 cuts in the capital programme.

A somewhat different perspective is offered by Castle's Ministerial colleague, David Owen (Minister of Health, 1974–6). While bemoaning the effects of the cuts, he nevertheless argued that in the early 1970s:

> the plain fact was that the hospital building programme ... was completely out of control. ... There was hardly a town of any size in the country that was not encouraged to believe that a new district general hospital was soon to be built. (Owen 1976: 43)

Somewhat contradicting this view, he was subsequently to complain of the '*grossly under-capitalised* hospital building programme – which, to be blunt, all of us have at various times used as a manipulator of the economy, cutting back on the construction industry for wider economic reasons'.[1] He called for the 'wise use of scarce resources' and for scaling the building programme to the point where it was 'within the capacity of the building industry'.[2] To put these comments into context, only in 1963 did NHS new building reach, for the first time, 2 per cent of *all* new building in the economy. Even in the years Owen complains about, the NHS absorbed barely 3 per cent of resources devoted to new building in the economy, quickly dropping to around 2.5 per cent after 1973.[3] This hardly suggests a programme that was beyond the capacity of the building industry, nor one that was completely out of control. Owen's remarks drew a response from Sir George Godber, who had recently retired as Chief Medical Officer, pointing to the continued disparity between the investment in hospitals *vis-à-vis* other public programmes: 'whatever else might be said about the programme it was clearly not out of control, but rather tightly controlled'; other states had invested far more.[4] What is at issue here is the extent to which the Labour government had any scope for manoeuvre. Whereas Owen believed that public expenditure was out of control, Castle argued that it was the process of *reducing* public expenditure which had 'got completely out of *political* control' (1980: 521). Put another way, the parameters of policy were being framed by a Treasury setting targets dictated by the perceived need to maintain the confidence of the financial markets (Panitch and Leys 2001: 107–18; see Webster 1996: 591–606 for discussion of the implications for NHS expenditure).

Figure A1, showing hospital capital expenditure in real terms, indicates that the impact of expenditure cuts was to reduce investment by about 20 per cent in real terms. Expenditure rose slightly at the end of the 1970s, then largely levelled out under the Conservatives, being maintained for most of the 1980s at slightly higher levels than had proved possible under Labour, though this was partly due to the contribution of land sales. Government spokesmen enthusiastically massaged the figures for presentational purposes, a good example being Norman Fowler's speech to the Conservatives' conference in 1986. Brandishing a lengthy printout, Fowler claimed credit for as many as 308 schemes, but over half of these were projects which, though firmly in the minds of RHAs, had yet to receive DHSS approval in principle. He claimed that 'the terrible days of "stop-go" in hospital building are behind us', a somewhat premature statement in the light of later problems with land sales.[5] Entrepreneurial RHAs did their best to maintain rapid progress and back up the Government. The West Midlands RHA was unexpectedly caught out when planned over-commitments did not materialise, forcing it to postpone schemes when the Treasury declined its request for 'unconventional' (private) finance. They were not alone.[6] The decade of steady post-1962 growth in HCHS capital investment was thus followed by a period of fifteen years in which there was limited growth in real terms (Figure A1). At 1961 prices hospital capital expenditure was generally around £80 million per annum in the period covered by this chapter, dropping to a little over £60 million per annum in the late 1970s. This can be compared with the Ministry's aspirations, when negotiating with the Treasury for the original Plan. The Ministry had pointed out that RHB submissions totalled some £800 million, implying a programme of £80 million per annum for ten years from 1962. At 1961 prices – for comparison with pre-Plan discussions – it took until mid-1976 for £800 million to be spent on hospital capital, and the Ministry had argued that even this would leave them short of a replacement level of investment. And expenditure then dropped back to 1970 levels in the latter years of the 1974–9 government, though the upward trend in capital spending resumed in the years prior to the reforms. While in terms of expenditure there are continuities here between Labour and Conservative governments, a more commercial and localist emphasis is evident in the policies of the latter, but neither government succeeded in accelerating the renewal of the hospital stock.

The implications of the foregoing events for the management of the capital programme can be explored through enquiries by government select committees, and through the records of individual health authorities. The 1973 cuts brought to a close a sustained period of expansion in the building programme. The pressures on the government required that these cuts be made quickly without detailed analysis of their social impacts. The Commons Expenditure Committee asked why they had affected the building programme at all, and suggesting that it had been an 'arbitrary decision ... (involving) no attempt at assessing priorities'. The government had, however, decided that the impact of the cuts should be 'even, proportionate ... on all programmes'. Nor had it proved possible to take account of the social impacts, especially the regional dimension of public expenditure planning: 'it would not have been possible to obtain the required reductions if we were to say that no reductions must fall on the assisted areas',[7] a comment of particular relevance to the Newcastle RHB, much of which was eligible for regional policy assistance. New capital development had already been subject to a moratorium from September 1973, and the effect of this and the cuts was that no new NHS schemes were started between then and March 1974. In any given year about two-thirds of the capital programme was committed to ongoing projects; cuts could therefore only be made by stopping new projects.

A corollary of the postponement of new starts was a substantial reduction in the proportion of capital devoted to new hospital construction (Figure A2). Only after the Hospital Plan had this figure exceeded 20 per cent; it rose to over 40 per cent by the early 1970s, peaking at 44.8 per cent of capital expenditure in 1976–7. Thereafter it fell swiftly back to around 25 per cent, reflecting cutbacks in capital programmes, and also (after 1980) a shift in policy aimed at the retention of physical assets.

The effects of such cutbacks on the hospital infrastructure included the retention of inefficient buildings, the diseconomies of being unable to bring new buildings fully into use, and wasteful small-scale capital expenditure incurred in 'titivating up Dickensian buildings'.[8] Cutting the long-term capital programme was 'electorally slightly less disadvantageous than cutting current expenditure' (House of Commons 1977: 105–7; see also Bosanquet and Townsend 1980: 210; Pliatzky 1982: 147–61). The ramifications were that a substantial maintenance backlog was building up, but as a witness to the Expenditure Committee explained, it would have been a 'false economy' to proceed with capital investments under tight revenue constraints: the situation was a 'choice of evils'.[9] By the late 1980s a succession of reports questioned whether sufficient investment was being made to avoid deterioration in the capital stock. The value of the NHS Estate was some £25 billion but new capital investment, at only £400 million, represented barely 1.5 per cent of this. One estimate put the maintenance backlog at some £2 billion (see NAO 1987, 1988; Audit Commission, 1991).

Management of the building programme was the subject of several inquiries during the 1970s.[10] Many projects were experiencing inordinate delays because of alterations even after contracts had been signed. Part of the difficulty was that, because capital allocations had been small, as soon as there was a chance of a major building project, 'everybody goes like mad' to get it underway. In face of the pressures on RHBs and BGs to produce results, schemes were often rushed through and problems only became apparent later.[11] For the same reasons, and also because of rising inflation, cost control was problematic. Contractor bankruptcies and industrial disputes did not help. Although the BMA had indicated a greater support for standardisation, there was a feeling that modifications and increased cost resulted from 'undue deference to local hospital opinion', especially in teaching hospitals where 'fairly large ideas' about hospital development could reflect the 'individual professional wishes' of senior hospital staff.[12] While these were legitimate aspirations it was recognised that, particularly in teaching hospitals controlled by Boards of Governors, not enough had been done to rein in capital expenditure.

Ambitious development proposals also caused difficulties. The redevelopment of the Liverpool Royal Infirmary exemplified the problems – it was criticised as being constructionally suspect, costly, and inflexible (Committee of Public Accounts 1977). Cuts in the capital programme rendered such large schemes – the hospital ultimately cost over £54 million at 1977 prices – problematic and led to large delays between schemes; it was not possible to build such developments at one fell swoop without delaying large numbers of schemes elsewhere. When hospitals eventually came on stream, planning assumptions had changed and they were sometimes excessively equipped, large catering and heating capacity being a case in point.[13] It was obviously preferable to build in as few phases of development as possible, but in the circumstances policy was modified so that large projects were broken down into more manageable schemes.

To what extent do these problems represent a form of 'state failure', as the New Right would have it? Looking back at this period, it sometimes appears that blame for these failings is laid at the door of the public sector. Yet inflation, contractor bankruptcies, and industrial disputes, which were responsible for many problems, cannot be blamed on the NHS. It is true that there were weaknesses in cost control but the NHS appeared to be making progress towards getting on top of this. Criticisms of the inherent deficiencies of public procurement, as subsequently articulated by defenders of the Private Finance Initiative (PFI) (see chapter 9), therefore require qualification.

Given the constraints on the capital programme, guidance to health authorities indicated that the objective implicit in the Hospital Plan – of single-site DGHs – was no longer the be-all and end-all of planning. The changed resource picture meant that the creation of a DGH was 'essentially an organisational act – the welding together of all the appropriate hospital services into an operational entity' (DHSS 1975) as long as the sites in question were close enough to make this work. The Labour government's 'Priorities' documents (DHSS 1976b) placed a broadly similar emphasis on the retention of physical assets and on assessment of the flexibility and practicality of locally agreed solutions. Prominent doctors called for more refurbishment of existing facilities.[14] Retention of high-quality hospital buildings would allow some scaling back of the capital programme but carried the risk of preserving the existing distribution of assets. In all this, policies can be read as adaptations to a more austere climate and as being designed to reduce expectations (Smith 1984a). Attention shifted to ways of using the NHS's capital stock more efficiently.

The more general question raised by these developments was the purpose of capital investment. A DHSS working party reported at length on this (1979). It argued that while the building programme had experienced difficulties this did not detract from the need for such a programme. It argued that further thought should be given to the essential features of the DGH, operational groupings of units, the role of small hospitals and the implications of reliance on single-speciality hospitals. The implication, given the changing resource climate, was a 'strategy based on development from the inherited stock, with less detail in central guidance and more local appraisal' (DHSS 1979: 69), and attention to investment appraisal to assess the possibility of meeting service needs through ways that did not always involve new investment. The Royal Commission on the NHS (1979: 141–3), however, pointed out that the mean age of the hospital stock was sixty-one years, and compared the replacement rate of British hospitals unfavourably with experience elsewhere. Despite this the report hesitated to endorse a 'crash programme' of construction, and declined to suggest a figure for a desirable rate of investment, merely calling for a 'planned programme of replacement and upgrading'. There is no sign that the Conservatives endorsed this. Instead, they endorsed the idea of much greater community support for hospitals and also the retention of physical assets. There is also some evidence that, following their election, they proved more willing to reject hospital closure proposals than Labour; most famously, there was a reprieve for the Elizabeth Garrett Anderson Hospital for Women (and staffed exclusively by women) which had obtained a letter of support from Mrs Thatcher while in Opposition (Rivett 1998: 338). There were several similar examples[15] leading one prominent manager to complain that 'NHS managers and the public are being conned when we are told to keep small hospitals open and balance the books'.[16]

One emphasis, forced by changed political and economic circumstances, was thus the retention of physical assets. Another was an attempt to generate resources internally by realising the commercial value of 'surplus' NHS land and buildings. The Davies Report (1983) identified a widespread problem of under-utilisation of space, the unnecessary retention of surplus property, and an accumulated backlog of maintenance expenditure. A key policy which flowed from this was the use of receipts from sales of surplus NHS property to fund new capital developments. Some would argue (Rivett 1998) that, for a time, land sales were the only source of real growth in the capital programme. Proceeds from this source grew rapidly, from £7.5 million in 1978–9, peaking at some £270 million, falling back to some £200 million in the early 1990s. Subsequently, steady economic growth and a further property boom drove receipts for England to around the £500 million mark by 1998. Occasional regional breakdowns (Health Committee 1991a: Table 11.4) showed that £150 million of the 1988–9 receipts of £265 million accrued to the four Thames RHAs, but the corresponding total a year later was £87 million and for 1990–1, £66 million. Such fluctuations had severe adverse impacts on planning; in the case of NW Thames, projected sales were roughly equal to the RHA's capital allocation;[17] the region was therefore critically dependent on sales to achieve service developments. The problems that could arise are exemplified by the redevelopment of the Chelsea and Westminster Hospital. This *in situ* project was to be financed largely by sales of surplus sites released by the closure of four other hospitals within the DHA. The Public Accounts Committee was concerned that, although the scheme relied substantially on land sales, there had been no attempt to analyse the implications of any downturn in land values. The decision to proceed had been taken at the height of the 1980s property boom, which collapsed in 1989. At the same time, the capital cost of the scheme had risen substantially. The combination of these two pressures meant that estimated net expenditure on the project rose by £52 million. The consequence was that the region had had to postpone 300 schemes in planning, twenty-four of which were major schemes costing, in total, £120 million. They included substantial schemes in suburban or shire locations (Barnet, Watford, Luton, Bedford) which were postponed for between six and twenty-seven months (Committee of Public Accounts 1993: Table 4). Furthermore, the projected revenue savings were far less than had been anticipated.

The PAC also drew attention to the apparent priority given to a costly project in central London when policy was to redistribute funds towards the shire counties. Although the scheme did not result in a net addition to hospital capacity, it was suggested that a more modest scheme ought to have been feasible, which might also have retained more of the existing buildings. Concern was therefore expressed that these broader strategic considerations had not properly been taken into account.

This case demonstrates rather graphically that there was 'no obvious connection between the state of the property market and the need for capital investment in the NHS' (Robinson and Appleby 1991: 17). An income source which could vary so wildly did not provide a sound platform on which to develop a hospital strategy.

As well as boosting the capital programme – though simultaneously increasing the degree of dependence on locally generated resources – these developments contributed to a reappraisal of the management of the NHS estate. In the absence of clear criteria for the valuation and use of NHS property, capital had been regarded as a 'free good' (Mayston 1990). Critics argued that this led to inefficiencies in the use of capital and this argument, which had been broached from time to time, was to feature strongly in the NHS White Paper.

Of equal importance, in terms of the process of hospital development, was the availability of revenue funds to commission new hospitals and to operate old ones. Chapter 7 has shown that, in the context of Powell's revenue 'straitjacket', this proved problematic. In an attempt to deal with this the DHSS compensated RHBs for the Revenue Consequences of Capital Schemes (RCCS) but this gave health authorities no incentive for economy, and was abandoned as an instrument of national policy by the mid-1970s (Smith 1984c: 1368–9), though individual RHAs continued the policy. Health authorities were therefore faced with the costs of commissioning new buildings in an inflationary and austere financial climate, in which revenue assumptions changed dramatically: real-terms revenue growth in the NHS declined from 3.75 per cent in 1973–4 to below 2 per cent after 1978 (Committee of Public Accounts 1981). Moreover, attempts were being made by central government to shift resources more firmly in the direction of priority services, at the expense of the acute hospital sector. These pressures also contributed to the growing maintenance backlog: forced to fund the revenue consequences of new developments from their own resources, the result was that health authorities cut back on maintenance expenditure.

The most visible result of revenue pressures was the mothballing of new buildings when health authorities lacked the funds to open them. Twelve hospitals featured in a Public Accounts Committee investigation of such delays, which had led to several thousand beds being unused as a consequence.[18] Other hospitals were affected as well, such as the Freeman Road Hospital in Newcastle, in 1981.[19] Such problems brought long-term planning into disrepute.

A further consequence of a constrained revenue climate was pressure on health authorities to close hospitals, whether or not alternative provision had been made available. The problems were especially acute in locations from which resources were being transferred as a result of recommendations of the Resource Allocation Working Party (RAWP) (DHSS 1976b). On the calculations made by RAWP, London (and various other urban locations) was deemed to be over-provided with hospital services, though opponents argued that high levels of hospital provision compensated for social deprivation and for poor primary care (the debate is expertly reviewed by Mays and Bevan 1987). By redistributing hospital revenue, in accord with various criteria of need, the aim was to even-up disparities in expenditure, between and within regions. The main losers were inner London health authorities and even in the financial climate of the late 1970s there were likely to be problems. There were efforts to coordinate and plan the city's hospital services, through various pan-London committees, such as the London Health Planning Consortium (1980), but lacking accountability and resources, these foundered (Rivett 1998: 334–6). The King's Fund (1987) echoed criticisms of an earlier era, in arguing that London's segmentation into four quadrants, controlled by separate RHAs, led to 'back-to-back' planning. As the RAWP recommendations continued to be implemented under revenue allocations which entailed real-term reductions in revenue budgets in some inner London areas, the result in many locations was a rapid run-down of hospital capacity (London Health Emergency 1987). Service rationalisation began to contribute proportionately more towards cost improvements; such savings increased from £28 million in 1985–6 to £69 million in 1990–1 (Mohan 1995: Table 1.2). Health authorities were having great difficulty in planning the development of their hospitals. Transfers from capital to revenue, deferrals of maintenance expenditure, and delaying of desirable service developments were all identified in surveys by the National Association of Health Authorities (1988) and inquiries by the National Audit Office (1989) and there was evidence that the problems were widespread, rather than being local difficulties (Mohan 1995: 84–6). In part as a response, the 1980s were characterised by an examination of alternative ways of organising the NHS, entailing greater competition between hospitals, the argument being that 'inefficient' hospitals had no incentive to improve their performance. Competition was also encouraged in the sense that health authorities were given greater freedom to generate income, one aspect of which was a degree of friction with the private health sector.

On the face of it this period was one in which hospital planning faced severe challenges. External circumstances and political decisions constrained both capital and revenue expenditure and, at times and in certain places, hospital development appeared a fraught and crisis-prone process. In response, there was eventually a questioning of the extent to which planning was really the problem, rather than the solution, and this resulted in pro-competitive policies which will be examined in the next chapter.

Policy by default? Localism, standardisation and centralisation

Can a consistent philosophy underpinning hospital policy be discerned in this period? Apart from a short-lived consultation paper (DHSS 1980a), and some general guidance to health authorities, there was no official statement of policy aims, but regional planning documents (NRHA 1979, 1986, 1991) affirm the centrality of the DGH concept. However, drawing on reactions to centralisation in the previous decade, the first point of note is a scaling down of ambitions, and proposals to retain small facilities as 'community' hospitals.

Reactions to the Hospital Plan indicated a strong desire to retain many local hospitals but it was not always clear where they would fit into the hospital service. There had been pioneering initiatives in the Oxford RHB, which saw community hospitals as extensions of primary care. In this sense the lineage of community hospitals went back to the Dawson Report with its emphasis on keeping patients out of expensive general hospitals. The Oxford initiative was adopted as a more general policy. An official circular explained that patients admitted to such hospitals had to satisfy three criteria: they needed care which could not easily be provided in their homes; they were not expected to require highly specialised care or special investigation; and they would benefit from care nearer home, to facilitate visiting and maintenance of links with the local community (DHSS 1974). While surgery, obstetrics and pathology were excluded, some general medical and short-term admission beds could be provided, as could outpatient clinics, and local GPs were to be given a role in management. The idea was to clarify the concept of a community hospital, rather than leaving it, by default, as the retention of existing hospitals. It was suggested that a size range of 50–150 beds was appropriate. The professional concern was that the underlying philosophy of community hospitals was not clear. Rather than saving money, it was possible that they could be filled by people who would otherwise have been nursed at home; they could therefore be an 'extravagance'. There was also scepticism – particularly from 1976, when capital cuts really hit home – that the purpose of the community hospitals policy was to provide a respectable argument for retention of old hospitals which should have been closed. The government was linking the community hospitals policy to their revised guidelines for standardisation in hospital construction. These limited the size of the first phase of new hospital building projects to 300 beds; the inference was that the rest could be found in community hospitals. There was potentially a 'dangerous confusion' between community hospitals as 'an extension of primary care and as a cheap way of bolstering inadequate hospital services'.[20] For some, the policy document did not clarify the role of the DGH and thus its definition of the community hospital was correspondingly vague.[21] Nevertheless, whatever the intellectual justification of the policy, health authorities now had the option of providing new community hospitals in locations previously lacking hospital services, as well as retaining threatened institutions in a new guise. Thus the Northern RHA established community hospitals in locations which had been identified as among the more disadvantaged within the region, such as Blyth, Penrith and Brotton (Cleveland). In the latter case the region was able to respond to pressure from the eastern part of Cleveland, where the Langbaurgh District Council had agitated for some years that a DGH should be located in this area. Even when agreed for a 1985 start, however, building of this hospital was delayed until the early 1990s (Townsend 1986). In Blyth, too, there had been considerable political reaction and pressure when hospital services had been transferred elsewhere.[22] But one of the first community hospitals to open in the region, a hospital which had actually been reopened with community fund-raising, closed again within five years due to revenue shortages.[23]

The period also saw the last statement of official policy on hospital size. Given some of the developments described in the previous section, the proposals of the Conservatives' consultation paper on 'the future pattern of hospital provision in England' (DHSS 1980a) did not come out of the blue.

This paper proposed to restrict the maximum size of acute general hospitals to no more than 450–600 beds, with up to another 200 beds in regional specialities where appropriate. Evidence was not presented for the rather vague generalisations offered. Small hospitals allegedly facilitated staff recruitment and had better relationships with the local community, whereas DGHs were said to be impersonal, relatively inaccessible and administratively complex. It was asserted that the NHS could not afford to lose physical assets – but compare the emphasis, within three years, on the identification and disposal of surplus land and property. Because of pressure on acute services, patients not needing the 'full panoply of investigation and treatment' could be catered for in peripheral hospitals. It followed that small hospitals were to be retained wherever 'sensible and practicable', and since this could lead to higher running costs (due to service duplication and movement of staff between hospitals) the DHSS urged that such financial consequences were 'properly assessed in advance'. Because the potential for increased expenditure had been admitted, it was claimed that the proposals were not a 'means to secure a reduction in planned capital expenditure'. Thus the emphasis had shifted from a concentration of services in a small number of single-site DGHs, to a more spatially decentralised pattern of provision.

Critics complained that the proposals were littered with non-specific observations and sweeping generalisations. The document relied heavily on the self-evident truth of its 'small is beautiful' case, and on tendentious propositions, such as the assertion that relationships with the community were better with small hospitals (e.g. Harrison *et al.* 1980). The claim that there was a maximum size above which diseconomies would develop was disingenuous, since the policy implied the retention of split-site hospitals, where presumably management and communication difficulties would be magnified. In addition, there were no references to providing hospitals in communities which presently lacked them, nor to the possibility of redeveloping existing facilities. The former could be seen as an inescapable consequence of the document's logic, while the latter would clearly be essential if future hospital policy was to be based on retaining the existing hospital stock. Such arguments lent weight to claims that the underlying motive behind the document was the restraint of capital expenditure, not a new departure towards a more flexible pattern of hospital provision. It was therefore an attempt to justify the *status quo*: hospital facilities had not been centralised, many single-speciality hospitals continued in existence, and staff worked on in decrepit surroundings (Smith 1984b: 1300). The National Association of Health Authorities criticised the document as a 'step back from 1962' and as a formula for 'perpetuating the haphazard supply of hospitals'.[24] The *British Medical Journal* dismissed the document as 'a dishonest response to a persisting lack of capital investment'.[25]

Analyses of trends in hospital size give some – albeit limited – insight into the impact of this policy (Figure A3). The logical outcome would have been a decline in the rate of closure of small hospitals, but the steady reduction in numbers of non-psychiatric hospitals continued, with the possible exceptions of 1981 and 1982. In the years 1977–80 the total number of hospitals with under 250 beds fell by between forty-two and sixty-five hospitals in each year, in 1981 by nineteen, and in 1982 by only three, but in 1983 the number in this size category declined by fifty-one and by sixty-three the following year. So if this policy had an impact, it was only evident for a couple of years before previous trends resumed, though the upward trend in 1983–4 may of course reflect a harsher revenue climate after the 1983 election.[26]

The local impact of the policy reflected the historical legacy of hospital provision in each area. In the Northern region, all the acute hospitals with over 600 beds contained regional or sub-regional specialities. Development proposals in some of these locations were constrained by the revised policy guidance. In Newcastle, proposals to extend the teaching hospital to 1,200 beds were scaled back to 700 beds, provoking substantial criticism because this would complicate the proposed relocation of two specialist hospitals on to the RVI site[27] and this meant retention of hospitals whose physical infrastructure was beyond the end of its useful life.[28] In some other locations proposals for DGH development were agreed only on condition that small hospitals, previously earmarked for closure, were to be retained.[29] This consultation document was the last formal attempt to spell out a national policy on the nature of acute hospital provision (Harrison and Prentice 1998: 3), but outlines of policy may be inferred from other sources.

First, there has been a move away from the idea of a national plan or blueprint, supervised bureaucratically from the centre. Following the decentralist philosophies of the Griffiths Report (DHSS 1983b), the Department of Health withdrew progressively from the detailed scrutiny of hospital building. From the late 1970s building plans were to be related to region's service-led strategic plans (as opposed, one might put it, to being purely a list of desirable building projects). From 1981, plans were required to integrate service developments with revenue, staff and capital assumptions. Put another way, individual health authorities had a responsibility to ensure that, when capital developments were proposed, the revenue was available to sustain them. Over-ambitious programmes would no longer be bailed out by devices such as RCCS (Paton and Bach 1990: 134–5).

Second, there was an increased emphasis on standardisation. The Department's original proposal – the 'Harness' concept – proved vulnerable to the changed economic climate.[30] The impetus for standardisation derived from the public expenditure cutbacks of the early 1970s which led David Owen to argue that 'the desirable will not always be obtainable'. Howard

Goodman, at the time chief architect at the DHSS, later stated that Owen was nonetheless determined to 'preserve every scheme in the building programme'.[31] This was achieved through the 'Nucleus' hospital. This was to comprise a first-phase development of *c.* 300 beds capable of expansion up to 900 beds. The intention was to limit provision (e.g. of ancillary or laboratory services) to what was needed to sustain the first phase, thus avoiding excessively large service departments. There was some, albeit limited, scope for variations in content. Nucleus would thus provide basic self-contained general hospitals in one phase, avoiding the lengthy multi-phase developments of the 1960s.[32] The cost advantages were substantial: first-phase Nucleus hospitals were estimated to cost only around £6 million at 1975 prices. Reflecting concern with economy, there have been criticisms that the accommodation in Nucleus designs left much to be desired (Smith 1984c). It was also suggested that an overtly centralist approach was pursued: one of 'Nucleus or nothing' (Smith 1984b: 1370). Nearly 60 per cent of suitable schemes adopted Nucleus designs (NAO 1990: paras. 3.17, 3.18), but following a Public Accounts Committee investigation, it became official policy to challenge *every* case in which a health authority chose not to use Nucleus (Committee of Public Accounts 1990: vii). Given that bed norms had in effect been abandoned as a means of planning, Nucleus thus represented the only element of national standardisation still in use in hospital development, and also one which hospital authorities had little choice but to accept. Development work on Nucleus was eventually abandoned after the NHS reforms, but the establishment of autonomous Trusts, responsible for their own capital programmes, made it logically impossible to impose standard designs anyway.

Thus, the period witnessed a mixture of standardisation and flexibility. Because of resource constraints, both Labour and Conservative governments sought to make maximum use of the existing building stock, opening up scope for greater local responsiveness. This apparent decentralisation was accompanied by greater central government control, in terms of hospital closure decisions and an insistence on standard design solutions for hospitals.

Developments in the Northern Region

Managing the capital programme

Much of the period was characterised by efforts to minimise the disruptive consequences of the foregoing fluctuations in the capital programme. The Northern RHA strove to retain as many of its highest priorities as appeared possible but there were lengthy delays in respect of some key projects. Comparisons between the 1979 and 1985 Regional Strategic Plans are instructive, particularly in the light of pre-1974 information on the progress of capital schemes. For example, Middlesbrough General Hospital was to have been superseded by at least one new DGH in South Cleveland; its inadequacies (and the impracticability of a comprehensive redevelopment scheme) had been recognised since at least the preparations for the Hospital Plan, but the start date of the promised South Cleveland Hospital was repeatedly put back, followed by delays in subsequent schemes. In Carlisle, the long-awaited second phase of the Cumberland Infirmary redevelopment, initially scheduled to commence in 1977, had not found a place in the 1979 Regional Strategic Plan (RSP) (Northern RHA, 1979). It was at 'approval in principle' stage when the 1985 version was drawn up, but had not been built by the time of the NHS reforms. Various public schemes formulated up to 1996 proposed refurbishment of existing buildings but the redevelopment finally took place under a privately funded scheme, nearly thirty years after originally planned. A similar story could be told of hospital redevelopments in Gateshead, where phase 3 was postponed for three years in 1976, and phase 4, scheduled originally for 1979, had not begun by 1985. The new DGH for North Tyneside (the former SE Northumberland HMC) was scaled back, in common with many projects coming on stream in the mid- 1970s; it eventually commenced in 1980. This meant the continued retention of the Preston Hospital (North Shields) which had been declared obsolete by the wartime surveyors; as a consequence, the Newcastle RHB spent over £1 million on this hospital between 1948 and 1974.[33] While the 1979 *RSP* envisaged completion of stage 3 of South Shields General by 1987–8, this had slipped to 1989 by the time of the 1985 *RSP* and less than one-third of the estimated capital cost had been spent by 1987.[34]

Perhaps more revealing is the statement in the 1985 *RSP* that likely capital resources would be short of total requirements by some £27 million over the period up to 1992–3. Among schemes for which no place could be found by 1985 were proposals for later stages of the redevelopment of the EMS hospitals at Durham, Bishop Auckland and Shotley Bridge. These had benefited to a degree from post-war capital investment, but complete redevelopment of these hospitals had not been possible. During the 1980s next to nothing was spent on upgrading these facilities.[35] One reason for the delay, which carried some echoes of debates in the 1930s, was uncertainty over where to locate hospitals against a background of a scattered settlement pattern and in the context of changing philosophies about hospital size. Again echoing the 1930s, the western area of County Durham experienced large-scale de-industrialisation in the 1970s and 1980s, leading to concerns that the population could not justify two DGHs, and only one was eventually built, in Durham, but intended to serve the catchment of the former Shotley Bridge General as well as the Durham area (Chapter 9). Given that, by 1989, the reforms were in the pipeline, it would have been rational for the RHA to put on hold schemes that, in the new marketplace, risked being unviable, and the result was yet more delay in the redevelopment of services in these locations.

Some of these delays might also be attributed in part to disputes about hospital configuration and strategy. This was the case in Durham, where there were ongoing debates about how best to serve the Easington district in the east of the county. Though located within the Durham AHA, this area fell within the catchments of – and was largely served by – hospitals in Sunderland and Hartlepool. In a bid for self-sufficiency the Durham AHA had proposed a two-DGH solution, one at Durham and one at Peterlee. Lack of agreement on this was only resolved in early 1980 but, for as long as the issue was in dispute, progress could not be made on redeveloping the EMS hospital, Dryburn, in Durham. There were also demands – including a petition, signed by 50,000 people – for a DGH in Washington New Town. This was under the jurisdiction of Sunderland health authority, and while the authority's intention had been to provide two DGHs, consideration of where best to locate them had to take account of demands from Washington. The decision eventually went against Washington but this was at the expense of some delay.

In what we might now see as a last throw of the dice for RHA-level capital planning, the RHA reviewed its capital strategy just before the NHS reforms (NRHA 1991). It analysed in considerable detail the distribution of actual and projected capital investment in the 1971–2001 period (making the assumption that schemes in the pipeline as firm commitments would actually be built). Between DHAs, capital investment at constant prices had varied substantially (Table 8.1). In this period, North Tyneside, Newcastle and South Tees led the way (column A), reflecting major expenditures on new or redeveloped DGHs. At the other end of the spectrum, *per capita* investment in Durham was the equivalent of 2 per cent of that spent in North Tyneside, while South West and North West Durham likewise received a fraction of the money spent in some more favoured locations. The data give East Cumbria a slightly anomalous ranking because they assume that the projected redevelopment of the Cumberland Infirmary (Carlisle) would proceed as planned. It eventually did, but under a PFI scheme (see Chapter 9) which meant that it was scaled down in size. The North Tees and West Cumbria figures are also somewhat anomalous, because these areas received new hospitals prior to 1971. The analysis by the RHA has therefore been extended by reaggregating pre-1971 capital expenditure at 1991 prices to the post-1982 DHAs, and adding this to the 1971–2001 figures. This gives a picture of the intra-regional pattern of investment from 1948–91 which includes projected expenditure to 2001. It reveals (column J) a fourfold variation within the region between West Cumbria and North Tyneside on the one hand, and the West Durham and Durham DHAs. Over a period of nearly fifty years five areas received (or were projected to receive) less than two-thirds the regional average level of investment. The Newcastle figures (which are underestimates: see Chapter 7) partly reflect investment in regional specialities; they also indicate the priority given to the city, which had exercised the Ministry in the 1960s. Thus the pattern of investment for the post-1971 period was a continuation of trends in the first two decades of the NHS. The comment that the RHA had pursued a 'clear strategy with a steady purpose' (NRHA 1991) over the past 20–25 years, with the aim of providing a DGH in every district, therefore had some justification, but extreme patience might have been added as a rider, given the delays experienced in some locations.

Nevertheless, the data presented provided ample justification, were it needed, for attaching top priority to developments in North and South Durham, followed by South Teesside and Hexham. Other developments, ranked slightly lower but no less important, in the RHA's view, remained as the completion of the Wansbeck DGH, a major redevelopment in Sunderland and a substantial investment at Newcastle General. The order in which schemes were to proceed was significant: the Sunderland scheme was so large that it would have pre-empted resources for the two Durham developments, pushing them still further back into the future. As it turned out those areas passed the fiftieth anniversary of the NHS without substantial renewal of their hospitals.

Impacts of revenue constraints on hospital development

In common with other health authorities in this period, the revenue budget was tightly constrained especially once cash limit control of expenditure had been introduced – and subsequently made legally binding. Moreover, despite the apparently decentralist philosophy of the Conservatives, in practice they centralised control over RHAs and their subordinates. Thus hospital capacity featured as an issue in regional and district reviews of performance. Thus, notwithstanding the scattered population and dilapidated hospital infrastructure the region was still required to explain its high beds-to-population ratio. DHAs were made aware of the need to consider withdrawal of entire areas of service, or the closure of whole hospitals, though one DHA objected that they had gone as far as they could towards a statistical norm.[36] Subsequently the 1986 version of the RHA's Strategic Plan envisaged reductions of some 8 per cent of acute beds by 1995 (Northern RHA 1986: 117).

The result of such pressures, in combination with a difficult revenue position, was that rationalisation of bed provision, and the pace of hospital closures, quickened. As is evident from Figure A4, a number of hospitals, often small and single-speciality units, were closed, mainly on Tyneside and Teesside, in this period. There were complaints that some of these closures were taking place in advance of the opening of new or replacement facilities. The debates can be illustrated with reference to events in Newcastle.[37]

The city's hospitals had actually been unified under one HMC from 1971; this was designed to facilitate integration of medical education and research with the work of the rest of the city's hospitals. The hospitals were of varying quality, the revenue budget proved to be above-target according to RAWP principles, and the health authority had a substantial commitment

Table 8.1 Distribution of capital investment within the Northern RHA, 1948–2001

	A Capital investment, 1971–2001, per head of 1991 population, 1991 prices £	B 1991 resident population (000s)	C Total expenditure at 1991 prices £	D Share of regional total %	E Share of regional population %	F Ratio of share of investment to share of population, 1971–2001	G Capital investment, 1948–71, at 1991 prices £	H Total capital investment, 1948–2001 at 1991 prices £	I Share of regional total %	J Ratio of share of investment to share of population 1948–2001
North Tyneside	469	149.2	69,974,800	10.18	5.1	2.0	9,448,000	79,422,800	7.78	1.52
West Cumbria	127	130.4	16,560,800	2.41	4.46	0.54	48,987,000	65,547,800	6.42	1.44
Newcastle	390	520.7	203,073,000	29.55	17.81	1.66	46,454,000	249,527,000	24.44	1.37
Darlington	269	120.1	32,306,900	4.7	4.11	1.14	23,047,000	55,353,900	5.42	1.32
Northumberland	251	211.4	53,061,400	7.72	7.23	1.07	35,342,000	88,403,400	8.66	1.2
East Cumbria	303	165.9	50,267,700	7.31	5.67	1.29	19,085,000	69,352,700	6.79	1.2
South Tees	311	297.9	92,646,900	13.48	10.19	1.32	25,661,000	118,307,900	11.59	1.14
North Tees	137	186.4	25,536,800	3.72	6.38	0.58	32,249,000	57,785,800	5.66	0.89
South Tyneside	222	139.6	30,991,200	4.51	4.78	0.94	12,089,000	43,080,200	4.22	0.88
Hartlepool	265	128.8	34,132,000	4.97	4.41	1.13	2,064,000	36,196,000	3.55	0.8
Gateshead	153	173.2	26,499,600	3.86	5.92	0.65	11,461,000	37,960,600	3.72	0.63
NW Durham	24	94.9	2,277,600	0.33	3.25	0.1	18,310,000	20,587,600	2.02	0.62
Sunderland	125	326.5	40,812,500	5.94	11.17	0.53	20,665,000	61,477,500	6.02	0.54
Durham	11	153.1	1,684,100	0.25	5.24	0.05	20,599,000	22,283,100	2.18	0.42
SW Durham	59	125.4	7,398,600	1.08	4.29	0.25	8,176,000	15,574,600	1.53	0.36
	235	2,923.5	687,223,900	100	100		333,637,000	1,020,860,900	100	

Source: Cols. A–C: Northern RHA 1991; Cols. D–J: author's calculations from Northern RHA (1991) and Newcastle RHB Annual Accounts (1948–71).

Note: This table does not include the South Cumbria DHA, which joined the Northern RHA at the 1974 reorganisation; pre-1971 data was not available for this area.

to commissioning the new hospital at Freeman Road. A central issue which required resolution was whether the city should have two or three main general hospitals. The view that a two-hospital solution was ideal had been evident throughout the debates in the 1960s. There ensued successive consultation documents, strategic plans and reviews, such as the 'one hospital on three sites' exercise of 1981, and the Hospital Services Review of 1988.

These exercises were driven by issues such as duplication and bed ratios. Newcastle was seen as over-provided in paediatric and general beds.[38] The most important issue therefore concerned whether or not Newcastle should have three general hospitals, but, among other things, children's acute services were provided in five sites and this was clearly unsustainable. Opponents of changes pointed to the evidence that Newcastle's residents still faced difficulties in accessing the city's hospitals. The counter-argument to this was that the pressures on Newcastle were due to inflows of patients from other parts of the region, and the prospective opening of new DGHs elsewhere in the region would eventually relieve the pressure. These arguments cut little ice, leading one union official to accuse the RHA of basing its arguments 'on facilities that had not been built',[39] such as the new hospitals in Northumberland and North Tyneside. The most vulnerable of the three acute hospitals in the city was Newcastle General. It was generally agreed that its buildings were decrepit and that, long-term, substantial investment would be required. The detailed Hospital Services Review (Newcastle DHA 1988: 12) envisaged that while '*ideally* Newcastle should have two hospitals rather than three, the current realities and future probabilities make it highly improbable that a reduction to two could be achieved' (emphasis added). As in the 1960s the probability of obtaining the necessary resources and support for a two-hospital solution was thought to be so low as to be not worth pursuing. The complexities of redevelopment and the associated transitional costs were deemed so great that this option was discounted. The review, therefore, argued against the gung-ho proponents of a two-hospital solution, and favoured three DGHs, each of which would offer general medical, surgical and paediatric treatment; otherwise, all other specialities would be concentrated on one site only, with one substantial Trauma Centre at Newcastle General. As late as July 1991, when the RHA considered its capital priorities, substantial funds were allocated to its redevelopment. As shown in Chapter 9, however, these arguments were swiftly undercut by the reforms.

In parallel with these arguments the health authority had to find revenue to commission Freeman Road and also persuade the Government to approve a crucial development – a new Ward Block (*c.* 400 beds) at the RVI. This was approved by the Conservatives but, as one of a number of decisions which followed their revised policy document on hospital size in 1980, the ultimate size of the redeveloped hospital was cut back from 1,200 to 700 beds. Moreover, a *quid pro quo* for the decision was that Freeman Road be fully commissioned. The combination of these two constraints was significant from the point of view of other hospitals in the city. It meant that proposals to relocate specialist units to the RVI involved an even more complex juggling act given the restrictions on the size of the hospital. And the commissioning of Freeman Road severely strained the revenue budget of the health authority.

We can relate the fate of several hospitals in the city to these changing circumstances. Initially there were closures of small, peripheral units in 1976 and 1977 – a small accident hospital (Walker Park) in the east end; the specialist Babies' Hospital; the Sanderson Orthopaedic (subsequently reopened for a different purpose). While such measures staved off insolvency up to *c*. 1979, the financial position then worsened dramatically because of an uncompensated increase in VAT, plus inflation running at around 16 per cent. The health authority was faced with simultaneously coping with commissioning a new hospital, balancing acute hospital provision across three main sites, and attempting to respond to demands for improvements in priority services, all against this sombre financial background. Unplanned, temporary closures were contemplated on several occasions, including the large Walkergate Hospital (a former isolation hospital, used almost wholly for geriatric patients), the effect of which would have been to reduce below acceptable minima the existing services for the elderly without providing replacement facilities. Pressures on revenue continued in the period up to the NHS reforms, resulting in repeated proposals for temporary and/or permanent closures of hospitals or parts thereof. These are described in some detail by Newcastle Health Concern (1986) and so this section uses selected hospitals to exemplify the general position. The Fleming Memorial Hospital for Sick Children was considered for closure on three occasions before succumbing in 1987; at various stages there were also proposals to close institutions such as the Princess Mary Maternity Hospital, Walkergate, Lemington and Ponteland.

It would, in fact, be difficult to argue a case against the closure of these hospitals, given the poor quality of their buildings and equipment, and their isolation from links with colleagues and from other specialist support. If these units had been retained, due to public pressure, with consequential closures elsewhere, this would mean that deliberate decisions had been made to support inefficient hospitals. However, regardless of the merits of these particular hospitals, closure proposals came forward in response to revenue pressures rather than as part of a planned process in which new capacity replaced old. The Fleming example is instructive, since the original intention was to close this hospital once a major redevelopment was commissioned at the RVI. That happy event eventually took place in 1992; Fleming had actually closed over four years previously and the decision to close it was taken before the contract had been awarded for construction of the Ward Block. As a further indication of this being a revenue-driven closure, it took place while the Hospital Services Review debate was taking place, and although there was no doubt that the Fleming would eventually close, there still remained issues to resolve, concerning the disposition of beds at the RVI, to which it was to move. A similar case could be made in respect of the Princess Mary Maternity Hospital. Again, no one contested the need to avoid duplication and integrate the facilities into the RVI, but dovetailing it neatly with the Ward Block development and the Hospital Services Review was difficult.

Although the hospitals closed in Newcastle in this period were difficult to incorporate into a long-term vision, the point made here is that, Freeman Road and the RVI apart, all the other eight non-psychiatric hospitals in the city were candidates for closure during this period, and with the exception of Walkergate, all eventually closed. Moreover, in common with DHAs elsewhere, closures were proposed and effected as a consequence of direct revenue pressures and (in some cases) before replacement facilities were available.[40] This was a process driven by financial, not clinical, criteria. In terms of the trajectory of hospital development, it appeared some distance from the ideal of a planned process in which new or replacement facilities smoothly superseded old ones.

Charity and commerce: voluntary fundraising and the expansion of the private sector

To what extent was the pattern of hospital provision influenced by developments external to the NHS, and what implications did this have for planning and regulation? This period was characterised by the growth of charitable funding for the NHS, and an expansion of the private sector. Both of these are bound up with political strategies towards, and policies for, the NHS. They can be seen, in common with developments elsewhere, as efforts to diversify the sources of capital for health care, and as responses to growing socio-economic differentiation.

Charitable fundraising for health care certainly had not disappeared in 1948 but it was largely confined to the promotion of medical research and patient welfare (for the development of policy see Mohan and Gorsky 2001: 91–102). However, the Conservatives envisaged an expanded role for charity, consistent with their emphasis on decentralisation, localism and disengaging the state. Hence, the Health Services Act of 1980 empowered health authorities to organise their own charitable appeals; these could, for example, permit communities to step in and rescue threatened hospitals.[41] In addition to financial advantages, this would 'stimulate community involvement and interest in the health service', and advantageous terms were considered, such as the possibility of transferring hospitals to voluntary organisations at 'peppercorn rents'.[42] Interestingly, Patrick Jenkin (Secretary of State for Social Services) at one point referred to the NHS as a series of local services, responsive to local needs and with a strong involvement from the local community (quoted in Klein 1985: 196). Despite this emphasis, the novel feature of the 1980s was the raising and application of charitable funds for major capital projects (Williams 1989; Lattimer 1996).

The most well known of these was the national 'Wishing Well' appeal for the redevelopment of the Great Ormond Street Children's Hospital. As a flagship for the charitable sector it could hardly have been more successful, raising far more than its target, but it was nevertheless criticised. On planning grounds it might have been more rational to sell the Great Ormond Street site and rebuild on a redundant (and more accessible) hospital site in the Outer Metropolitan Area, close to the M25. The appeal implicitly pitted hospitals in different areas in competition with Great Ormond Street for funds (Williams 1989: 104). Clearly, not all hospitals could be 'wished well' in this way. Those that possessed such pulling power began to use it both to raise funds and to leverage additional resources from government (Lattimer 1996; see also Chapter 9).

There were also various attempts to transfer hospitals to charitable ownership, motivated by the prospect of diversifying the funding base and also escaping constraints (such as nationally agreed wage rates) associated with the NHS. The first to do so was also connected with the Great Ormond Street Children's Hospital; its country branch, Tadworth Court in Surrey, reopened in 1983, as a Trust, drawing funds from a range of sources. Around the same time, at least one health authority (the then SE Thames RHA) actively investigated the possibility of returning some hospitals to community ownership as charitable trusts, but the idea never came to fruition (SE Thames RHA, 1985). There is no systematic data on such transfers of control, but the Community Hospitals Association (CHA) identifies seven hospitals which have transferred out of the NHS into the ownership of charitable trusts. These are small hospitals of a 'cottage hospital' character, generally located in relatively prosperous small towns (Brackley (Northants), Holbeach (Lincs), Hoylake and Tarporley (Cheshire), Odiham (Hants), Rye (E. Sussex) and Tetbury (Gloucs)) indicating some limits to a strategy of returning hospitals to community control. Some former NHS hospitals have transferred to charitable ownership but taken on a new role, such as the Mildmay Hospital, in London, which now specialises in the care of people with AIDS. Other examples, which have not involved a change of ownership but which have involved diversification of institutional funding bases, are to be found in the growing community hospitals movement (see Emrys-Roberts 1991; Higgins 1993; Tucker and Bosanquet 1991). The hopes expressed by Jenkin and other Conservatives, that numerous hospitals would transfer out of the NHS, were thus realised only on a small scale. Substantial community involvement in hospital finance nevertheless continued, evidenced by the number and scale of charitable appeals throughout the country. At the same time, of course, direct community representation in the NHS itself was being reduced through various organisational reforms. 'Active citizenship' was taking place without an extension of active governance (Kearns 1992).

The period also saw a steady expansion of the private hospital sector. This was partly a result of autonomous trends, such as greater segmentation in the labour market, so that companies were providing more benefits, such as health insurance, to their most-valued employees. It also reflected government action and inaction. These developments have ramifications for the acute hospital services. The private sector contributes substantially to elective surgery in certain areas; opportunities for private practice impact on the distribution of consultant staff, and private hospitals also compete with the NHS for other personnel. Growth in the private sector thus raises questions about how the public-private mix is regulated.

Perhaps the greatest single stimulus to private-sector growth was the 1974–9 Labour Government's attempt to eliminate private practice from NHS hospitals. This manifesto commitment did not extend to abolishing private medical care altogether; there was Cabinet concern that, if private hospitals were not allowed to develop, 'we should lose a lot of revenue from rich overseas patients' (Castle 1980: 704). The signal to the private sector was crystal-clear: the development of separate private hospitals would be essential. The issue became one of how best to regulate the public–private mix in any given locality. Labour established the Health Services Board (HSB), which oversaw the phasing-out of pay-beds, and sought to regulate private hospital development by requiring HSB approval for hospitals above a given size. The withdrawal of pay-beds was pursued steadily if unevenly; some rural areas were virtually exempt because pay-beds could not be withdrawn from NHS hospitals if there was thought to be insufficient demand locally to support a private hospital, while most of the beds withdrawn were under-utilised anyway.[43] The controls on private hospital developments affected very few hospitals – the great majority of hospitals fell below the size threshold above which HSB approval was required (Mohan 1986). Moreover, the HSB operated at the level of individual hospitals; it had no powers to regulate the *cumulative* effect of several developments in a locality notwithstanding negative effects on the NHS (e.g. competition for scarce staff) in locations containing several private hospitals, such as central London. Thus Labour's policies, perhaps paradoxically, produced a climate in which the private sector arguably knew exactly where it stood and the result was a steady expansion in private capacity outside the NHS, largely unaffected by the limited regulations that were put in place.

The Royal Commission on the NHS nevertheless concluded that the private sector was 'too small to make a significant impact on the NHS, except locally and temporarily' (Royal Commission 1979: 294). The Conservatives were apparently determined to change this, but the steps taken to encourage private sector expansion were limited and indirect, relating mainly to minor relaxations of regulations. While the Royal Commission had recommended that the HSB be empowered to assess the impact of the *total* numbers of private beds in a locality, the Government rejected this proposal, abolishing the Board and leaving only reserve powers to the Secretary of State to intervene if it were believed that the growth of private hospitals was interfering with the NHS in any given locality. Controls on private hospital development were thus largely neutralised after

1980 and this reserve power was removed with the 1989 reforms. Health authorities were also encouraged to take account of existing and planned capacity in the commercial sector (DHSS 1981). With hindsight, this might be seen as a first step towards an internal market, in which private and NHS hospitals compete with one another on the same terms. There were also some signs of partnerships, with private developers putting up capital for refurbishment of private wings of NHS hospitals.[44]

The expansion of private health care is well covered elsewhere (e.g. Griffith *et al.* 1987; Higgins 1988) so discussion here emphasises the implications for regulation and planning. The distribution of the private sector is skewed towards the most prosperous localities. While London remains dominant, there has been a relative shift of capacity to the Outer Metropolitan Area, an area benefiting more than almost any other in the UK from the economic growth of the 1980s. This concentration of opportunities for private practice has obvious ramifications for the distribution of consultant staff. In addition, the pattern of private facilities has the potential to influence the operation of the internal market, depending on where spare capacity is available, and the private sector is now a major player in terms of providing elective surgery. As long ago as 1986, some 30 per cent of the elective surgery in SW Thames took place in the private sector (Williams *et al.* 1989). Activity on this scale raises the question of how to balance public and private interests.

In the mid-1970s, the private sector had vigorously opposed the proposals of the HSB. While they could see its value in insulating them from competition by 'helping to secure a better distribution of private facilities' (Castle 1980: 557), they objected strongly to the actual size limitations above which independent hospitals would require certificates from the government (p. 695). Yet only a few years later there were requests for greater state intervention (Mohan 1986); this was implicit recognition that the absence of controls on private hospital location had contributed to over-capacity problems. A further criticism was that NHS authorities were not charging the full economic cost of pay-beds, because they were not obliged to cost their capital assets.[45] The continued existence of pay-beds was seen as a cause of over-bedding in the commercial sector, since private hospital developers had assumed that NHS pay-beds would be phased out. The reintroduction of pay-beds – about 600 were added during the 1980s, an increase of some 25 per cent (Laing 1993) – was unquestionably a response by health authorities to increasingly severe financial constraints in the NHS. It followed from the 1988 Health and Medicines Act, which freed NHS pay-bed units to charge commercial prices with a view to making profits, prompting several authorities to upgrade private wings and/or to develop dedicated pay-bed units.

Conversely there was growth in use of the private sector to treat NHS patients; just prior to the reforms, about half of all DHAs in England were believed to have made arrangements with the private sector for acute hospital treatment (Leadbeater 1990, quoted in Baggott 1998: 170). In these circumstances the map of hospital care in a locality would almost certainly include paybeds and a private hospital or two. Political and policy questions were therefore raised. Whether or not patients were treated publicly or privately was a matter of indifference to the Conservatives but the growth of private sector activity posed anew questions of regulation. In other countries, this might have taken the form of a certificate of need, as was the practice in the USA during the 1970s, in an attempt to reduce overcapacity. Such legislation was not likely to appeal to the Conservative government of the 1980s, and apart from attempts to monitor the extent of private practice by NHS consultants there have been no regulatory curbs on the private sector, either inside or outside the NHS. This contributes to overcapacity – and therefore waste of resources – and to pressures on local public health services (through migration of skilled staff). Neither of these problems have been satisfactorily resolved. The small scale of the private sector in the Northern RHA has meant that these issues have been posed with rather less urgency there, but that is not the case everywhere, particular concern being exercised about competition for staff.

Concluding comments

In this turbulent period for the NHS there was a struggle for supremacy between competing visions of how services would develop. There were severe frustrations with the hospital building programme, arising from delays in making the necessary funds available, but there was no overt challenge to the principle of DGH development, notwithstanding attempts to scale down commitments to large new hospitals and retain more assets. There were also policies which – in a climate of restricted resource growth – may be seen as harbingers of greater competition and localism, but equally there is evidence of centralisation, given the emphasis placed on standardisation.

To what extent does this period bear the hallmarks of an era of crisis management? Certainly the extracts from Castle's *Diaries*, and the evidence from individual health authorities, points to such a conclusion. The tight squeeze on the revenue budgets of health authorities meant that hospital development was a fraught process: many health authorities either failed to open new facilities or else closed old ones prematurely. Central government characteristically laid the blame for such developments on local health authorities, claiming credit, on the other hand, for illusory lists of building schemes.

For all these difficulties, nonetheless, planning remained in existence. The Northern RHA's 1991 review is an excellent example of a research-led strategy that made a serious analytical attempt at devising priorities. Reaggregating thirty years of data on capital investment, critically evaluating the condition of the estate, and assessing the accessibility and service implications of a range of options, this review presented a convincing case for capital investment. Through regression analysis, it was shown that, on past trends, capital investment had been a strong predictor of growth in caseload and, in fact, had had a stronger effect than growth in revenue expenditure. For every £100 spent, per head of population served, there would be an increase in caseload of some 4 per cent, over and above that expected with time (NRHA 1991: 21–2). It will be noted that this was a quite different justification for capital investment than that made in earlier decades. Revenue savings did not receive anything like the emphasis previously given to them though an estimate was made of them. It was also acknowledged that the real-terms cost of capital developments was rising; thus the scheme proposed for Durham entailed spending £460 per head of population, which if applied across the whole region would have presupposed a capital programme of over £650 million. As this would have been substantially more than the level of capital resources available to the RHA prior to 1991, the report perhaps wisely eschewed comment on the adequacy of the sums involved in its proposals, instead stressing that they would enable closure of the most important gaps. What was also missing was a discussion of how the increased caseload, which would result from new hospital investments, would be paid for, and also whether the hospital capacity thus created would be adequate. Such questions were to re-emerge with greater force after the reforms. This report nonetheless stands as a comprehensive region-wide analysis.

Though such analyses were still being conducted, the period was also one in which a different conception of planning came to be applied. Planning was now not about delivering specified lists of building schemes; instead, attention came to be focused on variations in utilisation and in health outcomes, and on variations in resource use by health authorities (with targets being set, for example, relating to bed turnover intervals or waiting times). Progressive though this no doubt was, there remained a need for the basic hospital infrastructure to be provided. Frustrations had emerged with the process of capital development which were only partly a function of the level of resources available to the NHS.

In such circumstances greater localism, pluralism and competition seemed to offer a way out. Health authorities and hospitals sought, with active state encouragement, to diversify sources of capital and/or to maximise the returns on their assets; this meant the growth of charitable and commercial fundraising, and the pursuit of opportunities for joint developments with the private sector. Given political and economic constraints on the NHS these can be read as attempts to depart from one of its defining principles, in the sense that market forces and local circumstances played a greater role in shaping the trajectory of hospital development. Nor was this accidental, given evidence of various measures by central government to encourage such initiatives.

If the 1960s were a period in which there was a shift from a Plan to a programme, the 1970s and 1980s look like a programme without a policy. A capital programme was pursued but there were so many sub-plots going on that no overarching logic can be detected. On the one hand, there was the continuation of central planning; on the other, the emergence of local initiative and proposals for competition between hospitals. This is where postmodern critics would contend the grand narratives of modernism – bureaucratic, centralised planning – have been brought into disrepute. Opponents of such arguments could equally point to the political management of welfare: localism and competition made a comeback precisely because of the failures of the state to deliver resources. Imposition of a grand template on this period, such as the argument that policy developments reflect an attempt to restructure state welfare so that it corresponds more closely to emergent economic structures following the demise of Fordism, oversimplifies a complex period of experimentation in service delivery. The mix of developments in this period thus created something of a policy vacuum – the old paradigms of planning were distrusted, but nothing had been put in their place. On the other hand the seeds of many post-1991 changes had been sown, which is why the NHS reforms can be characterised as a change of pace, not of direction. The pattern of health care would no longer be determined as part of a centralised, hierarchical plan; instead it would depend on the competitive qualities of individual hospitals.

9 Hospitals after the 1991 reforms

Markets, hierarchies or networks?

The NHS reforms drew inspiration from a range of sources and, as a consequence, they had multiple ramifications for policy. First, looking westwards, it was suggested that market forces could be reconciled with the public purposes of the NHS and thus eliminate inbuilt inefficiencies and perverse incentives. The ideas of the American health management specialist, Alain Enthoven (1985) were particularly important here, because they appeared to render feasible the introduction of markets without the electoral suicide of a fully competitive (i.e. insurance-based) system proposed by the New Right (e.g. Adam Smith Institute 1981, 1984; Letwin and Redwood 1988; Whitney 1988). Second, looking backwards, government advisers drew inspiration from traditions of voluntarism and, specifically, the autonomy enjoyed by voluntary hospitals before 1948 (Timmins 1995: 462); there began a search for ways of liberating hospitals from the dead hand of bureaucracy. Third, looking eastwards, the collapse of state socialism presented the government with an ideological reservoir on which to draw. They represented the NHS as a monolithic bureaucracy, born out of the same post-war circumstances in which communism had triumphed, but a system which was ultimately doomed. Malcolm Rifkind put this case well, claiming that when the NHS was established, it was believed that:

> the best way to administer resources was through a form of rigid, centralised planning. ... That view was shared in Eastern and Western Europe as well ... (but) a structure established 40 years ago does not necessarily make sense in the dramatically changed circumstances of the 1980s and 1990s ... in this country and elsewhere we have seen a growing disillusionment with central planning and control.[1]

In fact, having made such ringing declarations of intent, the Government were soon forced into their partial retraction. Thus, Health Secretary Virginia Bottomley declared, on the one hand, that the NHS must not slip back into the old ways of 'monolithic, oppressive over-planning',[2] but on the other hand, that 'the NHS is not a market, where the outcome is allowed to fall where it will, because it is a managed public service' (quoted by

Wistow 1992). The Conservatives were thus simultaneously implementing market reforms while denying they were doing so. After the 1997 election, Labour arguably had the opposite problem of insisting that it was not implementing market reforms, while actually relying on them (e.g. through private finance of hospital development). These tensions arise from the difficulties of grafting market incentives on to the existing structure of the NHS.

The NHS review, launched in the winter of 1987–8, quickly ruled out a fully fledged, insurance-based market system (because of the technical difficulties as well as the likely electoral consequences: Timmins 1995: 458–64) and instead sought to introduce an internal market. This meant that while the NHS's global budget was to be fixed, how it was spent was to be determined by competition. The White Paper which introduced the reforms (Secretary of State for Health 1989) proposed that the purchasing and providing responsibilities of health authorities should be separated. In future, health authorities (and budget-holding GPs) would place contracts with those hospitals they judged to provide the best quality services at the lowest price. This would be more responsive to need than a system in which patients were simply and unquestioningly referred to their nearest hospital. On the provider side, NHS Trusts were created; these would be autonomous organisations, independent of the direct control of health authorities, which would stimulate innovation. They would compete to attract business from purchasers, which was intended to produce an efficient and responsive service. [3]

The diagnosis of the NHS's problems thus emphasised several enduring themes in Conservative social policy: performance and efficiency, consumerism, and managerial autonomy. It was suggested that although the NHS had reduced inequalities in service provision, there remained apparently chance variations in the 'performance' of hospitals. The inference was that these betokened inefficiency in resource use, which would be corrected by the 'sanitising discipline of the trusty market' (Pollitt 1986). The problem was that this market was highly unequal. Despite substantial capital investment, there remained disparities in service provision and the condition and age of the capital stock. Moreover, differential levels of investment, and the state of the local labour and property markets, meant that the playing field was uneven. In short, grafting the notion of an internal market onto the service was likely to be problematic. Consumerism would be facilitated by allowing purchasers to choose the hospitals to which patients were to be referred, but this presupposed that a choice of hospitals existed, which was far from being the case everywhere. Managerial autonomy was presented as a guarantor of responsiveness and efficiency.

In sharp contrast to the era of top-down planning, management were to be free to react locally to whatever difficulties arose in their district or hospital. They could draw on the resources available in the local community to provide a wide range of services and devise their own strategies for service development. For the first time the health service would also have to build in the cost of capital into its pricing structure, through the system of capital charging. This was central to the creation of competition between providers of care. A corollary, which is particularly relevant to this book, was that capital investments were to be funded out of the revenue budgets of NHS Trusts, and it was also initially proposed that Trusts be permitted to borrow to fund new investments.

In terms of the broader themes of this book, the NHS reforms were presented as replacing a hierarchical, command-and-control organisation with one driven purely by market signals. They also appeared emblematic of a shift from government to governance – from state bureaucracy, to a more diffuse and decentralised set of partnerships and relationships. However, such bipolar contrasts oversimplify what actually happened; substantial elements of pre-reform organisational structures and modes of coordination were to remain in place.

What were the implications of the reforms for policy towards the acute hospital sector? First, there is a discussion of the impacts on the extent of competition and monopoly, followed by an assessment of the rationalisation of the acute hospital stock. Second, there is the question of the character of NHS trusts. To what extent have they drawn on new sources of resources and diversified their activities, and to what extent has this had implications for the planning of health services? The discussion of Trusts is framed in relation to broader arguments about the corporatisation of health care, which is seen as a response to an increasingly competitive financial climate. Third, a key innovation has been the increased reliance on the Private Finance Initiative for funding of hospital development and the ramifications for the process and pattern of capital development are therefore explored.

Creating and operating the internal market: the demise and return of 'planning'

The crucial innovation in the NHS reforms, the purchaser–provider split, had significant ramifications for the distribution of resources in the service. In the first three decades of the NHS, revenue resources largely reflected the historic pattern of service provision, and were not closely matched with population distribution. The attempts to redistribute funds under the RAWP system (DHSS 1976b) had had some effect on this, but there remained imbalances. The post-1991 system simply gave funds to health authorities in relation to their resident population, making no assumptions about where those people were to be treated. Even on a relatively unsophisticated analysis this was likely to imply substantial net transfers of funds, from inner-city areas (notably in, but not confined to London) to suburban and rural localities (Mohan 1990). This was because, broadly speaking, purchasers could now choose between high-cost urban hospitals and local, cheaper facilities, whereas previously their residents might have been locked by inertia into referral linkages to urban hospitals. In order to attract patients, hospital trusts were competing largely on price and also (insofar as it could be judged) quality. It was widely expected that this would demonstrate the variations in costs between hospitals, with the result that purchasers would naturally redirect patient flows to cheaper hospitals. For Trusts, insecurity resulted because purchasing of health care was fragmented as much of it was devolved to budget-holding GPs. The difficulty this posed was that, as contracts were being negotiated on a hospital-by-hospital and annual basis, the loss of contract income could place elements of a hospital's activity in jeopardy. It could also threaten cooperative links between hospitals, links not susceptible to price calculations; medical research links, which often depended on collaboration between dispersed teams working across several hospitals, are an obvious example. Concerns as to the combined effect of the switch of purchasing power and competition between hospitals led to several measures designed to minimise the likely impacts.

The first year post-1991 was to be a 'steady state' year, of minimal disruption to the pattern of contracts (and therefore patient flows). The freedoms available to Trusts were also constrained; they were prevented from borrowing money, from making investments that could not be recovered from contract income, from cross-subsidising between services, and from using surpluses. Other interventions included imposing (or, alternatively, refusing to sanction) mergers between providers, preventing purchasers switching contracts where this might threaten provider viability, and officially endorsing informal agreements between providers not to compete (Iliffe and Munro 2000: 314–15; Le Grand 1999: 33). Constraints on access to capital prevented creation of spare capacity, although most economic theorists would regard this as a pre-requisite for competition. All this took place in a political environment characterised by a succession of centrally imposed targets, and by a procession of initiatives which ring-fenced elements of expenditure for specific purposes (albeit often allocated on a competitive basis: Griffith 1999: 47).

The language of the reforms therefore softened over time (Ferlie 1994; Baggott 1998: 191–209). Short-term contracts were replaced by longer-term ones; the threat of competition, rather than the reality, was used to ensure the 'contestability' of the negotiating process (Ham 1996; Dawson and Goddard 2000). More recently, there are now partnerships operating within local strategic frameworks, and collaborative networks, some of which, oxymoronically, have been mandated as a result of Labour's 1997 White Paper (Department of Health 1997) with its 'duty of partnership'. The market may never actually have been a competitive, Darwinian entity, and in some respects it has operated within such a centralised climate that Paton (2000: 27–8) regards current policy as command-and-control by another name. Light (1997: 315) refers to this as 'dictated competition'; this was 'perhaps a contradiction in economic theory, but not in politics'. This does not mean that markets have not had substantial effects on the pattern of hospital provision but it does suggest that there are more elements of continuity with previous policy than is sometimes acknowledged.

One reason for this is that investments in the hospital stock had partially undermined the scope for competition. The aim, from 1962, was to develop a network of district general hospitals to close gaps in the service and to even up the distribution of qualified medical staff. Subsequent reorganisations sought in part to redraw the map of health authorities so as more closely to approximate hospital catchments (and also to achieve coterminosity with local government, to facilitate coordination of hospital and community services). The corollary was that patient flows were largely confined within health authority boundaries and a key aim was developing self-sufficiency in hospital care. Where local hospital capacity did not exist, health authorities would come to agreements, outlined in regional strategic plans, to assign patients to hospital catchments; this also meant that hospitals would have a catchment population large enough to justify provision of a particular range of services.

What health authorities saw as desirable self-sufficiency, others saw as objectionable monopoly. For the New Right, not only was the NHS anti-competitive on principle, it was also anti-competitive in practice since there was limited scope for reallocating patients to a hospital other than the one in whose catchment they lived.

If hospitals were, henceforth, to compete for patients, rather than serving a defined area, what would the implications be? Exworthy (1998) pointed out that for most health authorities and trusts, there was little scope for substantial switching of contracts from one provider to another, reflecting the extent to which most DHAs had inherited, or had acquired, a DGH. This does not mean that there is a monopoly in every district. Appleby *et al.* (1994: 43–6) found that, using an index of market contestability based on American anti-trust legislation, only one-quarter of acute trusts in the West Midlands RHA were in a monopoly position with respect to their local market (the figure would be higher for less-urbanised regions of the UK). This indicated that there was some scope for competition. Nonetheless, purchasers and providers were often in a mutually dependent relationship. Where a single purchaser accounted for a substantial proportion of the income of a Trust, switching this to another provider could destabilise the position of the first Trust, in effect putting it out of business. The situation in many localities was therefore one of bilateral monopoly and we might expect such local embeddedness to reduce the potential for sudden switching of contracts. The position was rather different in major conurbations, where there were obvious problems in coordinating purchasing decisions across several health authorities, and where a Trust might have a relationship with several purchasers. In such circumstances withdrawal of small amounts by several purchasers could have severe cumulative consequences for Trusts.

The Newcastle region has not witnessed the instability experienced in some localities, such as inner London. With the exception of Newcastle-upon-Tyne, most trusts rely very substantially for contract income on their local health authorities. Insofar as the pattern of contract placement can be inferred from trust and health authority documents, there has been little change in the pattern of referrals. The exception to this general rule is on Tyneside where there is some evidence that contracts have been switched from hospitals in Newcastle, to the new DGHs commissioned during the 1990s in North Tyneside and Wansbeck (Northumberland).[4] The issue here, of course, is whether one can separate out the effects of market forces from those attributable to new hospital construction. But the general point to draw from this section is to emphasise that the degree of 'localism' and embeddedness in the quasi-market has constrained its effects on the hospital system. In many parts of the country, Exworthy (1998) suggests the pattern of monopoly and catchments – the geography of patient referrals – will have changed little.

Over-capacity, mergers and rationalisation

There were, of course, exceptions. The large-scale transfers of purchasing power post-1991 from urban to suburban locations clearly had the potential to threaten the viability of hospitals, especially in circumstances where there were several potential competitors. The likely implications for London were pointed out by the Health Committee: 'given the acknowledged overcapacity prior to the introduction of the reforms, to say that financial viability is likely to prove "difficult" for many London hospitals after the introduction of the reforms is likely to prove an understatement'.[5] This was because health authorities in the suburbs and home counties, previously locked in to relationships with urban hospitals, could (and did) decide to switch contracts around. Consequently, the announcement of a 4 per cent floor in revenue growth to all RHAs in 1991 indicated that the implementation of the reforms was being diluted on political grounds,[6] as transitional protection was provided for pressurised localities. Market forces could not be unleashed wholesale; some intervention was needed. Their minds concentrated by the impending general election and the possible closure of at least one teaching hospital in London, the Government announced (during the 1991 Conservative Party conference) an inquiry into the problems of the London hospitals, chaired by Professor Bernard Tomlinson (former Chairman of the Northern RHA). Some form of coordination would be required if *ad hoc* closures were not to undermine a comprehensive acute hospital service and seriously weaken key provider units and centres of medical excellence. Of course the announcement of the Tomlinson Inquiry represented a major volte-face for the government. If there existed surplus capacity (which opponents questioned), London was the one place where competition would exist due to the proximity of so many alternatives with which to place contracts. Furthermore, the whole point of the market was to rationalise hospitals, in a situation where the implacable opposition of the teaching hospitals and professional elites had blocked change for nearly 100 years (Rivett 1986). The government had clearly backtracked, implicitly acknowledging the political consequences of its reforms and attempting to minimise their costs.

The Tomlinson Report (1992) argued that residents of inner London were overprovided with hospital beds, which they used at above-average rates; the situation was therefore inequitable. Critics challenged the basis on which these conclusions had been drawn, pointing out, for instance, that a key reason for this was the poor quality of primary care. If areas comparable to inner London were examined, there were no significant differences in hospital provision or use, and London's acute hospital services were no less efficient than the national average (Jarman 1993: 982). Nevertheless, change was inevitable – purchasers were already withdrawing funds (totalling approximately £50 million in 1992–3) from central London's hospitals, and still greater reductions were anticipated in subsequent years. The problem of reconciling planning and markets was acknowledged by Tomlinson:

> It has indeed been said [that] *the best thing that could have happened was to allow the internal market to carry on and destroy a few hospitals* and then people would have put their problems right very quickly. ... The danger in the process of *indiscriminate reduction* of hospitals in London is so great ... that we believe the process ... has to be a carefully and ... *a firmly managed process'.*[7]

In subsequent questioning, Labour MP Hugh Bayley argued that the 'big strategic decisions need *something more than market forces'*; responding, Tomlinson acknowledged the 'philosophical difficulty' of having 'managed change in a market that is intended to produce change'.[8]

The managed rundown was to be overseen by the London Implementation Group (LIG), which established reviews of specialist services and agreed sets of principles for consolidation. The threatened closure of some of the London teaching hospitals, notably St Bartholomew's, provoked enormous public reaction, centred around the hospital's symbolic significance (Moon and Brown 2001). Despite the high profile of this case, arguably the most important consequence of the rationalisation of London's services was progressively to rouse Conservative backbench MPs to protest, hoping to exploit the dwindling Parliamentary majority for constituency advantage. Enraged by the threatened closure of the casualty department at Edgware Hospital, two members representing North London seats, Hugh Dykes and Sir John Gorst, threatened not to support the government unless the unit was reprieved. When, despite these protests, the closure was announced in late 1996, Gorst 'withdrew his cooperation', ensuring that the government's majority was wiped out; it became a minority government with the loss of a subsequent by-election.[9] On returning to office Labour's Health Secretary, Frank Dobson, took the opportunity to differentiate New Labour from the Conservatives, calling for a moratorium on rationalisation. Specifically, he declared that he wished to see Bart's remain open, in an obviously populist gesture. The subsequent Turnberg Review (1998) departed from Tomlinson in disputing the view that London had an excess of beds, and calling for a slackening in the pace of closures. It noted that Tomlinson's dire predictions of falling referrals to London had not been borne out – nearly one-sixth of London's acute beds were still used by non-Londoners. But Turnberg was still criticised for vacillation – for example, in failing to take tough decisions about the future of teaching hospitals.

The unpalatable market medicine, then, was repeatedly sweetened with a dose of political intervention. There was something of a regression from a 'pure' market, which reduced the scope for wholesale destabilisation of services. At the same time, Trusts have had to operate under a more stringent regime. The requirement to cover capital charges, and demands for high levels of efficiency savings, have combined with the purchaser–provider split to force reconfigurations.

To some extent this has been a managed process. Annual reviews by the Institute of Health Service Managers allow some general lessons to be drawn (Turner 1994–6). Public resistance had caused hospital closure programmes to 'grind to a halt', forcing health authorities and Trusts to be 'less radical'. A 1996 review, therefore, noted a trend towards greater collaboration and away from 'unproductive' rivalry, and argued that purchasers and providers were both willing to be more 'realistic' about changes. When one adds to this the idea that significant and long-term purchaser commitments are needed for capital developments to be viable, the market appears much less Darwinian than is sometimes thought to be the case. In fact the negotiation of large-scale, block contracts is arguably not so different from the process of defining hospital catchments associated with an earlier era of planning.

Tracking effects on the hospital stock is not straightforward. Once Trusts were created, it became impossible to obtain separate data on any component units of a Trust which incorporated more than one hospital. Bed numbers in acute hospitals did, however, continue their steady decline – on average, there has been a decline in acute bed capacity of 2 per cent a year since 1980 (Hensher and Edwards 1999). A highly visible effect of the reforms has been a rapid process of hospital mergers.

Seventeen mergers of NHS Trusts took place between 1991–7; a further twenty-three came into effect in 1998 (Garside 1999; note that Goddard and Ferguson (1997) regard these figures as substantial underestimates). Some, such as certain post-Tomlinson changes, were imposed; others have been voluntary, designed to achieve economies of scale and scope, or else to deal with alleged excess capacity. Other 'drivers' of mergers are the belief in a significant link between better outcomes and greater treatment volumes, and professional criteria, such as those relating to training of medical staff or policies on doctors' working hours, cause pressure for greater concentration. Still other reasons relate to quite specific post-reform developments. Merger may help Trusts raise capital for new developments especially when site rationalisation is possible; this might offer opportunities to build new developments which would not be viable for a single Trust. A larger Trust could also spread risk over a greater volume of activity. Such factors are perhaps more relevant for Trusts exploring private finance. Merger may also be a response to uncertainty, giving a Trust greater control of its local market. But there is scepticism over the benefits achieved (Ferguson *et al.* 1997).

It is perhaps a sign of the times that the Department of Health, in seeking to regulate mergers, drew on American competition legislation, proposing that mergers be scrutinised if they would result in joint market shares in excess of 50 per cent of total market activity (Dawson 1995). An interesting point here is the horror of monopoly, given that the aim of policy from 1962 had been to create it. More fundamentally, perhaps, conventional markets rely on spare capacity, but given the expense of creating spare capacity, the pressure to minimise it probably exceeds the desire to see real competition (West 1997: 139). The point is that mergers are taking place to minimise spare capacity even though many would now question whether it exists.

The experience of the Northern region includes some significant mergers. First, there are hospitals separated by long distances such as Hexham and Newcastle. Perhaps Hexham never was a serious candidate for DGH status, but it was ultimately merged with Newcastle Acute Hospitals. Durham and Shotley Bridge merged as part of the North Durham PFI deal (see below), leaving the latter very much as a community hospital in this depressed part of County Durham. Other substantial mergers took place in Sunderland, where the intention was that acute services provided on five hospital sites would be rationalised on to two, and Teesside. Figure 9.1 shows the main acute hospital trusts in the region in 2000. Several Trusts incorporate more than one general hospital, and some mergers have involved hospitals separated by some distance as well as hospitals located close to each other in large urban centres. Comparisons with the Hospital Plan are instructive: there are several locations where DGHs or scaled-down general hospitals were proposed – Bishop Auckland, Wansbeck, Hartlepool, Shotley Bridge and Hexham. They have all been developed (or are under construction; see Figure A5) apart from Shotley Bridge. But they have also all been merged with other, larger hospital trusts. Geographically this could be read as signalling a concentration of general hospital provision into the main estuarine conurbations, involving a process of even greater rationalisation than that envisaged in the Plan. There is an interesting historical twist here. The Newcastle RHB's reactions to Bonham-Carter indicated that Ashington (later superseded by Wansbeck), Shotley Bridge, and Bishop Auckland should all 'lean on' neighbouring DGHs – not unlike the eventual outcome of hospital mergers and Trust reconfigurations illustrated here.[10]

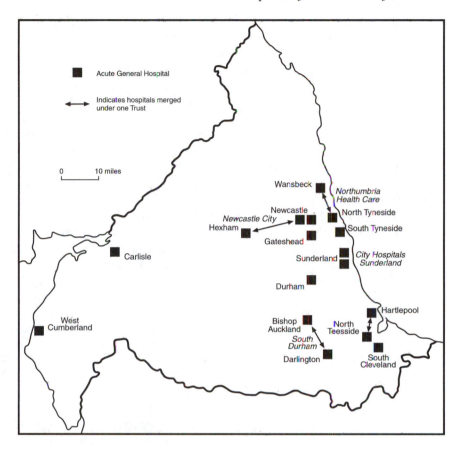

Figure 9.1   Major acute hospital trusts in the Newcastle region, 2001

Source: Institute of Healthcare Management Yearbook 2000–1

As in previous generations, however, events in Newcastle were perhaps the most controversial. The issue of whether the city should have three or two general hospitals had never been properly resolved. The addition of the new Freeman Road hospital was heavily criticised (Chapter 7) but, that hospital having established itself over a twenty-year period, attention switched to the Newcastle General Hospital as a candidate for downsizing.

This hospital's future had periodically been in doubt, and one corollary was that it had not benefited from the substantial capital investments that had gone into the other general hospitals in the city during the 1970s and 1980s, though it had substantial investment in the first two decades of the NHS.[11] Within a month after the 1991 reforms, the General dropped its initial plans for an application for Trust status. There ensued something of a power struggle in the city for ascendancy.[12] Over the next two years, it became clear that – as in London – purchasers were beginning to withdraw some contracts from Newcastle in general, not just the General in particular.

It was also evident that, of the three, the General was bound to be the most vulnerable: the RVI was inseparable from the medical school and there were restrictions on disposal and redevelopment of the site; the Freeman, barely 15 years old, was a flagship new development. This is not to say that the other main hospitals did not suffer in the new marketplace (see, for example, Kingman 1994), but it was evident that something would have to give.

The consequence was the third review of the city's acute services in barely a decade (Newcastle Health Authority 1993), though one which did not engage in a direct comparison with the 1981 and 1988 reviews. It rested its case primarily on the likely impacts on Newcastle of new DGHs outside the city, pointing out that of the 125,000 patients treated each year in the city's general hospitals, only half were from Newcastle. The inference was that the 20,000+ residents of Northumberland and North Tyneside being treated in Newcastle would all obtain treatment locally when their new general hospitals were completed. The other sources of major inflows to Newcastle were from locations where substantial new DGH investment was not anticipated. These assumptions, though plausible, needed to be tested against the availability of sufficient capacity in the surrounding DHAs to carry real weight, given the use to which they were to be put. For the central proposition of the 1993 review was that the General cease to be a DGH, losing 500 beds and its casualty department, though retaining regional cancer services, and instead developing as a day hospital and community health centre for the immediate locality.

Opponents criticised the implicit assumptions in these proposals. Over 100,000 inpatient and outpatient visits needed to be redirected and there were queries as to whether other hospitals could cope with the volume of redirected caseload. A comparison with previous strategic plans for the area is instructive. The 1993 review appeared to discern rather more surplus capacity than had been visible only five years earlier and which would not have been predicted from analysis of long-term trends in bed numbers. Moreover, the review was written and published in only the second year of the reforms. Rather than the market deciding the future configuration, this could be viewed as a pre-emptive strike, the effect of which was to secure the Freeman and the RVI while ensuring that if there were to be major switches in purchasing intentions, the General would bear the brunt. There is some evidence that contracts were indeed switched[13] producing difficulties for all three hospitals, and the major purchaser, Newcastle and North Tyneside, was also steadily switching funds from acute services to primary care.[14] The acute services review was presented by the main protagonists as an example of having 'bitten the bullet' and resolved a problem which had plagued the city for fifteen years. Adding to the challenges of contracts being switched, the Newcastle trusts, in conjunction with the rest of the NHS, were subject to a remorseless squeeze for greater efficiency savings of around 2 per cent per annum (Kingman 1994). In these circumstances a merger began to look inevitable. Reflecting the relative position of the three hospitals, the RVI and Freeman eventually merged in 1998 and as acute services began to move from the General, its demise as an acute centre became a self-fulfilling prophecy, because those services remaining there were clinically exposed, lacking support from the presence on-site of physicians and general surgeons. This might be seen as just another provincial mini-Tomlinson, and one which accurately reflected power structures and political constraints, such as the ability of medical school interests to shape the reform agenda, and the political impossibility of writing-off one of only five totally new general hospitals built in the region since 1948. The logic of the acute services review also contrasted with pre-reform plans, and it appeared inconsistent for the Health Authority to use as part of its case the argument that Newcastle GPs were having difficulties getting patients admitted to hospital, when the review's aim was to remove the local capacity that might have made it possible to overcome those difficulties. These developments seem entirely of a piece with a wider downsizing agenda in the NHS, driven by financial criteria and constraints, and which ruthlessly eliminates hospital capacity without guaranteeing a shift of resources into other areas of the health service. But it is notable that, rather than the market determining the shape of future developments, key strategic decisions were made before market forces had had a chance to work. Such decisions have been characterised by Dawson (1995: 10) as 'shotgun' reviews.

Summary

The developments described exemplify the ways in which the operation of market forces has been modified in practice. Indeed the context in which markets operate – the cumulative outcome of previous rounds of investment – has heavily constrained the outcomes, because of the limited scope for competition. The mutual dependency of purchasers and providers, and the extensive public reaction to reconfiguration proposals, has meant that there has been considerable intervention in the process of service reconfiguration. Moreover, the creation of new capacity, a requirement for more competition, has been tightly controlled. The management of reconfigurations has thus been a rather less brutal process than might be thought but it has nevertheless led to dramatic downsizing. In some cases it has been the threat, rather than the reality, of the market which has been used to justify change. This adds grist to the mill of those critics who argue, as Leys (1999) does, that the process is finance-driven, not needs-based. The result was a continued reduction in hospital capacity, with acute beds falling (in England) from 117,000 in 1990–1 to 108,000 in 1998–9 (Department of Health 2000a: Table 3.1), while accommodating a continued rise in inpatients through swifter discharge and treating more day cases. The decline in bed numbers was eventually halted following the report of the National Beds Inquiry in 2000.

Self-governing trusts: the corporatisation of health care?

Several commentators have argued that health-care provision is undergoing a 'corporate transformation' (e.g. Salmon 1995). The implication is that health care is now a solidly corporate endeavour, driven by the profit motive. The analytical focus of such arguments is on developments in the for-profit sector of health care, especially the ways in which competitive pressures force restructuring, hospital closures, expansion into new areas perceived to offer potential for profit, and exclusion of needy populations. Such developments have, of course, had knock-on effects, on not-for-profit hospitals, many of which have become 'virtually indistinguishable' from the for-profit chains, in that they have become far more entrepreneurial. These arguments were, of course, developed in the context of the USA under Republican administrations, during which pro-competition strategies were pushed forcefully, and where for-profit and not-for-profit hospitals compete with one another. In these circumstances hospitals faced a straightforward fight for survival and were forced to diversify into new markets. Broadly the same process has been noted in New Zealand, where hospitals were reconfigured as Crown Health Enterprises (CHEs); these were limited liability companies which were required to make surpluses and return a dividend to their shareholding ministers (Barnett 1999). To what extent are such arguments valid in the British case?

Two key points can be made. The first relates to the implications of the transition to Trust status for the character of hospitals, their *modus operandi*, and their accountability. The second relates to the boundary between public and private sectors and the extent of corporate transformation within the private sector.

A key rationale for the establishment of self-governing hospital trusts was to liberate them from the bureaucratic constraints of accountability to local communities, thereby enhancing '*local* (my emphasis) ownership and pride', and stimulating 'local initiative and greater competition'. Opponents argued that hospitals were 'opting out' of the NHS, and stressed the organic links between hospitals and the communities of which they were a part. Whatever the historical validity of such claims, which were partly deployed as rhetorical devices to enlist support, they were dismissed by the Government. These hospitals were not 'opting out' of the NHS; they were simply being given greater managerial freedom. Extensive consultation on proposals for trust status was impossible, according to Kenneth Clarke, because there was no way of identifying the 'natural constituency' of a hospital; 'hospitals do not belong to any particular section of the public'.[15] The lack of consultation, and the brusque manner in which protests were dismissed, had echoes of the modernist rhetoric of Powell twenty-seven years earlier. But it is striking that, having in earlier policy statements laid great stress on the need for community support of hospitals, the Conservatives were prepared to ride roughly over such protests. And although the intention was originally to liberate Trusts from bureaucratic intervention, and in particular to downplay the significance of the regional tier in NHS management, it soon became necessary to reinvent an intermediate layer of governance. Some Trusts clearly objected strongly to supervision by RHAs but there remained a need for a regional tier, in order to preserve a degree of regulation, for example of Trust business plans and capital aspirations.

Having promulgated a localist justification for the formation of Trusts, the Conservatives reduced local representation on them, and local involvement in consultation about their strategic development has also been steadily reduced. NHS Trusts were criticised for taking more of their business in private session on grounds of commercial confidentiality, and for containing fewer representatives of local communities, to the point where they were seen as part of an unaccountable quangocracy (Jenkins 1995). These changes have not been reversed by Labour, whose most recent approach to consumerism in the NHS, its National Plan, will still further reduce the scope for open public debate about the future of hospitals.

It could, of course, be argued that hospitals *are* accountable to the public, in the sense that they draw the great bulk of their funds from contracts placed by public purchasers of health care. However, given that commentators from both left and right now speak of an urgent need to revive democratic participation in the core institutions of the welfare state, the insulation of Trusts from democratic influences may be judged regrettable (see Chapter 10). The creation of Trusts has thus limited democratic input into hospital management, but it has not established them (as is the case in, say, New Zealand) as commercial organisations. However, by being granted more autonomy, Trusts have been able to diversify their sources of capital, which is another feature of the corporate transformation of health care (Kuttner 1996; Smith *et al.* 1995; Brown 1996). Charitable fundraising and private patient income are notable here.

The recent growth of charitable income in the NHS has been discussed by several authors (Lattimer 1996; Mohan and Gorsky 2001; Pharaoh and Mocroft 2001). Major variations are evident between individual trusts and, therefore, between places. For the 1998–9 year, fifty-seven Trusts or special trustees had income from charitable sources in excess of £1 million, and the total for these organisations was £220 million, or nearly 75 per cent of NHS charitable income in England. Five institutions – Guy's (£32 million), Great Ormond Street (£23 million), St Bartholomew's and the London (£15 million), the Christie Hospital, Manchester (£15 million) and the Royal Marsden (£10 million) – had a total income of £95 million from charitable sources. The remaining Trusts with income over £1 million were generally teaching or specialist institutions, or large urban general hospitals. In contrast there were 133 Trusts with a charitable income of under £100,000 and the great majority of these were providing community health, mental health, or ambulance services. This pattern clearly reflects the ability of such high-profile, glamorous institutions to capture the public imagination.

We can compare these figures with the revenue budgets of their 'parent' NHS Trusts. For three institutions (Christie Hospital (21 per cent), Great Ormond Street (11 per cent) and Guy's (10 per cent)) charitable income equated to over 10 per cent of their total income; for a further twenty-four NHS Trusts, charitable income was equivalent to over 2 per cent of total income.

This impression is reinforced if we consider the scale of the asset base held by individual trusts. The teaching hospitals were permitted to retain control of their endowments after 1948, through their Special Trustees. As of 1998, assets valued at £575 million were controlled by the Special Trustees of St Thomas's Hospital (£256 million), St Bartholomew's (£114 million), Guy's (£111 million) and Great Ormond Street (£92 million).[16] The Special Trustees of hospitals in London held assets valued at a combined total of £860 million in 1997–8 and, as an indication of recent growth in these funds, a previous estimate for 1996–7 was £639 million (Holly 1997).

The resources generated by charity, and the charitable asset base, thus remain heavily skewed towards high-profile institutions with a preponderance in central London. Not much has changed here in fifty years to alter the basic contours of this pattern. This might have profound consequences for equity, if it meant that hospitals had differential access to capital, and for planning, if the availability of charitable funds were to influence the trajectory of hospital development.

To exemplify the issues, charity featured strongly in redevelopment proposals in London in the 1980s and 1990s. At St Bartholomew's, £18 million in government support matched £30 million in charitable donations, and at Guy's £100 million had been committed by government to match £40 million from charitable sources (Lattimer 1996: 45). The very success of charitable appeals in London made the planned rationalisation of the capital's acute hospital services much harder to achieve. This happened partly because some of the resources available to the Special Trustees were put to use in resisting hospital rationalisation (Holly 1997), and because of the political contacts made through fundraising (Lattimer 1996: 123). Debates after the Tomlinson Report illustrate this issue very well. Some of the report's recommendations directly threatened the future of several hospitals which had spent substantial charitable resources on redevelopment or refurbishment. Tomlinson's view was that 'such sunk costs, however recently incurred, are small compared to the revenue costs of the NHS; they should not dictate strategic development in London' (Tomlinson 1992: 30). Thus, Tomlinson proposed that despite the scale of charitable spending at Guy's, most clinical services would relocate from Guy's to St Thomas's Hospital. The reaction by several charities was either to withhold donations previously agreed, or to demand repayment.[17] The final decision on Guy's involved the preservation of most of phase III of the Guy's redevelopment, in which charity had played a key role. Other hospitals, such as the Royal Marsden and the National Hospital for Neurology and Neurosurgery, were reprieved on similar terms. These and other cases (Webb and Hanley 1997) indicate the potential for decisions to be influenced by considerations of the availability of funds. They illustrate the difficulties of planning a hospital system in which the availability of charitable funds varies so substantially and gives the beneficiaries of charity considerable scope to use funds to defend the interests of a particular hospital. Moreover, funds given for a particular purpose cannot always be transferred to other uses, so that hospital endowments cannot be used to invest in primary care, for example (Pharaoh and Mocroft 2001).

A final illustration is the announcement of a fundraising campaign to construct a new children's hospital in Cardiff entirely through charitable largesse. This is said to be the first attempt since 1948 at such a project.[18] In the 1950s, a key argument used against such appeals was that decisions on the allocation of scarce NHS capital could in effect be pre-empted. If appeals failed to reach their targets, it was suggested, there would be pressure on the state to close any funding gaps.[19]

The scale of resources from non-statutory sources gives certain hospitals considerable scope in terms of financing capital development. Charitable resources can also reduce a Trust's requirement to obtain capital either through the public sector or through the Private Finance Initiative. These developments therefore raise the issue of where the boundary between public and private responsibility is to be drawn.

In terms of diversifying sources of capital, Trusts have also steadily expanded their private facilities. This is particularly associated with some major acute hospitals in London, an activity which also involved an international dimension. Freed from their ties to the local, they sought to go global, in a manner which has echoes of the American health empires (Ehrenreich and Ehrenreich 1972). Quantitatively, sixty-one dedicated NHS pay-bed units were established between 1991–5, representing an addition of 985 beds. Inpatient and outpatient revenue almost doubled in this period, from £113 million to £215 million (Hassell 1995: 5). By 1998–9, private patient revenues for NHS Trusts in England reached £331 million (*Laing's Review* 2001). It is interesting to compare revenues from private practice for the first wave Trusts in the first post-reform year with more recent figures (for 1997–8). For the thirty-two (of fifty-seven) first-wave Trusts which were either specialist or general acute hospitals, private-patient income had increased from £29.6 million to £56.6 million, with several hospitals more than doubling income from this source over this period. This is a small number of Trusts but by 1997–8, of the 173 Trusts in these two categories, ninety-seven showed a rise in private-patient income over the previous financial year. For the specialist hospitals, private income amounted to 7.5 per cent of revenues. When we add private-patient and charitable income together, there are eleven Trusts where these sources equate to over 10 per cent of total income, led by the Christie Hospital, Manchester (31 per cent), Royal Marsden (30 per cent), Great Ormond Street (24 per cent) and the Brompton (17 per cent). These, like the other institutions raising large sums privately, are specialist hospitals. These figures suggest the possibility that certain of the most prominent hospitals in the UK will develop a much more diversified funding mix, drawing on commercial and charitable resources as well as receiving the bulk of their income from public funds. However, this would impart a rather different dynamic to the process of health-service development, in which access to health care depended to a growing degree on locally available resources. In fact, in the Northern region, such income sources contribute much less to the finances of most Trusts than is the case in the examples shown.

However, in terms of the trajectory of hospital development, these activities by Trusts raise the question of the balance between public and private provision. Trends noted by Rayner (1986, 1987) towards commercialisation of the private acute sector have continued. Although the steady expansion of the sector in the 1980s seemed to stall in the 1990s it has now resumed its upward trend. Some 11 per cent of the population have private health insurance and there are quite predictable social and spatial variations (ONS 1997), though the proportion of operations purchased privately has remained roughly constant, at around 13–14 per cent, since the late 1980s (Williams *et al.* 2000). To what extent does the private sector influence the overall trajectory of hospital development?

One argument is that private and NHS hospitals are competing for the scarce time of consultant staff, because expanding the supply of medical personnel is a slow process. There have consequently been arguments, over the years, about how to regulate private practice, the latest twist in this being a proposal to limit the amount of private practice that can be done by doctors in their first seven post-qualification years.

A more general issue concerns regulation of the private sector, and its relationships with the NHS. Whereas the Conservatives introduced certain tax breaks for private care in 1991, these were abolished by Labour and an expansion of private insurance and greater charges was firmly rejected in Labour's NHS Plan (Department of Health 2000b). Other issues have been more contentious; the private sector believes that private beds in the NHS are unfairly subsidised, and argues that the NHS does not make enough use of private hospitals. NHS-funded patients remain a very small proportion of the private sector's business. Labour seems to be attempting to conciliate the private sector, emphasising the need to move away from a reactive approach (i.e. using independent-sector providers on an *ad hoc* basis) towards a more collaborative relationship. This reflects winter beds crises in their first term of office; the private sector offers spare capacity, on which the NHS can draw. Labour's recent 'concordat' with the private sector envisages that health authorities will enter into local partnerships which will maximise local capacity. The issues here will relate to the sharing of information, on capacity and costs, and to the regulation of the private sector. It remains to be seen whether partnerships can be developed which are any more effective than those of the inter-war era. The NHS has not, however, been slow to take advantage of market opportunities, having taken over a specialist unit (the London Heart Hospital) in central London in the summer of 2001. And spare capacity might get some PFI-funded deals off the hook of inadequate bed numbers. But the success of this policy will depend on local circumstances. The regional disparities in the distribution of private-sector beds remain substantial; there is approximately fourfold variation in private acute bed availability between regions.[20]

To summarise this section, the UK has not experienced the kind of corporate transformation of health care charted by Salmon (1995) in the USA. Nor have hospitals been completely severed from connections with their local communities, in a contractual if not a democratic sense. There is evidence of a small number of Trusts using their position to diversify their funding base, though on the figures available this is largely confined to specialist and teaching hospitals in London. In the region with which this book has been mainly concerned, such income sources have contributed far less. However, the small scale of such developments does not mean that they can be easily dismissed, because a feature of the past decade has been the entrepreneurial character of health care, in which the pursuit of income sources almost becomes an end in itself, possibly to the detriment of NHS patients. There are also implications for planning if, as suggested here, hospital development comes to depend on locally available resources. In this sense these developments may serve to distort the NHS's priorities. As an indication of the extent to which this competitive logic will be pushed, the government's system for monitoring and rewarding NHS Trusts is one of 'earned autonomy'. Those deemed successful gain additional freedoms, including greater financial autonomy and the scope to invest surpluses; those deemed 'failing' are subject to evermore managerial scrutiny and direction. And, as discussed in the concluding chapter, the present government has proposed granting NHS Trusts greater autonomy, including the possibility of being handed over to non-profit agencies.

Capital charging, private finance and hospital development

There are long-standing criticisms of the problems associated with valuation of and charging for NHS capital assets (see Chapter 5 above, and Mayston 1990). The 1989 White Paper argued that, because capital costs are 'not fully taken into account when comparisons of performance are made between different parts of the NHS or with the private sector' (Secretary of State for Health 1989: para 2.23), a capital charging system would be introduced. This would encourage health authorities to 'use assets efficiently and to invest widely', as well as putting NHS hospitals on a 'level footing with private hospitals, which have to meet the costs of capital on a normal, commercial basis' (para 2.24). Trusts were initially required to build into contract prices what were termed capital charges, equivalent to 6 per cent of the replacement cost of their assets. The logic of the policy was clear: Trusts would have incentives to dispose of surplus assets and rationalise their estate to minimise the impacts. In the abstract, this is unobjectionable but the question is whether the policy has put unsustainable pressure on Trusts to rationalise capacity. There is little doubt that capital charges were crucial in tilting the balance of financial advantage away from high-cost urban locations and that this was behind the pressures on hospitals in London and other large cities. It has also been suggested that the capital charging system was a deterrent to necessary investment in maintaining the asset base, leading to a rise in the NHS's maintenance backlog.

The way capital was to be financed also changed. Trusts were now expected to meet the cost of new capital developments through resources generated internally. Thus capital charges were recycled within the NHS in order to cover new capital expenditure. It was initially proposed that Trusts could take out private-sector loans to circumvent constraints on public capital expenditure, though this was then prevented. The possibility of private finance was explored and initiated somewhat tentatively by the Conservatives but its enthusiastic adoption under Labour requires some explanation. Under the Private Finance Initiative (PFI), private corporations design, build, own and operate services in return for an annual fee for the duration of a contract, typically twenty-five to thirty years. PFI has been promoted as a means of bringing private sector finance and skills into major capital developments throughout the public sector. The government have tended to present PFI as another example of their pragmatism, but critics contend that this conceals fundamental issues about how the NHS is organised. One account would see PFI as part of a broader revolution in governance and public-service delivery, in which the state is no longer responsible for the delivery of services, but instead hands them over to a range of partners (Chapter 1; Rhodes 1997; Osborne and Gaebler 1992). What matters is not who delivers services, but ensuring that they are delivered. One (potentially teleological) view is that PFI simply represents the logical endpoint of a marketisation process which began with competitive tendering for ancillary services, extended through the internal market, and concluded with the *de facto* privatisation of everything but the salaries of nurses and doctors.

The unspoken assumptions of the PFI are primarily microeconomic. While the government may need to be responsible for delivering a particular service which is financed through taxation, PFI allegedly permits an element of risk to be transferred to the private sector, and allows efficiency gains through the private sector's enterprise and discipline. If there are cost overruns, the private sector would pick up the bill. This was to give it an incentive to deliver on budget and on time, and Ministers enthusiastically peddled the myth that public procurement had inevitably failed to do this, arguing, as Frank Dobson did, that the only thing being privatised under PFI was the 'cost overruns'. However, the NHS's performance in controlling building costs and contracts had unquestionably improved, so the argument was less clear-cut than Dobson (and others) would have liked.[21] However, what makes PFI different from other forms of privatisation is that the private sector retains a substantial role in PFI projects; moreover, unlike contracting-out of ancillary services, for instance, the private sector provides the capital asset, as well as the service. Some prominent advocates have therefore suggested that PFI is the 'Heineken' of privatisation, reaching hitherto untouched parts of the government machine (Kerr 1998: 18). Allegedly, there is a 'win-win' situation since the NHS gets improved services, the private sector gets new opportunities to make profits, and, furthermore – and this is the macroeconomic justification – projects funded by PFI do not feature in the public-sector borrowing requirement. Hence private finance was attractive to the Conservatives in the 1990s because they were trying to restrain borrowing in an attempt to meet the convergence criteria for European economic integration, but recessionary conditions were pushing up government debt. These arguments no longer applied, due to the improving state of the economy, by 1997, but Labour nevertheless enthusiastically embraced PFI (Clark and Root (1999) document the development of Labour's attitude), swiftly removing obstacles to it. Although Labour has famously strict policies on borrowing, the Treasury Select Committee (2000a) recently observed that public investment could be raised substantially without breaching the government's declared policies on public debt. If the macro-economic arguments are not clear-cut, what of the micro-economic issues, concerning the cost of individual projects?

Impacts of the PFI on hospital development

The level of capital investment in the NHS in England since 1991 has been analysed by Sussex (2001: 31–4) who distinguishes between government-funded capital, the contribution of land sales and the impact of the PFI. At constant prices capital investment in the early 1990s was about 40–50 per cent higher than the previous peak attained in the early 1970s, though there was a substantial fall of about 20 per cent between 1995 and 1998. Since then total investment has grown substantially. Even allowing for the PFI deals which have been signed, Exchequer-funded capital investment will contribute about 75 per cent of total spending, and will reach about £2.6 billion in 2003–4. On its own this would still constitute the 'largest capital building programme in history', as Labour are fond of claiming and as the Department of Health's *Investment Strategy* (Department of Health 2000c) makes clear, which will contribute substantially to renewing the asset base. So why are PFI deals often the subject of such controversy? The reason is that for new hospitals and substantial rebuilds, the PFI is often the only option available, whereas Exchequer-financed expenditure is largely spent on smaller-scale projects.

Critics argue that PFI-funded projects are associated with significant increases in capital costs for buildings which often entail substantial reductions in hospital bed capacity. Cost increases arise because of the need to structure deals in such a way that they are attractive to the private sector. This often implies greenfield or edge-of-town sites, which generate more certain returns, more quickly. It also reflects the costs of financing the project; because the private sector is said to be bearing risk, a higher interest rate is usually charged, compared to the cost of government borrowing. Critics dispute the need for, and the size, of such risk premiums, on the grounds that hospital development is ultimately underwritten by commitments to funding the NHS, which future governments would be unwise to repudiate. Because of the expense of PFI schemes, annual interest payments to the private sector absorb a larger proportion of Trusts' incomes than do capital charges. In addition, payments made to the private sector appear to be higher than those made to government under capital charging. Two forms of payment are made: an availability fee, and a service fee. The former includes construction costs, rolled-up interest, and life-cycle maintenance, and is equivalent to the rental charge. The service fee covers facilities management (cleaning, lighting, laundry). In the first wave of PFI schemes, the rental payments/availability fees ranged from 11.2–18.5 per cent of construction costs (compared to the 6 per cent capital charge). It follows that the proportion of trusts' incomes spent on charges for capital will more than double in PFI-funded hospitals; trusts are unable to replace like with like for the same annual cost (Gaffney *et al.* 1999a). The consequences can be exemplified by reference to two major PFI developments in the Northern region, at Carlisle and Durham (Price *et al.* 1999; Gaffney and Pollock 1999b).

The Carlisle Hospital scheme replaced Cumberland Infirmary, the City General, and the City Maternity Hospital with a new purpose-built hospital on the Infirmary site. The North Durham scheme built a new hospital at Durham to replace the Dryburn Hospital (Durham City) and the acute facilities of the Shotley Bridge Hospital, in the north-west of the county. Shotley Bridge was to be redeveloped as a community hospital through a separate PFI deal. Substantial increases in capital costs took place in the move from public to private finance. The Carlisle scheme's capital cost rose from £41 million to £67 million, partly because the scheme was a new build rather than merely the completion of the protracted redevelopment of the existing hospital. However, the capital cost of both schemes rose by over 20 per cent as a result of financing costs which would not have occurred with public finance, and the Durham PFI consortium appeared to be raising more money on the capital market than was strictly necessary to meet construction costs. It was able to do this on the basis of a guaranteed stream of future income from PFI availability payments, and Gaffney and Pollock (1999b: 12) suggested that very low interest rates had been secured, reflecting the perceived lack of risk in the project. In another case it was reported that a PFI consortium, having secured finance at one rate of interest, refinanced the development at a lower rate, and pocketed the surplus.[22] This leakage of money from the NHS demands greater attention.

Even without these cost increases, the effects of PFI on the finances of these Trusts are substantial. In both Durham and Carlisle, the annual cost of capital equated to around 7.5 per cent of Trust income in 1996–7. However, the PFI schemes were to cause these proportions to more than double, creating a gap between current and projected annual capital costs of over £5 million (Durham) and £3.55 million (Carlisle). These figures are not dissimilar to ones calculated for other PFI developments in Edinburgh (16.2 per cent of Trust income), Bromley (14.5 per cent) and Worcester (15.8 per cent) (Gaffney and Pollock 1999a; Pollock *et al.* 2000). One response is that this reflects the relative quality of the buildings: it would be surprising if capital charges for new hospitals were not higher than the substandard facilities they were replacing, but the gap is nevertheless substantial. This 'affordability gap' clearly has an adverse effect on Trusts. What are the effects on services?

Effects on staffing

The implication of PFI is that substantial savings need to be made in the costs of labour.[23] Evidence from both Carlisle and Durham indicated a significant reduction in clinical staff expenditure, in both absolute and proportionate terms. In Durham, clinical staff costs were projected to fall as a proportion of Trust income, from 64 per cent to 47 per cent (Gaffney and Pollock 1999b: 13). In both locations these cuts fell disproportionately on nursing budgets: in Durham qualified nursing staff were to be replaced with unqualified health-care assistants; in Carlisle large cuts in nurse numbers were envisaged. This did not appear entirely compatible with other elements of trust strategy, which appeared to envisage that the dependency levels of patients admitted to the new hospitals would be higher – yet they were to be cared for by less-qualified personnel.

Effects on hospital bed provision

PFI schemes appear to be associated with reductions in bed numbers (on average, 28 per cent in a selection of schemes) that are substantially greater than long-term trends would indicate; nationally acute bed numbers fell by just over 1 per cent per annum during the 1990s. In the Carlisle case, total planned beds had fallen from 520 (in 1995–96) to 465 (1999) and further reductions (to *c.* 440) were anticipated. In Durham, more substantial reductions were proposed. A 1992 'Approval in Principle' document had proposed a 910-bed DGH for the North Durham area. This proposal was overtaken by events, however, as the internal market forced a reappraisal, leading to a proposal (1994) for a 565-bed general hospital, later reduced to 454 beds in 1996, when the case for a PFI development was presented. The emphasis had also changed: the PFI Business Case proposed that the dependency levels of patients would increase, and implicitly assumed that lower-dependency care would be provided for in community-based facilities or in the home. The contrast is significant. The initial (910-bed) proposal was based primarily on service considerations whereas the PFI bid was constrained by the need to structure a financial package which was commercially viable. This argument is not based on the kind of uncritical bed worship which Kemp (1964) criticised long ago, or indeed on an attachment to hospital provision *per se*. The government has argued that bed numbers in PFI deals have been decided on clinical grounds, but Pollock *et al.* (1999) suggest that the reverse is true, and that projected capacity has to be brought in line with the income that will be available to cater for it. In fact, within weeks of opening, the North Durham health authority was contemplating deals with a local private hospital in order to deal with the projected caseload.[24]

Effects on hospital workload

A further option is to increase the productivity of the clinical workforce. PFI business cases incorporate targets and efficiency measures (in relation to lengths of stay, throughput and bed occupancy) which are acknowledged to be 'challenging'. Others do not always include data on throughput or caseload, or information on the relationship between provision and need. The Durham proposals, for example, appeared to suggest that purchasers had agreed to fund only the trust's 1996–7 caseload into the future. The implication – that patient numbers would remain stable – was at variance with demographic projections for the area which would have suggested a rise in admissions. Future patient numbers are treated 'as a variable, which can be adjusted to fit the financing of the development' (Gaffney and Pollock 1999b: 24).

These assumptions about level caseload were somewhat contradicted by the prediction that the Trust could increase its activity levels by up to 20 per cent. Unless the Trust could reduce lengths of stay below the national average (unlikely in an area with relatively poor health status), this increase in caseload could be accommodated only if occupancy levels were to rise above 100 per cent, which was absurd. Lengths of stay could be reduced only if there were a parallel expansion of community care, but, according to critics, vagueness in the Durham PFI business case did not suggest that the necessary shift of resources to community care was likely to take place. The same could broadly be said of the Carlisle proposals (Price *et al.* 1999). The community services, on which throughput targets depend, are not the responsibility of the Trusts. In this respect, Trusts, acting in a rational (but self-interested) way, are externalising their costs. The result was that substantial developments were taking place without a clear specification of the type and volume of cases to be admitted, or of the relationship between admissions and need for hospital services. Thus, when the Carlisle hospital was criticised for being unable to deal with its caseload, an inquiry argued that this was not a problem of insufficient hospital capacity but rather one of inadequate community services.[25]

However, this was unsatisfactory, because there was no guarantee that the necessary community-based services *would* be made available.

Income generation

The affordability gap might be closed (or reduced) in other ways too. Swift rationalisation of the asset base of the trust is one possibility here. Most PFI developments have two features in common: centralisation of inpatient services on single sites, and disposal of remaining sites. Handing over to the private sector parcels of land with development potential has clearly been attractive. This argument could equally apply to land sales under a non-PFI financial regime but it leads to a preference for greenfield sites and new-build schemes, with developers largely avoiding *in situ* redevelopment. The resulting accessibility consequences have exercised opponents of schemes (e.g. Edinburgh, Norwich) especially when developers appear to be presented with opportunities for profitable property development. Other options have involved writing charitable fundraising into bids for capital, as at Carlisle (Price *et al.* 1999), the bid not being viable without charitable support,[26] and increasing income from patients, whether private or not. PFI bids have assumed that the generation of external income from such sources is integral to financial viability. Thus, business cases make reference to the incidence of private medical insurance. This option is not likely to generate the same benefits in the Northern region as elsewhere but a sample of PFI bids nationally shows that in all cases the proportion of private beds has increased (Pollock *et al.* 1999: 182). Hospitals may also generate additional income through selling other services to inpatients; the North Durham hospital hit the headlines immediately on opening, when charging patients £25 per week for television rental.[27]

Summary

The ramifications of these developments are significant. PFI deals have been predicated on staff reductions, more rapid throughput and the availability of community care to prevent bed blocking. Critics suggest that on all these counts, implausible targets are assumed, and that hospitals will have difficulties balancing the books. In these circumstances, there have been various subsidies to 'smooth' the process of implementing a PFI deal, and, occasionally, additional payments have been required from purchasers of health care so that contractual obligations to private consortia can be met. This raises the question of whether PFI provides value for money. Hospital developments should proceed under the PFI only if it can be shown that they offer better value for money than public procurement. Critics have argued that the criteria used to compare public and private finance are skewed in favour of the private sector, and that a more balanced approach should be adopted (Sussex 2001). Finally, the initiative has been determinedly forced through, being presented by politicians as the 'only game in town' (see Ruane 2000, 2001).

A final point concerns the implications for strategic planning of a capital development process based on decisions of individual Trusts. Initially, once the financial viability of a PFI scheme was determined, there was no basis for deciding between hospital development schemes. Thus, schemes were being considered at the level of the individual hospital or trust, a process which failed to consider how hospitals relate to each other or to other parts of the health service (Boyle and Harrison 2000: 55). One reason for this was the weakening of regional governance in the NHS after 1991 which left inadequate strategic planning capacity in place. Recognising this, the Health Minister, Alan Milburn, announced in December 1997 the establishment of a Capital Prioritisation Advisory Group (CPAG) to regulate the flow of PFI deals. The public presentation of this was interesting, Milburn saying that: 'Previously the whims of the market determined capital development plans in the NHS. In the future hospitals will be built where they are needed most and where they will deliver the greatest benefit to patients.'[28] Yet this anti-market rhetoric was not accompanied by any softening of the priority given to PFI. Acknowledgement that a crucial criticism of PFI was correct was followed by reaffirmation of commitment to the policy (Gaffney and Pollock 1998). Contrary to Milburn's assertion that 'need' was to be the key determinant of priorities, CPAG guidance on 'service need' included nine weighted criteria. The largest single weight was given to the more effective use of resources and the scoring system also gave far larger weights to service reconfiguration than it did to access or service development. The message is clear: it is financial criteria which are to lead to a scheme gaining preference under CPAG, and these criteria reinforce an emphasis in planning on whether or not a scheme can obtain private finance.

In turn, this raises the question of just how hospital provision ought to be planned. Gaffney and Pollock (1998) make several relevant points about the methodologies used by health authorities to project future levels of demand. They are highly critical of modelling which simply deflates projected caseload on the basis of assumed reductions in hospitalisation rates and lengths of stay. Boyle and Harrison (2000) also point out that the government has still sanctioned some £1.5 billion of capital investment without a clear indication of what they wish to achieve through it, and Dawson (2001: 485) suggests that there remains virtually no evidence as to the long-term effects of PFI on service delivery. Yet again, echoes of the 1962 Plan are relevant: we know much about the ultimate pattern of facilities, but rather less about how they relate to one another. Boyle and Harrison (2000) contend that the Department of Health does not yet have 'an adequate strategic framework for investing in hospitals' (p. 62) nor one for investing in complementary services. The National Beds Inquiry could help provide such a framework, though this has been criticised, on the grounds that much more is required than 'a view on likely bed numbers' (Harrison 2000: 5).

Concluding comments

The post-1991 period has witnessed substantial changes in and reconfiguration of acute hospital provision in the NHS. However this does not mean all the changes can be attributed to the internal market and this raises several questions about the intentions and outcomes of policy changes.

A case can be made that in fact the various restrictions on the operation of the internal market meant, in practice, that it was arguably never tried. This led Enthoven, whose ideas underpinned the reforms, to conclude on a return visit that market forces had not been properly implemented. He emphasised the absence of investment to create spare capacity, scathingly described moves towards cooperation as 'coddling the inefficient' and argued for a much stronger line against Trust mergers (Enthoven 1999). What this would do to the configuration of hospital services can only be surmised but the pre-Tomlinson chaos in London, though short-lived, gives some clues.

Health authorities and Trusts in most locations wanted to avoid such disruption and numerous reviews of acute hospital configurations have occurred, in which initially adversarial relations between providers and purchasers have developed into more collaborative relationships. The threat rather than the reality of market forces may be what matters here, and the outcomes have been contingent on local networks of power in the NHS. The Newcastle case illustrates this well – the (likely, but unquantifiable) threat that new DGHs would remove resources from the city's hospitals led to a swift resolution of the two/three hospital issue. One could argue, however, that the full commissioning of proximate DGHs would have had similar, though negotiated, effects on referrals to Newcastle's hospitals, in the absence of reforms. Newcastle would have suffered from this process, though it would also have facilitated access to Newcastle's hospitals for Newcastle's residents, an issue which has bedevilled the city since before the inception of the NHS (Chapter 2).

The widespread destabilisation predicted at the time has thus not occurred; nor, with the limited exceptions noted above, have hospitals disengaged from the NHS in pursuit of more profitable opportunities. This has led to the suggestion that competitive relationships between hospitals were short-lived and have been superseded by collaboration which is not all that different from the planning of the pre-1991 NHS. There is some descriptive validity in this but it neglects the wider context in which hospitals are operating. Broadly speaking, New Labour accepts globalisation and international capitalist competition as inevitable (Panitch and Leys 2001), albeit with greater (if targeted) redistribution within those parameters, such as the substantial growth in NHS resources. This means that there continues to be pressure, driven by what Leys (1999: 1155) termed a 'Treasury – NHSE – hospital management nexus' for 'downsizing acute care, shedding costs, and shifting to private provision'. Examples of this are the relentless pressure on Trusts to achieve savings in management costs via mergers, and, most recently, the system of 'earned autonomy', which extends greater freedoms to the most successful (including freedom to invest surpluses) while threatening the least successful with takeover or even closure. The commitment to the PFI is part and parcel of this approach, because deals are concluded on the basis of criteria of affordability, which means configuring bed provision in ways which externalise costs so as to make the hospital a viable proposition. Reflecting on the PFI one is reminded of Keynes' comment that 'when the capital development of a country becomes a by-product of the activities of a casino, the job is likely to be ill-done' (quoted in Hutton 1995: 243).

The implied problem here is that reconfiguring the hospital in the manner implied by the PFI may also redraw the boundaries around the NHS. Achieving the required throughput of patients in PFI hospitals means speedy discharge once they no longer need acute facilities. This requires better community care or nursing home provision. Forty years on from the 1962 Plan, access to these remains variable but the key point about recent legislation on nursing home care is that eligibility criteria for it (in England) have been tightened. Critics therefore contend that discharged patients will bear costs which ought properly to be borne by the NHS (Pollock 2000: 393–4). This problem is not unique to PFI-funded hospitals, because of secular trends towards quicker discharge, but it is more acute in such hospitals, because of the substantial reductions in bed provision.

Turning to the broader theme implied in the title of this chapter, it can be argued that elements of all three (markets, hierarchies, networks) can be detected in this period. Hospital hierarchies may not have been completely established by the Hospital Plan but in many areas they exist and have not been destabilised by competition. Markets were certainly evident post-1991 even though their impact became somewhat blunted in practice, and market criteria are certainly evident through the PFI. Networks and partnerships might be a characterisation of the processes by which hospital rationalisation has been managed, but these networks have been established within a system which remains hierarchical and closely managed from the centre (Paton 2000), and which offers little scope for community involvement. This may be one reason for a number of large-scale protests against hospital downsizing, as communities object to decisions being taken by bodies with no local roots and (perhaps more fundamentally) to the administrative logics behind those decisions (Barker 1997; Moon and Brown 2001; Tuohy 1999). Arguably this reached a peak in Kidderminster, Worcestershire, where several councillors were elected on an anti-PFI platform and a local doctor was returned as MP in the 2001 General Election. These developments are part of a wider disenchantment with electoral politics and a search for single issues around which to campaign, particularly in the context of a government with an impregnable majority. But they carry echoes of the warnings of civil servants, in the 1940s, of establishing a system of 'mechanical perfection' in which the public could take no interest. These protests are not without paradoxical elements: the absence of community control does not prevent large numbers of individuals voluntarily committing money, time and physical effort to support their local hospital. Despite protests against the bureaucratic state, citizens thus seem willing (consciously or unconsciously) to accept new forms of what Rose (1996) terms 'governmentality', in which localities play an increasing part in generating their own resources for welfare provision. It will be interesting to observe whether the new generation of privately financed hospitals are successful in terms of generating community attachment, in the way that their predecessors did. The evidence of a desire for such participation is one reason why government proposals for community control of hospitals strike a responsive chord.

Finally, some relevant comparisons with earlier periods in this book are in order. First, the reactive and *ad hoc* character of post-1991 policy formulation is notable; there was not so much a grand design as what Harrison and Wood (2000) term 'manipulated emergence', some broad contours of policy were known but not the precise details. Given this, an obvious comparison is that the launch of the reforms, and the subsequent endorsement of PFI, had as much – or as little – of an evidence base as the 1962 Plan. However, one might have more sympathy for the Permanent Secretary's description of the Plan as a 'mix of caution, faith and determination' than for Kenneth Clarke's insouciant insistence that reform could not wait for pilot schemes: 'change cannot be conditional on a protracted academic appraisal'. Whereas in 1989 Conservatives at times appeared to imply that the precise nature of change was a matter of indifference, at least in 1962 there was a commitment to a defined outcome, in terms of a list of hospital projects. Second, how convincing is the implied characterisation of the pre-reform NHS as a command bureaucracy? Moran (1995), for one, is sceptical: he argues that while the state did secure resources for the NHS through taxation and largely became a monopoly employer of doctors, this did not mean that health policy was necessarily implemented at the periphery in the manner envisaged at the centre. Given the (at best) partial implementation of the Hospital Plan, characterisation of the reforms as the supersession of hierarchies by markets is thus oversimplistic. Third, the repertoire of post-reform attempts to regulate the internal market demonstrates both the absence of planning capacity in the NHS and the continuing importance of hierarchical organisation in some form.

10 Conclusions

The aim of this book has been to contrast various forms of regulation of hospital provision over a long time period illustrated, where possible, through the experience of one region. What wider lessons can be drawn from this chronological study? The general themes raised at various stages by this book concern the future role of the hospital, and the appropriate level of hospital provision; the interpretation of the changes described herein; and the financing and governance of hospital care.

The future role of the hospital

The pace of change in the health sector, and the extent of reductions in acute beds, has led some to project a scenario in which there is a continual, inevitable and market-driven reduction in acute hospital provision. There are several developments which may lead to a continued reduction in the significance of the hospital in health-care delivery (on this, more generally, see Vetter 1995; Mistry 1997), and therefore some reconfiguration will be inevitable. Earlier chapters have highlighted continuing disagreement over the question of the optimum size for hospitals and such debates will continue, for various reasons.

First, technological advance in medicine will permit more procedures to be undertaken either in non-hospital settings, or as day cases. Improvements in diagnostic techniques and anaesthetics, and the development of keyhole surgery and other less-invasive methods, have combined to reduce the 'collateral damage' from which patients must recover (West 1998: 41), and thus lengths of stay have diminished greatly. Second, moves to evidence-based health care have led to proposals for some procedures to be discontinued on grounds of clinical effectiveness, while purchasers are shifting resources towards prevention, primary and community care. The combination of all these has led the government's health-care Technology Foresight panel to speak of 'rolled-back' health care, though this may concede too much to the beneficial effects of technological change.[1]

A third factor, medical staffing, is also crucial (West 1998: 72). Training requirements are usually specified in terms of the minimum number of cases that must be treated on a hospital site to provide the requisite experience for doctors in training. Reductions in the working hours of junior doctors have meant that, in order to maintain cover, more juniors need to be employed at each hospital. Because the supply of junior doctors is relatively fixed, any move to reduce their hours and employ more doctors on a rota means that any given speciality operates from fewer hospital sites. Trends towards specialisation compound this process, because of the connection between volume, expertise and quality of service. West (1998: 85–96) suggests several possible models which might develop as a result.

First, by projecting trends in bed use forwards, and by making inferences about the likely development of technology and medical practice, scenarios have been suggested in which considerable rationalisation takes place. The BMA's Joint Consultants' Committee (1999) argued that the DGH would continue to be the basic unit of hospital provision. Echoing the Bonham-Carter report (Chapter 7), it suggested that a minimum of two consultants were required in each speciality and major subspeciality, and that acute medicine and surgery were interlinked, and should not be practised on one site. Considerable centralisation was thus inevitable but, echoing controversies of the 1960s, the foreword to the report stated that 'the public is ambivalent in wanting the highest standards of clinical care but opposing closure of even the smallest hospitals. Frankly *the two ambitions are incompatible*'; the physical closure of one-third of the hospitals in the UK would be 'politically unacceptable'. West's (1998) alternative scenarios therefore envisage partial centralisation, with supporting facilities in community hospitals or in Elective Resource Centres (the latter would provide a limited range of relatively straightforward procedures). Such developments might be more feasible in urban settings where the acute bed requirement for a community might be provided across two or more sites, but in rural areas, smaller populations might, on present trends, generate the need for limited numbers of beds which would not be viable. On the whole, though, trends towards concentration will continue, creating larger local monopolies than envisaged in 1962, unless there are changes in policy – for example, attempting to preserve competition in hospital markets (Harrison and Prentice 1998: 172). However, the Government's recent proposal for 'diagnostic and treatment centres', offering fast-track surgery, is indicative of new thinking in hospital provision.

The question of just how many beds are needed was given salience by a number of large-scale protests against hospital rationalisation and the PFI. Critics argued that the PFI led to above-average reductions in bed provision. Health authorities and trusts retorted that this was not the case and that PFI deals reflected planned decisions about the adequacy of future hospital capacity. Still others argued that the culprit was to be found in the higher echelons of the NHS, because regional offices were refusing to approve hospital strategies unless they entailed significant reductions in bed numbers. Indeed one health economist argued that the whole debate was futile because there was no 'right' answer to the numbers of beds needed by the NHS; supply would influence demand and admission thresholds would rise or fall accordingly.[2]

Against this background the government launched a National Beds Inquiry, to test the hypothesis that bed closures had gone too far. Its report (Department of Health 2000a) pointed to growing pressures on the acute hospital system, which had increased bed occupancy to 83 per cent. Bed provision was below the levels found in most OECD states. The Inquiry laid particular stress on the rise in emergency admissions to hospital, especially among the elderly population, and the report pointed to the failure of community-service provision to expand and to the reduction in home-care support. Because of this, around 20 per cent of bed-days occupied by the elderly could have been avoided if alternative facilities had been in place. Forty years on from the Hospital Plan, and eighty years after the Dawson report, the provision of complementary community facilities was still a constraint on developments in the acute sector. The Inquiry resulted in three scenarios; the general emphasis was on stabilising, or slightly increasing, the number of acute beds, and expanding the availability of intermediate care. The latter was justified on the grounds that areas with higher rates of long-term care provision and district nursing appeared to have lower rates of acute admissions. The emphasis on intermediate care was welcomed, although concerns remained about how it would be financed (Mallender 2000; Pollock and Dunnigan 2000). However, Harrison (2000) contended that the Inquiry had missed an opportunity to review hospital policy more generally. The fact that the Inquiry had been set up in the first place reflected a failure on the part of the NHS to maintain an appropriate framework for considering the future of service provision. The capacity at regional level to think strategically had been dismantled during the 1990s, and thus, Harrison (2000: 4–5) argues, the ability to take a system-wide view of hospital developments was very weak. The Department of Health's capital investment strategy did not do that (Boyle and Harrison 2000), nor did the incentives facing individual agencies in health and social care necessarily encourage collaboration. And, as Pollock and Dunnigan (2000) observe, although the National Beds Inquiry's recommendation of a halt to bed capacity reductions has been welcomed by many observers, more and more PFI deals are being approved which almost inevitably lead to reductions in capacity, and involve externalising costs. There is another parallel here: debating the 1962 Plan, Denis Howell criticised the way 'a colossal amount of money will be transferred from the taxpayer to the ratepayer',[3] because the Plan was predicated on an expansion of community care. Once again, an expansion of investment of hospital services is predicated on complementary services which may or may not exist and which, if provided by local authorities, may be means-tested. Both the Hospital Plan and the PFI therefore redistributed the costs of change in the service because of assumptions made about capacity and complementary facilities.

Interpreting change in hospital policy

There are two central issues here: the extent to which a periodisation in terms of markets, hierarchies and networks is appropriate, and the value of commentaries which stress broader epochal transitions in the economic or cultural spheres. An easy periodisation – a succession, from voluntary failure, to planning, to state failure, markets, and finally to some form of networks – must be rejected. Elements of markets and networks, if not hierarchies, certainly co-existed before the NHS. The extent to which they were superseded under the NHS is doubtful, given the difficulties of implementing even the commitments of the Hospital Plan. The Hospital Plan only partially implemented its implicit vision of regional hierarchies and, of course, while the Plan was being progressed the extent to which there was integration between hospitals and other health services was highly variable. The externalities associated with market-led reforms after 1991 posed anew (in a British context, at least) the dilemma of how best to regulate hospital development. Certain elements of planning thus remained in place. Thus, a meltdown of hospital capacity was avoided by strategic intervention and management of the restructuring process in ways which were not entirely without resemblance to 1970s-style strategic planning. Softening of pro-market rhetoric, and emphases on greater stability in placing contracts, gave the NHS something of the appearance of collaborative networks, in which alliances formed between partners with a shared interest in the quality of health services in a locality.

However, such relationships have developed in the context of an NHS which remains strongly centralised, in terms of national targets for service delivery and demands for efficiency savings. These are coupled with systems for rewarding the successful, implying that a dynamic of inter-hospital competition still rules the service, notwithstanding substantial increases in resources. And the financing of hospital development is not just a technical adjunct to that: private finance determines the character of the NHS, downsizing it even as the National Beds Inquiry calls for a halt to hospital rationalisation.

These ideal-typical models, then, were never found in a 'pure' form. If so, to what extent can they be said to have failed? This is important because of the claims made as to the superiority of different ways of managing hospital development by politicians and others. One argument might be that they have never been properly tried, as in Enthoven's (1999) claims about the NHS reforms, or the view that the Hospital Plan was never resourced at the level needed to make a real impact. A different view is that the definition of failure depends on circumstances and context: thus, the claim that the pre-NHS system was defective because of its substantial inequalities may be a case of evaluating it by post-hoc collectivist criteria, which would not have been recognised at the time. A third view might be that it is inappropriate to condemn institutions or organisations for circumstances beyond their control. Criticisms of 'state failure' need to separate innate problems of state intervention from the difficulties of implementing policies in a turbulent economic and political climate. Selective appropriations of history may be being presented here, in which particular weaknesses are exaggerated into generalised critiques.

If the markets/hierarchies/networks triad is an over-simplification, how do these trends in hospital policy relate to debates which have attracted much attention from social scientists such as transitions from modernism to postmodernism? Superficially there is a fair degree of correspondence. For Giddens (1990) the consequences of modernity include the application of scientific principles, the formation of states which govern social life through bureaucracies, and a vision of modernity as *progress*: an attempt to make a clean break with a problematic past.[4] Clearly such arguments were implicit in the nationalisation of hospitals and in the Hospital Plan: Eckstein (1958: 262–3) thus suggests the aims of the NHS were to 'make subject to calculation what had previously been left to chance ... [and] replace spontaneous adjustment with deliberate control'. Whether what has subsequently happened may be characterised as 'postmodern' is much more open to question. We might best regard postmodernism as a critique of modernism, rather than a coherent alternative to it. Postmodernism is sceptical of grand narratives and, thus, of centralised solutions imposed upon diverse localities. This is not so far removed from a fairly standard conservative critique of bureaucracy and planning, which lends itself to a politics of deregulation, and a denial of the possibility of 'planning' for a better future. These developments are reflected in the demise of state regulation based on planning blueprints, and the rise of flexible decision making, based on partnerships between a variety of stakeholders (Cooke 1990). In these circumstances, local initiative and economic circumstances will, to a greater degree, determine the trajectory of welfare state development, and Chapters 8 and 9 indicate ways in which these issues have come to the fore in recent decades.

Responding to such developments, it has been argued that in many areas of social policy, new 'governmentalities' have emerged, in which citizens are led to realise that it is part of their duty to support local welfare services (Murdoch 1997). However, this is not an autonomous trend, but one which has been carefully managed: there is no alternative to PFI; hospitals must henceforth be planned on the basis of economic realism, and so on. There are connections here to debates about whether welfare state developments simply reflect wider changes in the organisation of production, the alleged transition from Fordism to post-Fordism being frequently cited here (Burrows and Loader 1994). On this view the NHS would merely mimic changes going on around it, but this seems an oversimplification in the context of hospital policy. Even if the NHS had really corresponded to Fordist logics, other than superficially, it is not clear that current developments reflect post-Fordist forms of organisation (e.g. in terms of flexibility, networks, etc.). In fact PFI deals appear to involve some familiar practices of intensification of throughput, externalisation of costs through faster discharge, and cutting labour costs as far as possible in order to maximise returns to shareholders. Hospital development might therefore more simply be regarded as another element of the corporate takeover of Britain (Monbiot 2000), in which the character of the services that are delivered is reconfigured along commercial lines. Current policies appear agnostic about such developments, and the growing contribution of the private sector is presented as something that is inevitable, because of constraints imposed by global economic competition. The funds available to the NHS have undoubtedly increased, but there are concerns that greater private-sector involvement may change the character of the NHS as a public service. Key issues here relate to NHS finance and governance.

Hospital finance and governance

In the course of the lengthy timespan covered in this book, state intervention substantially improved access to health care. Disparities in bed provision under the voluntary system had narrowed only slightly over a long time period (Gorsky *et al.* 1999) but public provision eventually closed many gaps: as Kenneth Robinson reminded a medical audience in 1966, he was certain that places such as 'Carmarthen, Swansea, Swindon or Whitehaven' would not have been beneficiaries of new investment if 'these things depended on charity, benevolence and ratepayers' money'.[5] New and substantially remodelled hospitals were eventually built in needy locations, although (as indicated in Chapters 6–8) there were also lengthy delays. This was also, by and large, a planned process, with norms of desirable levels of bed provision being used to identify gaps to be closed by new investment. Until comparatively recently under the NHS, charitable and private sources of funds have had little impact on the trajectory of hospital development. With some limited exceptions, such sources of income still account for only small proportions of Trust budgets, but they have the potential to distort a planned allocation of resources. Moreover the availability of capacity in the private sector, and the government's agnostic concordat, may mean that NHS-funded care takes place to a growing extent in – and thus will come to depend upon the commercial viability of – the private sector. The private finance initiative continues this trend: it brings private capital into the NHS and is thus about creating opportunities for profit within a sphere which was distinctive precisely because it was decommodified; that is, services were provided for use, not exchange. It is true that a substantial public-sector hospital capital programme remains in place, but critical analyses of PFI show the way private finance is being used to redraw the boundaries of what is available on the NHS. Short-term, high-volume interventions, in hospitals operating at maximum capacity, are what the PFI demands, and costs are displaced on to the remaining local health services.

Defenders of the PFI point to the difficulties experienced with public procurement and imply that private finance is innately more efficient. This does not explain why difficulties (such as those discussed in Chapters 7 and 8) are not still encountered in the rest of the public capital programme. One wonders whether valid criticisms are being made here. Sir George Godber's riposte to David Owen (Chapter 8) is highly apposite: the hospital programme was not out of control, it was subject to too much control. Given the scale of resources available, relative to the problems facing them, the Ministry needed to ensure that priorities were being set and adhered to, leading to delays while hospital strategies were checked. Many of the high-profile problems in the hospital building programme resulted from specific local circumstances, rather than from public procurement *per se*. Some failings of public procurement may also be partly attributed to circumstances over which the NHS had little control: inflation, industrial relations, and the state of the construction industry, to say nothing of radical changes in revenue assumptions. These could of course be wrapped into a 'new right' critique of overload and ungovernability, but the point is that the inherent superiority of private finance needs to be demonstrated and founded on an evidence base (Dawson 2001; Sussex 2001). Moreover the PFI unquestionably redistributes the cost of financing health care into the future, and as it expands it will absorb a growing proportion of NHS expenditure. The short-term advantage of an expanded building programme may therefore have long-term costs.

The question of governance is related to that of finance because a persistent criticism of the NHS has been a failure to promote public involvement. This view features in recent pronouncements from various points of the political compass. When proposals for a national health service began to be debated the Ministry of Health indicated a preference for a mixed economy, supervised by local authorities. The concern was expressed that a separate, unelected organisation was inappropriate, because services would be delivered through a 'mechanically perfect' body in which citizens could take no interest. Participation and community support would best be assured through local government control. Forty years on and the boot was on the other foot; by 1989 the problem in the NHS was deemed to be too much democratic input, not too little, according to the Minister of Health. Hospitals did not belong to any section of the community, so Trusts did not need local input, and they became part of a centrally appointed quango state. This aspect of the NHS reforms was not reversed by Labour. The question of the relationship between hospitals and their communities therefore continues to attract attention in the form of proposals for greater community control of hospital services. The aim here is to reconcile the equity of public provision with the flexibility and responsiveness of the market (Ham 1996; Hirst 1994). Thus, Green (1998: 58–62) makes proposals for much greater individual choice in health care, which he contends would force providers of services to respond to consumer preferences. Hospitals would be removed from 'political control' by being privatised as non-profit, voluntary hospitals. There would be no planning agencies under this system;

presumably, where they did not exist, hospitals would come into existence on the basis that communities anticipated sufficient revenue flowing to them from the purchasing cooperatives to which individuals would subscribe. Given the scale of the resource commitments involved, the obvious problem here would be guaranteeing availability of services in all locations since the pre-NHS evidence indicates under-investment. Nor is it clear whether, if hospital development continued to be financed privately, Green's hospital trusts would be more accountable to community representatives than to private shareholders. Bosanquet (1999) similarly endorses a mixed economy although his proposals mainly discuss community and nursing home care, and they do not really indicate how the substantial investment needed to create additional capacity would come about.

These proposals would still leave unresolved the question of how best to reconcile the best features of planning and competition. The latest proposals from Labour indicate that NHS Trusts will be allowed to earn greater autonomy: the better a Trust does, the more freedom it receives. The implication is that standards will in this way be ratcheted up, across the board, but the question is whether it is possible – if it's not logically contradictory – to raise the performance of every Trust to that of the best: not all can win in this game. Moreover, by accepting that investment for the creation of replacement capacity is to a significant degree funded privately, Labour is further emphasising competition between hospitals. Finally, such autonomy is not likely to be accompanied by more participatory management arrangements.

Reconciling equity and choice: looking backwards and forwards

It seems appropriate to conclude this assessment of hospital policy with three vignettes from different periods, including contributions by two individuals with North Eastern roots and long commitments to the NHS. The contrasting attitudes to the problem of extending access to hospital care are of interest.

The first illustration is from the 1930s. The Ministry of Health's declared policy involved a gradualist approach, building on the activities of local authorities but largely relying on persuasion, not compulsion. The surveys of local authorities showed 'variation in the standards achieved' but the Minister was relaxed about this because he had no desire to limit the activities of local authorities to the 'maintenance of a mechanical efficiency'. Progress in public health would depend on the 'liveliness of the interest taken in it'.[6] The implication was that a degree of inequality was tolerable. However, the evidence (Chapters 2 and 3) shows that if left to themselves, some local authorities would have achieved very little, and a levelling-up of standards would have been unlikely. There were also major problems of articulating a collective interest as a basis for collaboration, and the wartime debates, in which advocates of voluntarism and municipalism fought to a standstill (Chapter 4), indicate the difficulties of overcoming such obstacles. Extension of public–private partnerships also presumes the existence of partners – but these did not exist everywhere prior to 1948, and the same is true of the private sector today.

The second illustration is from the 1960s. Having nationalised the hospitals governments then faced the problem of satisfying demands for a modernisation of the infrastructure. Chapters 5 and 6 show that the response was very limited, and that only in the late 1960s was the situation beginning to change. During the 1960s the slow pace of change led to a growing chorus of criticism, exemplified by Henry Miller's indictment of the failure to resource the hospital plan at realistic levels (featured in Chapter 7). In 1967 Miller commented that one HMC in the Newcastle region would have to make do with its 'antediluvian' facilities until 1997. The reason was that government expenditure priorities limited the resources committed to hospital building while HMCs had to await their place in a regional programme which itself depended on and was constrained by the exigencies of the national economy. While the Hospital Plan could give some guarantees that something would be done to modernise the hospital stock, its frustration potential was enormous. As a result, unfortunately, Miller was optimistic. Two PFI-funded developments have recently opened (Carlisle, North Durham) and in two other areas (Bishop Auckland, Hexham) comprehensive reconstruction of the local general hospital has only recently begun. These are localities where the hospital stock inherited by the NHS was minimal and of poor quality (Chapter 2) yet for a combination of reasons, complete reconstruction was delayed for half a century. In these circumstances private finance of course appeared attractive but questions about the adequacy of hospitals provided in this way have yet to be resolved.

The final comment here comes from Alan Milburn, the current Health Secretary, whose recent speeches, exemplified by an address to the Fabian Society[7] may indicate the future trajectory of policy. Echoing familiar criticisms rehearsed elsewhere in this book, Milburn argued that the 'top-down model of the 1940s cannot deliver in the twenty-first century', an argument which echoes those of Conservatives when introducing the NHS reforms. His argument was couched in the language of consumerism, choice, decentralisation and empowerment. As well as giving patients scope to turn to the private sector, the emphasis on reconnecting public services with the communities they serve seems to imply a greater degree of local funding for health care, as well as greater autonomy for NHS Trusts. This is acknowledged in statements such as ensuring that 'public control means something more than simply state control', or speaking of an NHS which has 'more plurality of providers'. The proposals for 'foundation hospitals', announced in January 2002, put this into practice, by loosening some financial and management control over hospitals, and by granting them greater commercial freedom. Milburn argued that the NHS was born into a world where 'everyone was given the same rations'; the NHS therefore strove for equity for the population, at the expense of choice for the individual. Today, he contends, unprecedented investment gives the NHS a chance to 'reconcile equity and choice'. This elusive philosopher's stone is to be attained through strengthening the levers available to 'consumers' by removing obstacles to patient choice. In the absence of spare capacity in the NHS, however, patient choice can really only be exercised if there are private-sector alternatives within reasonable travelling distance. Given what we know about the distribution of such resources, the benefits of such relationships will be more easily available to certain places than others. One inference would be that Milburn is trying to bind the middle classes and the upwardly mobile into supporting Labour's programme (not unlike earlier suggestions by Hutton (1995: 310–11), though Hutton would not endorse the expanded use of the PFI). Labour is acutely aware of the possibility of defection to the private sector: 11–12 per cent insurance coverage nationally translates into some substantial proportions of voters locally, which could lead to growing reluctance to support public services. Baldwin's (1994: 29) analysis of welfare state development is relevant here. He argues that explaining solidarity 'only in terms of the needy's ability to wrest concessions' ignores the 'acquiescence of the self-reliant' which is an equally necessary requisite of reform – or, for that matter, of sustaining existing welfare arrangements. But sustaining this acquiescence – preventing middle-class defection – may well have as its corollary greater diversity, at least at the margins, and especially in those localities with a large private sector and with strong voluntary support for health care. Although it is undeniable that the funding available to the NHS has increased substantially under Labour, Milburn's proposed vision may well be found wanting in hard economic times: reconciling equity and choice may be impossible to achieve on a national basis.

A future hospital service needs to avoid the inequities of the pre-NHS system, the frustrations of the maligned era of top-down planning, and the problems posed by competition within the public sector and pressure to configure hospitals in ways that are fiscally acceptable to private financiers. New Labour has attempted to reconcile two arguably contradictory positions, denying that it is pursuing market-led policies while simultaneously encouraging private finance and competition. It is now determined to decentralise, while simultaneously rolling forward its National Plan. Like the Ministry of Health in the 1930s, the government seems willing to accept a degree of localism and variability in order to continue to secure continual support for the NHS. If the implication of the current trajectory of policy is that the NHS will become a much more diverse collection of services than in its history to date, the issue then will become the degree of inequity that is tolerable.

Appendix A

Figures

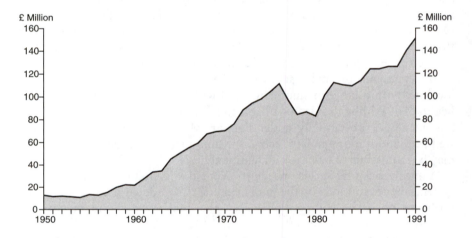

Figure A.1 NHS capital expenditure, England and Wales, at constant 1962 prices
Source: Summarised Accounts of Health Authorities

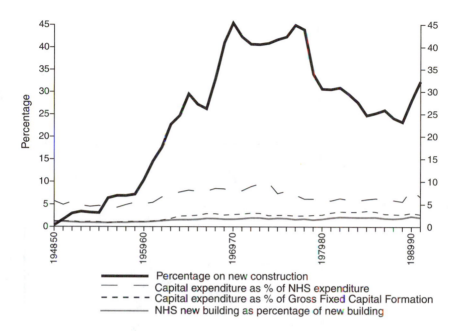

Percentage on new construction
— — Capital expenditure as % of NHS expenditure
- - - - - Capital expenditure as % of Gross Fixed Capital Formation
——— NHS new building as percentage of new building

Figure A.2 Indices of change in NHS capital expenditure, 1950–91
Source: Summarised Accounts of Health Authorities (annual)

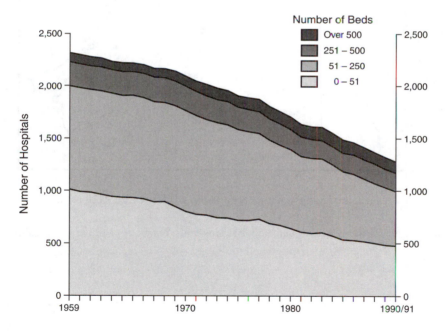

Figure A.3 Nonpsychiatric hospital size trends, England and Wales, 1959–91
Source: Health and Social Service Statistics; Digest of Health Statistics

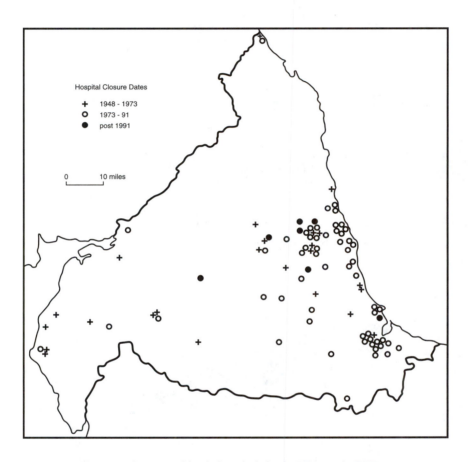

Figure A.4 Closures of nonpsychiatric hospitals in the Newcastle RHB area,
      1948–2001

Sources: Newcastle RHB Annual Reports; Hospitals Yearbook; Ministry of Health,
      1962a.

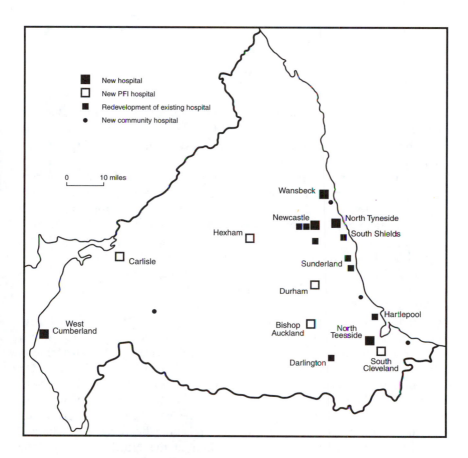

Figure A.5 Major investments in new hospital provision, Newcastle RHB area, 1948–2001

Appendix B
NHS organisational structures

Reference is made at various points to the administrative entities that ran hospitals under the NHS. For those not familiar with these there are good guides to the changes in these since 1948 in texts such as Levitt *et al* (1999), but a brief summary is given here:

1948–74 Hospital management was the responsibility of Hospital Management Committees, which consisted of groups of hospitals in a defined geographical area. Psychiatric hospitals, and hospitals for those with learning difficulties, were run under separate HMCs. Above the HMCs, Regional Hospital Boards (RHBs) were responsible for planning regional hospital services, including strategic decisions on the allocation of capital resources and hospital development. Teaching hospitals were given autonomous status under Boards of Governors (BGs), reporting directly to the Ministry of Health.

1974–82 In an attempt to secure greater integration with local authority services, Area Health Authorities (AHAs) were created, bringing together a greater range of services including those health services which had formerly been the responsibility of local government. The new authorities had a substantial degree of coterminosity with local authorities, to facilitate cooperation; in addition, local authorities had rights to nominate members to them. Below them, in the larger AHAs, there were health districts which were the operational arm of the service. Teaching hospitals were merged with their local health authorities although in the Northern region, the Board of Governors and the Newcastle HMC had merged from 1971. Regional Health Authorities (RHAs) took over the role of RHBs and in the case of the Newcastle region, there were modifications to boundaries mainly on the south-western fringe of the region.

1982–91 The post-1974 structures were perceived as unduly bureaucratic and therefore the 1982 reorganisation removed one tier of administration. RHAs remained in place but below them there were 192 District Health Authorities (DHAs); within these emphasis was placed on the delegation of power to units of management. Districts generally approximated to the areas served by general hospitals and one consequence was a loss of coterminosity with local authorities.

The next formal reorganisation took place in 1991 with the NHS reforms. The key innovation was the separation of the purchasing and providing roles of the health service. This meant that health authorities were to commission care from hospitals, on the basis of price and quality, rather than simply sending patients to the local hospital or the hospital to which, historically, they had always gone. For this to happen, autonomous NHS Trusts were established as providers of health care; eventually, all of the provider units within the health service were established as Trusts. There ensued a process of permanent revolution in the configuration of health authorities. First, Regional Health Authorities did not really have a role in the new system but there were concerns that Trusts could pursue their aspirations without restraint and so a regional tier was reinvented, in the form of regional outposts of the NHS Management Executive. Insofar as regional authorities had ever been subject to democratic influence locally, this was no longer the case. The purpose of the outposts was to ensure a degree of coordination of Trust activities and business plans. These were superseded by eight regional offices of the Department of Health, which oversee the development of the service sub-nationally, and which are responsible for issues like prioritising business cases for hospital investment. Second, health authorities were now responsible solely for purchasing care, not providing it, and in contrast to pre-1991 arrangements, they have a mixture of executive and non-executive members and unlike the post-1974 reorganisations, there are no direct nomination rights for local government to health authorities. The purchasing plans of health authorities are supervised by the regional offices who ensure they follow national priorities and guidelines. In order to acquire greater levels of bargaining power in negotiations with Trusts, there has been a steady process of merger and concentration, so that health authorities have become larger over the past decade, approximating to counties in many parts of England.

Notes

1 Planning, markets and welfare: debates about hospital policy and the welfare state

1 Select Committee on Estimates, 1970, Evidence, Q.1687–91.
2 In the Northern region this question arose in locations such as SE Northumberland, east Durham, and east Cleveland, where populations fell on the margins of, or in between, the catchments of existing general hospitals. After the 1974 reorganisation there were also discussions about flows in and out of the region on its southern boundary, to and from hospitals in Darlington and Northallerton. While provision of new facilities often reduced such flows it did not always eliminate them, but doing so would have involved confronting the referral and admission practices of GPs and consultants. Regional Strategic Plans typically contained discussions of how best to delimit hospital catchments, although one has to consult internal memoranda and planning documents to obtain a flavour of the arguments over these and the political obstacles to change.
3 This applied not just in NE England, of course; the absence of hospital facilities from the new towns around London provoked persistent Parliamentary criticism during the 1950s.

2 Legacies, donations and municipal priorities: the development of the hospital services prior to 1948

1 H.C. Deb., v.422, *c*. 44–7, 30 April 1946.
2 Reg Race, H.C. Deb., v. 980, c. 1256, 11.3.80.
3 This committee was set up to distribute grants to the voluntary hospitals (see Chapter 3) and its remit therefore required assessment of the existing distribution of hospital capacity.
4 Source for these figures is Onslow Commission, 1925.
5 These figures actually underestimate the parlous position of some boroughs; Gateshead's only voluntary hospital was a small institution for children, for instance.
6 Ministry of Health, *Hospital Surveys*, vol. 10, 87.
7 Ministry of Health, *Hospital Surveys*, vol. 9, 115.
8 Elsewhere there are substantial proportions of patients whose area of residence was not available for hospitals in Birmingham, West Suffolk, Herefordshire, Worcestershire and Lancashire; in the fuller analysis referred to some allowance is made for this. Note also that this analysis is not possible for South Wales, nor for Scotland, because the survey reports do not present the data in the necessary form.

9 A densely populated county like Buckinghamshire had numerous small hospitals but no towns of the required size; conversely most hospitals within the boundaries of Lancashire and Yorkshire were located in the respective CBs of those counties.

10 MH 58/173, Hospital Accommodation Report No. 8, Northumberland. Note, of course, the comment in the Onslow Report that waiting lists could indicate the *success* of a hospital in attracting patients due to the quality of facilities, or the presence of medical staff of high repute.

11 *Ibid.*

12 TWAS, HO/RVI/72/160, *Annual Report*, 1919, quoted in Gorsky *et al.* 1999.

13 For example, the adequacy of hospital accommodation in Newcastle repeatedly attracted the attention of the City's Health Committee in the 1930s; e.g. TWAS, MD/NC/99/15, 16, 18, meetings on 4 July 1930, 17 October 1930, 28 November 1930, 23 March 1934. See also Mess (1928: 115–17) and Hadfield (1979: 134).

14 TWAS, MD/NC/99/23, 15 June 1939.

15 Author's calculations from data in wartime Hospital Surveys.

16 Ministry of Health 1946, vol. 10, 44.

17 TWAS, HO/PMH/3/4.

18 TWAS, HO/PMH/1/4, Governing Body minutes, 18 June 1934.

19 Ministry of Health 1946, vol. 10, 54.

20 DCRO, H/SWD/152–60.

21 DCRO, H/DU/13. Overdrafts are not a totally reliable index of distress. Several large hospitals ran six-figure overdrafts but were allowed by their bankers to carry on doing so because of the size of their endowments (Gorsky *et al.* 2002). That option was not available to many institutions in the North East.

22 TWAS, 1130/23, Tynemouth Victoria Jubilee Infirmary, *Annual Reports.*

23 TWAS, 1381, Monkwearmouth and Southwick Hospital, *Annual Reports.*

24 TWAS, 1381, Sunderland Royal Infirmary, *Annual Reports.*

25 TWAS, HO/RVI/72, Newcastle RVI, *Annual Reports.*

26 MH 61/65, Thompson–Tribe, 10 January 1938; for similar comments, Gillett–Brown (Minister of Labour), 14 January 1938.

27 MH 61/73, file note, n.d., probably October 1936; MH 61/68, Memorandum on the financial position of Durham County Hospital, 20 December 1935.

28 MH 61/72, Letter from House Governor, Sunderland Royal Infirmary, to the District Commissioner of the CSA, 17 January 1936.

29 MH 61/68, 'Memorandum on the financial position of Durham County Hospital', 20 December 1935.

30 MH 61/73, 5 August 1936.

31 MH 61/65, 27 July 1937; several other voluntary hospitals made similar points.

32 Ministry of Health 1946, vol. 10, 13.

33 Ministry of Health 1946, vol. 10, 73.

34 Ministry of Health 1946, vol. 10, 87.

35 Ministry of Health 1946, vol. 10, 91.

36 Ministry of Health 1946, vol. 10, 37, 39, 41, 55, 68, 71, 83, 91.

37 Ministry of Health 1946, vol. 9, pp.111–12.

38 Ministry of Health 1946, vol. 9, 13, 26.

39 Ministry of Health 1946, vol. 10, 13.

40 MH 55/624, 'England and Wales: Summary of Hospital Accommodation'.

41 The reason for this is that the geographical breakdown of area of patient residence is given for individual hospitals, not for beds within them; we cannot therefore infer whether the patient was attending for general, or specialist treatment, except by allocating patients in proportion to the distribution of beds between specialities within hospitals. And the classification of beds introduces major problems of comparability: many 'special' beds in municipal hospitals

were, in fact, for the chronic sick or the tuberculous, and such provision was largely absent from the voluntary sector.

42 Cumberland CC, Medical Officer of Health, *Annual Report*, 1935, p. 10, quoted in MH 61/05, file note, March 1937.

43 MH 61/67, Minute by Mr Francis, 17 May 1938.

44 An application for loan sanction to construct at least one infectious diseases hospital was turned down by the Ministry on grounds of financial stringency: MH 61/05, 'Special Areas: Medical Services of Local Authorities'.

45 *Ibid.*

46 *Ibid.*

47 MH 66/12, Durham CC, *Survey Report*, p. 41.

48 MH 66/182, Northumberland CC, *Survey Report*, p. 76.

49 MH 55/624, 'England and Wales: Summary of Hospital Accommodation'.

50 Ministry of Health 1946, 9, 114–15.

51 Ministry of Health 1946, vol. 10.

52 Ministry of Health 1946, 62, 70.

53 Ministry of Health 1946, vol. 10, 89.

54 Ministry of Health 1946, vol. 9, 22, 112, 113; vol. 10, 40, 41, 49, 51, 55, 71, 79, 92.

55 Ministry of Health 1946, vol. 9, 112; vol. 10, 13, 40, 42, 44, 47, 48, 54, 70, 81, 91.

56 Ministry of Health 1946, vol. 10, 51–2, 61–5, 72, 92.

57 The EMS involved the *de facto* nationalisation of hospitals and an effort to make facilities available where they had not previously been provided. It also involved the dispersal of hospital capacity from major cities. See Dunn 1951, for more details.

58 TWAS 672/146 (Minutes of the Hospital Centre Committee, 1933–45), and 672/151 (Board of Governors of the RVI – Reorganisation Committee minutes). These show that at various stages in the 1930s, small voluntary hospitals (the Princess Mary Maternity Hospital, Fleming Memorial Hospital) had all sought land within the RVI site. The principle of a unified Hospital Centre in Newcastle had been agreed by late 1942 (Hospital Centre Committee, 29 September 1942 and 9 December 1942).

59 Ministry of Health 1946, 10, 14.

60 Ministry of Health 1946, 10, 14.

61 Ministry of Health 1962, 6.

62 Ministry of Health 1946, 9, 114–16; 10, 14–15, 96–9.

63 Ministry of Health 1946, 10, 15–16, 22–8.

3   Regionalism: a positive or negative consensus?

1 *Hospitals Yearbook*, 1940, xlviii, 'Regionalisation'.

2 Originally the Prince of Wales' Hospital Fund, this body gave grants to support London's voluntary hospitals and, in doing so, attempted to secure a degree of coordination in hospital development.

3 Source: calculations based on statistics in Ministry of Health 1925: 18–26.

4 MH 58/165, Robinson–Chamberlain, 28 February 1925.

5 Onslow Commission, *Final Report*, p.7: see also MH 58/172, Brock–Newman, 6 August 1924: 'subscribers (to contributory schemes) resent any suggestion of cooperation with the Poor Law. They seem to take the view that they have paid insurance premiums for treatment in a voluntary hospital, and they are determined to have what they have paid for'. A North Eastern example is provided by Durham County Hospital: in 1921 the Workmen's Committee rejected proposals

for amalgamation with a neighbouring Poor Law infirmary on precisely these grounds: DCRO, H/Du/13, *Minutes*, 10 October 1921.

6 MH 58/172, Brock–Newman, 6 August 1924.

7 MH 58/165, Robinson–Chamberlain, 28 February 1925.

8 MH 137/25, 'Memorandum on the Finances and Work of the Voluntary Hospitals, 1911–38', p. 6.

9 Cave Committee 1921: 15. The witnesses were Sir Napier Burnett (British Red Cross Society) and Mr G. Verity (Chairman of the Governors of Charing Cross Hospital), respectively.

10 A. Pyon of the Royal Waterloo Hospital for Women and Children: *Hospital and Health Review*, 1922, 1 (4): 137.

11 *Hospitals Yearbook*, 1923: 8–9.

12 Sir A. Stanley, 'The Function of the Voluntary Hospital in Relation to Public Health Services', *Hospitals Yearbook*, 1929: 95.

13 MH 58/164, Orde–McLachlan, 17 April 1935. Orde had previously worked as Secretary of the Newcastle RVI.

14 *Ibid.*

15 In this respect the BHA's proposals went nowhere near as far as those of the Cathcart Committee (1936) on the Scottish health services, which advocated a degree of compulsion.

16 However, an anonymous Ministry of Health note dismissed this as 'utterly impracticable' because it would 'destroy that local pride and patriotism that, if kept within bounds, is not without its advantages' (MH 80/24).

17 MH 80/24, Macgregor, 'Future Development of the Hospital Service', 24 May 1938.

18 MH 80/24, note by Pater, 14 November 1940.

19 Martin Gorsky's (2001) work on Aberdeen confirms the PEP verdict.

20 'Regionalisation', *Hospitals Yearbook*, 1940: xlviii–lxiii.

21 TWAS, HO/1381, Sunderland RI Annual Reports, 1923, 1924, 1925, 1935.

22 MH 66/917, Sunderland CB, *Survey Report*.

23 MH 66/993, Hartlepool CB, *Re-survey*.

24 MH 66/41, Cumberland CC, *Survey Report*.

25 TWAS, MD/NC/99/20, Health Committee, 21 February 1936.

26 TWAS, MD/NC/99/21, Health Committee, 9 September 1936.

27 TWAS, MD/NC/99/19, 25 June 1936.

28 Current work in progress, with Martin Gorsky and Tim Willis, is addressing the role of contributory schemes in promoting the regional integration of hospital systems.

29 MH 71/52, Menzies–MacNalty, 15 December 1937.

30 MH 80/24, note by Pater, 14 November 1940.

31 MH 80/24, Pater, 'Notes on Hospital Policy', 18 December 1940.

32 MH 58/165, Robinson–Chamberlain, 28 February 1925.

33 CAB 27/577, CP (220), 34, para. 137.

34 See Mohan (1997). However, apart from some exchanges between local authorities and the Commissioner for the Special Areas on this point (see discussion of Durham CC, below), there is little direct evidence that health capital projects were *rejected* by the Ministry due to the financial position of local authorities. Rather the Ministry's approach was more subtle, seeking to emphasise the high costs of developments.

35 MH 66/41, Cumberland CC, *Survey Report*, pp. 41, 96.

36 Northumberland CC: MH 66/183, Ward–Neville, 25 October 1935.

37 MH 66/285, North Riding CC.

38 MH 66/890, survey letter, 1 March 1932.

39 MH 66/993, West Hartlepool, *Re-survey*.

40 MH 66/41, Cumberland CC, *Survey Report*, p. 83.
41 MH 66/79, extract from *Medical Officer*, 24 August 1935.
42 MH 66/12, Durham CC, *Survey Report*, pp. 54–5.
43 MH 55/4, Robinson–Hill, 19 May 1933.
44 Ministry of Health, *Annual Report, 1933–34*, Cmd. 4664, 56.
45 MH 66/917, Sunderland CB, *Survey Report*.
46 MH 66/923, Sunderland CB, *Coordination of Health Services: Resurvey*.
47 MH 66/1069, Carlisle CB, *Survey Report*.
48 *Ibid.*
49 MH 66/1069, Carlisle CB Survey letter, 19 April 1932.
50 Ministry of Health 1946, vol. 9: 52.
51 TWAS, MD/NC/99/13, 10 January 1930, 21 February 1930.
52 TWAS, MD/NC/99/22, 1 June 1937.
53 MH 55/4, Note on interview with the BMA, J. C. Wrigley, 19 December 1932.
54 MH 71/52, 8 April 1938, recording a discussion about competing proposals in Bournemouth and Poole, and noting the Ministry's reluctance to refuse to sanction both.
55 MH 80/24, Macgregor, 'The future development of the hospital service', 24 May 1938.
56 MH 80/24, Pater, Notes on hospital policy, 18 December 1940.
57 *Ibid.*
58 MH 61/64, file note, 31 May 1935.
59 MH 61/64, memo to Ryan, 23 August 1935.
60 MH 61/64, file note, 9 September 1935.
61 MH 61/64, Ryan–Stewart, 11 September 1935.
62 MH 61/64, Tribe–Orde (British Hospitals Association), 30 October 1935; see also MH 61/64, Dalton–Ryan, 15 October 1935: 'a press notice by Government might produce a flood of applications from the type of voluntary hospitals, e.g. small cottage hospitals, which we are not too anxious to assist but which a general invitation to apply might make it difficult to refuse'.
63 MH 61/73, Commissioner to Tribe, n.d. but probably November/December 1936 – emphasis added.
64 MH 61/73, Ryan–Forbes Adam, 24 December 1936 – emphasis added.
65 MH 61/12, 'Schemes for Which it is Important that Grant Should Still be Available', 1938.
66 MH 61/64, Forbes Adam to Commissioner, 5 December 1935.
67 MH 61/65, Ryan to Ministry of Health, 15 November 1936.
68 MH 61/65, Letter from Newcastle Voluntary Hospitals to Forbes Adam, 16 December 1937.
69 MH 61/65, Ryan to Ministry of Health, 15 November 1936.
70 MH 61/65 , Orde–Ryan, 20 November 1936.
71 MH 61/65, Meeting between officials of the Ministry of Health and the Commissioner, 23 December 1936.
72 MH 61/65, letter to District Commissioner, 4 August 1939.
73 HLG 30/19, Macgregor–de Montmorency, 30 November 1937.
74 MH 61/73, Ryan to Tribe, 20 November 1936.
75 MH 61/72, note to Holloway from the Ministry of Health, 12 February 1936.
76 MH 61/33, file note, 9 March 1937.
77 This discussion draws on a much fuller examination of the CSA's role in making grants for health purposes: see Mohan (1997).
78 MH 61/12, de Montmorency–Thompson, n.d., probably late 1938. These figures include beds regardless of ownership (i.e. Poor Law and municipal institutions) and type (i.e. long stay, mental illness and mental deficiency) as well as acute facilities.

79 *Commissioner for the Special Areas, Annual Report*, 1936–37, Cmd. 5595, para. 183.
80 *Commissioner for the Special Areas, Annual Report*, 1937–38, Cmd. 5896, para. 235.
81 MH 61/64, file note, 31 May 1935; source is Commissioner's own written comments on a press cutting.
82 MH 71/53, Carnwath – Chief Medical Officer, 22 November 1938.
83 This was John Pater, who joined the Ministry of Health from university and was heavily involved in post-war planning. His published account of the establishment of the NHS is written with some circumspection (Pater 1981); his unpublished autobiography, from which the above quote is extracted, is more candid: Churchill College, PTER 1/6, pp. 36–7.

4 Wartime hospital policy: attractions and limitations of public-private partnerships

1 MH 77/25 'Hospital Policy in London', August 1941.
2 MH 77/25, 'Suggestions for Post-war Hospital Policy', August 1941.
3 Churchill Archives, PTER 1/6, p. 51.
4 MH 80/24, MacGregor, 'The Future Development of the Hospital Service', 24 May 1938.
5 MH 80/24, 'Areas in which there is a Known Need for Additional Accommodation for the Civilian Sick', n.d. but probably mid 1939.
6 MH 80/24, MacGregor, 'The Future Development of the Hospital Services', 24 May 1938.
7 MH 80/24 'Finance', n.d., but late 1939.
8 MH 80/24, 'Future Development of the Hospital System', n.d., 1938.
9 MH 77/25, 'Suggestions for a Postwar Hospital Policy', August 1941.
10 There were conflicting views on this; for instance, the Medical Practitioners' Union argued that membership of a contributory scheme actually helped secure a priority in admissions which was 'not based on medical need': MH 77/26, 'The Transition to a State Medical Service', August 1942.
11 MH 77/25, Brock–Maude, 4 September 1941.
12 MH 80/24, 'EMS Finance', n.d., late 1939(?).
13 MH 77/25, NPHT, *Memorandum on the Coordination of Hospital Services*, 1941.
14 MH 77/26, 'Post-war Hospital Policy', June 1942.
15 MH 80/24, 'Note on Hospital Regions', May 1942.
16 MH 80/24, Ministry of Health, 'Note on Regionalisation', 18 August 1942.
17 MH 77/26, MPU, 'Transition to a State Medical Service', August 1942.
18 MH 80/33, 'Planning a Hospital Service', n.d.
19 MH 77/25, 'The Emergency Hospital Scheme as a Starting Point for Future Development', 2 September 1941.
20 *Ibid.*
21 MH 80/24, 'Notes on Post-war Policy', 8 May 1940.
22 MH 80/24, 'Notes on Hospital Policy', 18 November 1940.
23 D.S. Murray, *The Future of Medicine*, quoted in Stewart 1999: 136.
24 MH 77/25, 'Office Committee on Post-war Policy', 24 January 1941.
25 MH 77/25, Wrigley, 'Hospital Policy and Regionalisation', n.d.
26 *Ibid.*; MH 77/26, 'Notes on the General Administrative Structure', March 1943.
27 MH 80/24, Pater, 'Notes on Hospital Policy', 18 December 1940.
28 *Ibid.*
29 MH 77/25, 'Suggestions for a Post-war Hospital Policy', August 1941.
30 MH 77/25, LP (41) 167, 'Post-war Hospital Policy: Memorandum by the Minister of Health', 14 October 1941.

31   MH 80/30, notes for [Bevan's] Second Reading speech, 1945; this document reviews several different proposals.
32   MH 77/28, Rock Carling–Jameson, February 1944.
33   MH 80/24, 'Future Development'.
34   MH 80/24, Forber–Chrystal, 23 November 1939.
35   MH 77/25, de Montmorency–Maude, February 1941; Brock, 4 September 1941, noted the 'far from favourable experience' of joint boards with respect to mental illness services; and Wrigley deplored the lack of collaboration between local authorities due to the 'separate and conflicting interests' of county councils and county boroughs.
36   MH 77/25, Wrigley, 'Hospital Policy and Regionalisation'.
37   MH 80/24, note by Macgregor, 9 January 1941.
38   MH 77/25, office committee on post-war hospital policy, 24 January 1941.
39   MH 80/24, Pater's note on Macgregor's minute of 14 November 1940.
40   MH 80/27, note by Macgregor, 9 January 1941.
41   MH 77/25, C. Latham 'Voluntary or Municipal Hospitals: The Case for Public Control', *The Star*, 12 August 1941; F. Menzies, 'Hospital Policy in London', MH 77/25, August 1941.
42   There is some evidence for this from the *Hospitals Yearbooks*; the specialist voluntary hospitals generally received a much higher proportion of their income from payments for public services than did voluntary general hospitals, though the picture is somewhat clouded, as public payments to voluntary general hospitals could well have been for the provision of specialist, rather than general services.
43   MH 80/34, comments by Pater on King's Fund memorandum, ? spring 1944.
44   MH 80/34, 'Comments on Nuffield Memorandum', July 1944.
45   MH 80/28, 'Comments on the Report of the Conservative Party Committee on Health Services', May 1945.
46   MH 80/33, NHS(44)7, comments by Rucker and Maude.
47   MH 80/34, 'Reform of the Voluntary Hospital System', n.d.
48   MH 80/24, 'The Future Development of the Hospital Services'.
49   MH 80/24, comments on Pater's paper on 'Hospital Regions', December 1940.
50   MH 80/24, note by MacIntosh, 28 January 1939.
51   MH 80/24, 'Meaning of "Regions" in Connection with the Proposed Hospital System'.
52   MH 80/34, Rucker–Wetenhall, 16 November 1944.
53   MH 80/34, Rucker–Wetenhall, 3 November 1944.
54   MH 80/34, various papers.
55   MH 80/34, 'Voluntary Hospitals and Payments from Rates', n.d.
56   Churchill Archives, PTER 1/6, p. 51.
57   MH 77/25, de Montmorency, 12 February 1941.
58   MH 80/24, Forber–Chrystal, 19 September 1939.
59   'The Voluntary Hospitals are Dead – Long Live the Voluntary Hospitals', *The Hospital*, January 1944: 9–12.
60   MH 77/26, MPU, 'Transition to a State Medical Service', August 1942.
61   MH 80/34, note by Sir A. Anderson, Royal Free Hospital.
62   MH 80/24, MacNalty, 'Proposed National Hospital Service', 21 September 1939.
63   MH 80/24, MacNalty–Forber, 'Regional Organization of Hospital Services', 18 December 1939.
64   MH 80/24, Office Committee on post-war hospital policy, 10 January 1941; McNicholl, 'Post-war Hospital Policy', 24 October 1942; Forber–Chrystal, 17 September 1939.
65   MH 77/22, Memo by Daley, 28 February 1941.

66 Note that extensive searches in the PRO have failed to reveal records of inter-war applications for loan sanctions for hospital development. See Chapter 3 and also Mohan (1997) for such evidence as has survived.

67 MH 80/24, Forber, 'Regional Organisation', 23 November 1939.

68 MH 80/24, de Montmorency, 29 August 1941.

69 MH 80/24, MacNalty–Chrystal, 22 September 1939.

70 MH 80/29, Secretary's minute 'NHS – Hospitals Scheme', August 1945.

71 The foregoing paragraph has summarised the arguments contained in *Ibid*.

72 CAB 129/3, CP(45) 205 – *The Future of the Hospital Services*.

73 *Ibid*.

74 *Ibid*.

75 Lord President of the Council; former Leader of the LCC, which had the most extensive system of local government health services in the country.

76 PRO CAB 129/3, CP (45) 227, 12 October 1945.

77 *Ibid*.

78 MH 80/34, note by Rucker, summarising objections to nationalisation, 22 September 1945.

79 CAB 129/3, CP(45)205, 'The Future of the Hospital Service'.

5 'False hopes and frustrations': the absence of a capital programme, 1948–59

1 MH 137/227, Newcastle RHB, oral evidence to Guillebaud Committee, GC(53)7, November 1953.

2 CAB 128/15, CM 37(48)1; CAB 129/34, CP(49)105.

3 *Ibid*.

4 CAB 128, CM 10(50)3, 13 March 1950.

5 CAB 134/447, IPC (47) 6, 28 August 1947.

6 T227/955, Gilbert–Bridges, 3 August 1949.

7 MH 90/30, *Memorandum on Hospital Building Work*, August 1948.

8 C (51) 45, 17 December 1951.

9 T227/402, 'Investment in the Social Services Sector', 16 March 1954.

10 T227/402, Lucas–Blaker, 23 November 1953; Mitchell–Clarke, 24 November 1953.

11 T227/402, Marre–Clarke, 16 December 1953.

12 T227/402, Ministry of Health Investment Programme submission, 1954–5 *et seq.*, November 1953.

13 T227/402, Macleod–Butler, 26 April 1954.

14 CAB 134/783, CCE (54) 5; CAB 129/69, CC (54)20 – both quoted by Bridgen and Lowe 1998.

15 C (54) 348, 17 November 1954.

16 CAB EA (54) 25th meeting – quoted by Webster 1988a: 217.

17 T227/403, Macleod–Brooke, 24 January 1955.

18 T227/403, Brooke–Macleod, 4 February 1955.

19 H.C. Deb., 9 February 1955, *c.* 1907–13.

20 *Daily Telegraph*, 'Crisis in the Hospitals', 15 February 1955.

21 T227/403, Macleod–Butler, 19 September 1955.

22 T227/415, 'Five Year Survey of Social Services', various dates, November 1955–June 1956.

23 T227/415, Brooke–Macmillan, 16 May 1956.

24 T227/1300, Brooke, 14 July 1956.

25 T227/485, Workman–Turnbull, 21 January 1957.

26 CAB 129/94, C(58)158, 18 July 1958; see also T 227/1169, Marre–Turnbull, 14 October 1958.
27 T227/1169, Turnbull–Marre, 18 November 1958.
28 MH 137/38, Graham–Turnbull, 27 November 1958.
29 T227/414, Marre–Thorley, 1 October 1955; Clarke–Marre, 7 October 1955.
30 T227/62, 'The Financing of Capital Expenditure out of Loan: Memorandum by the Minister of Health', 24 June 1950.
31 T227/62 'The Financing of Capital Expenditure out of Loan', 26 June 1950.
32 T227/403, Treasury evidence to Guillebaud Committee.
33 T227/403, Workman–Rigby, 14 July 1955.
34 T227/403, Treasury evidence to Guillebaud Committee.
35 T227/1132, Thorley–Clarke, 30 September 1954.
36 T227/1131, Report of Treasury Investment Committee, n.d., probably early 1954.
37 T227/1142, 'Government-controlled Investment', n.d., probably mid-1956.
38 T227/402, Binning, 23 November 1953, emphasis added.
39 T227/955, Kelley–Workman, 2 November 1954. See also papers in MH 137/30, referring to the futile and nugatory expenditure incurred by RHBs as a consequence of financial restrictions.
40 T227/956, Kelley–Workman, 30 April 1955.
41 T227/957, Rossiter–Turnbull, 24 June 1958.
42 T227/957, Marre–Turnbull, 13 March 1959.
43 MH 137/41, Russell-Smith–Fraser, 15 July 1960.
44 T227/333, Moberly–Mitchell, 8 December 1952.
45 T227/333, Figgures–Workman, 18 July 1955.
46 T227/403, Treasury evidence to Guillebaud Committee.
47 T227/403, draft of Treasury evidence to Guillebaud Committee.
48 T 227/402, Investment in the Social Services sector, 16 March 1954.
49 T227/1300, Turnbull–Petch, 23 July 1956.
50 T227/402, Clarke, 18 March 1954.
51 T227/402, Clarke, 29 April 1954 – emphasis added.
52 T227/402, Macleod–Butler, 26 April 1954; memo to Butler, 30 April 1954.
53 T227/402, e.g. Kelley–Workman, 2 December 1954.
54 T227/403, Clarke, 4 January 1955.
55 MH 137/31, Bavin–Pater, 23 September 1954.
56 See, for instance, T 227/955, Mitchell–Owen, 24 December 1952; Turnbull–Owen, 31 December 1952.
57 T227/955, Haddow–Owen, 6 January 1953; Marre–Owen, 4 February 1953.
58 T227/956, Workman–Turnbull, 26 May 1956; Brittain–Turnbull, 16 August 1956; Workman–Thorley, 8 January 1957.
59 T227/957, Kelley–Dubery, 15 February 1958.
60 T227/957, Simon–Walker-Smith, 23 October 1958.
61 T227/1225, CPE (SC)16, Improving Control in the Health Service.
62 T227/402, Kelley–Workman, 2 December 1954.
63 T227/402, Workman–Clarke, 2 December 1954.
64 T227/403, Investment Review 1955: Memorandum by the Ministry of Health.
65 T227/415, Turnbull–Playfair, 5 December 1955.
66 T227/1142, Marre–Turnbull, 6 February 1956.
67 T227/1168, 20 July 1956, 27 July 1956, 2 August 1956.
68 T227/402, Clarke, 29 April 1954.
69 T227/402, Clarke, 20 December 1954.
70 T227/403, Clarke–Couzens, 28 January 1955.
71 T227/1142, Workman–Jarrett, December 1955.
72 T227/1142, Workman–Thorley, 22 May 1956.

73 T227/402, 'Distribution of Money for Capital Expenditure to RHBs', n.d. but probably 1953.
74 T227/402, Bavin–Workman, 30 January 1954.
75 *Ibid.*
76 MH137/31, Pater–Godber, 25 November 1954.
77 MH137/31, Godber–Pater, 10 December 1954.
78 MH137/33, note to Secretary, 19 November 1956.
79 MH137/33, Gregson–Pater, 30 April 1955.
80 T227/1304, quoted in Boys–Robertson, 12 October 1959.
81 T227/402, Kelley–Workman, 2 December 1954.
82 MH137/32, Gregson–Bavin, 20 April 1955.
83 MH137/39,Gedling–Pater, 20 August 1959.
84 MH 137/32, Macleod, 7 June 1955.
85 TWAS, HA/NR/20/3, RHB, *Annual Report, 1951–52,* p. 73.
86 TWAS, HA/NR/20/2, RHB, *Annual Report, 1950–51,* pp. 49, 15.
87 For example, Irene Ward (Tynemouth), H.C. Deb., v. 498, c. 1371–80; Frederick Peart (Workington), H.C. Deb., v. 517, c. 549–58; Arthur Blenkinsop (Newcastle East) and Joseph Slater (Sedgefield), H. C. Deb., v. 600, c. 879–914.
88 TWAS, HA/NR/20/1, RHB *First Report*, 1948–50, pp. 31–4.
89 TWAS, HA/NR/20/1, RHB *First Report*, 1948–50, p. 45.
90 TWAS, HA/NR/3, *Planning Committee*, 23 May 1949.
91 TWAS, HA/NR/3, *Planning Committee*, 22 November 1948.
92 RHB(48)54, *Hospital Building Work.*
93 TWAS, HA/NR/3, *Planning Committee*, 13 December 1948.
94 TWAS, HA/NR/3, *Planning Committee*, 24 November 1950; see also Guillebaud Committee papers, e.g. MH137/227 GC (53)5.
95 TWAS, HA/NR/1/1, RHB, *Board*, 3 December 1948, minute 6. The Special Area received £76,000 in the 1949–50 financial year whereas on the basis of its number of beds it should have received some £45,000.
96 TWAS, HA/NR/3, *Planning Committee*, 13 December 1948. The Hospital Surveys had in fact noted the absence of good quality hospital provision in the Bishop Auckland area; see p. 25.
97 TWAS, HA/NR/3, *Planning Committee*, 11 April 1949.
98 TWAS, HA/NR/3, *Buildings Committee*, 5 April 1949.
99 TWAS, HA/NR/20/1, RHB *First Report*, 1948–50, p. 10.
100 TWAS, HA/NR/20/3, RHB *Third Report,* 1951–52, pp. 61–3.
101 TWAS, HA/NR/20/2, RHB *Second Report*, 1950–51, p. 49.
102 TWAS, HA/NR/3, *Planning Committee*, 26 November 1951.
103 TWAS, HA/NR/3, *Planning Committee*, 27 October 1952.
104 TWAS, HA/NR/20/4, RHB *Fourth Report*, 1952–53, p. 78.
105 TWAS, HA/NR/3, RHB *Planning Committee*, 8 December 1952.
106 H.C. Deb., v. 494, c. 1375, 1377, 31 March 1952.
107 TWAS, HA/NR/3, *Planning Committee*, 12 June 1953.
108 TWAS, HA/NR/3, *Planning Committee*, 15 October 1954.
109 TWAS, HA/NR/3, *Planning Committee*, 10 March 1952.
110 The problems of redeveloping the EMS hospitals were discussed, *inter alia*, at meetings of the RHB *Planning Committee* on 22 November 1948, 11 April 1949 and 24 November 1950.
111 TWAS, HA/NR/3, *Planning Committee*, 28 October 1955.
112 TWAS, HA/NR/3, *Planning Committee*, 17 July 1953.
113 HM(55)19, *The Hospital Building Programme.*
114 TWAS, HA/NR/19/51, notes and correspondence, 19 March 1952, 12 October 1953, 2 March 1954.

115 By 1954 Peterlee was 'high on the list' but it would 'not be included at present' in a list of priority schemes: RHB, *Board*, 2 April 1954.
116 TWAS, HA/NR/19/52, 'Hospital Services for Peterlee New Town', 10 February 1961.
117 TWAS, HA/NR/19/52, 'Notes of a Meeting between the RHB and Peterlee Development Corporation', 3 December 1959.
118 For the political pressures on the Ministry, see T227/402, Macleod–Butler, 26 April 1954.
119 TWAS, HA/NR/3, *Planning Committee*, 18 December 1953 – emphasis added.
120 TWAS, HA/NR/3, *Planning Committee*, 16 December 1955; 15 June 1956; 18 January 1957; 19 December 1958.
121 Newcastle RHB Review of Groupings of Hospitals for the purposes of management by HMCs – report to RHB Planning Committee, 18 January 1957.
122 TWAS, HA/NR/3, *Planning Committee*, 18 January 1957.
123 MH 88/262, Collingwood–Powell, 1 December 1961.
124 TWAS, HA/NR/3, *Planning Committee*, 20 July 1958.
125 TWAS, HA/NR/20/7, RHB, *Seventh Report*, 1956–57, p. 7.
126 T 227/402, Macleod–Brooke, 26 April 1954.
127 T 227/403, Evidence to Guillebaud Committee, p. 6.
128 Author's calculations from Ministry of Health *Hospital Building Progress Reports* and RHB *Annual Accounts*.
129 T227/957, Marre–Turnbull, 24 November 1958.

6 Explaining and reappraising the 1962 Hospital Plan

1 *The Times*, 24 January 1962.
2 CLRK 1/3/1/1, Clarke–Robertson, 29 June 1960.
3 An early example is MH 80/33, 'Planning a Hospital Service'. Godber also wrote various articles relating to bed norms and the DGH concept.
4 T291/22, CPE (SC3), 6th meeting, 22 February 1960.
5 T227/1305, e.g. Marre–Robertson, 14 December 1959; T291/22, CPE (SC3), 12th meeting, 1 June 1960.
6 T291/23, e.g. Boys–Rossiter, 26 January 1960; T291/24, Robertson–Douglas, 8 December 1960.
7 T291/23, Boys–Rossiter, 26 January 1960.
8 T291/27, Robertson–Douglas, 8 December 1960.
9 T291/24, drafts of report of Plowden subcommittee on health services.
10 MH 137/41, Hodgson, 14 July 1960.
11 MH 137/41, Russell-Smith–Fraser, 15 July 1960.
12 T227/1310, Robertson–Clarke, 4 November 1960.
13 T227/1311, Robertson–Clarke, 9 January 1961.
14 T227/1310, Ministry of Health, investment programme submission, 1960.
15 T227/1310, supplementary note, marked 'for Treasury files only' of Treasury/Ministry of Health meeting, 4 April 1960.
16 T227/1310, Rossiter–Robertson, 27 April 1960.
17 T227/1311, Douglas–Robertson, 13 November 1961; Robertson–Douglas, 11 December 1961.
18 For example: MH 90/64, minutes of meeting of RHB Chairmen, 21 March 1961.
19 MH 88/325, letter from Secretary of United Bristol Hospitals to Ministry of Health, 25 November 1961.
20 T291/23, HM Treasury, 'Control of Government Expenditure on Building', May 1959.

21 T227/1170, Kelley–Boys, 15 January 1960.
22 T291/22, CPE(SC3)2, 26 November 1959; CPE(SC3)6, 22 February 1960.
23 MH 90/83, Meeting of RHB Chairmen, 15 September 1961; MH 137/42, Fraser-Clarke, 23.10.61.
24 Reported in the *Supplement* to the British Medical Journal, 1959, p. 71.
25 MH 137/41, Gedling–Hodgson, 5 August 1960.
26 MH 137/41, note of meeting at Treasury, 8 November 1960.
27 MH 137/41, Fraser–Clarke, 17 November 1960.
28 *Ibid.*
29 MH 137/42, Gedling–Douglas, 16 October 1961.
30 MH 137/42, Fraser–Clarke, 23 October 1961.
31 MH 137/42, Powell–Brooke, 26 October 1961.
32 Powell, H.C. Deb., v. 633, c. 988, 1 February 1961.
33 HC Deb., 4 June 1962, c. 104, v. 661.
34 MH 88/27, note by Dr Oddie, 3 July 1958.
35 MH 88/27, Tatton-Brown–Davies, 3 March 1960.
36 Ministry of Health circular, HM(61)4.
37 MH 88/325 – South West RHB ten-year hospital programme.
38 MH 88/262, 'Notes on Visits to Newcastle, Liverpool and Manchester RHBs', March 1961.
39 Ministry of Health circular, RHB (48) 1, Development of Specialist Services.
40 MH 99/120, Aldridge–Boys, 1 October 1959.
41 MH 123/278, proceedings of joint conference on hospital planning, 30 June 1960, paper by Dr N. Goodman.
42 *Ibid.*
43 MH 99/121, Fraser–Powell, 4 July 1961; Gedling–Russell-Smith, 30 June 1961.
44 MH 88/325, file note, 7 July 1961.
45 MH 88/325, file note, 15 July 1961.
46 MH 88/325, 'Bed Norms', 16 June 1961.
47 MH 99/121, Fraser–Powell, 4 July 1961.
48 MH 123/231, various dates.
49 MH 123/242, Robinson–Douglas, 16 November 1960.
50 RUSM 1/21, 13 November 1961.
51 MH 88/343, Alton–Hedley, 19 October 1961.
52 MH 88/262, 'Notes on Visits to Newcastle, Liverpool and Manchester RHBs', March 1961.
53 MH 137/42, 'Memorandum for those who will be discussing with RHBs the preparation of proposals sought in HM(61)4', 15 March 1961.
54 These comments are based on material in MH 88/343, MH 88/262 and MH 88/325.
55 T227/1311, Russell-Smith–Robertson, 27 January 1961.
56 Maclay, HC Deb., v. 661, *c.* 35–6, 4 June 1962; also Ministry comments on RHB draft plans in MH 88 file series.
57 Denis Howell, HC Deb., v. 661, *c.* 62–3, 4 June 1962.
58 T227/1311, Douglas–Robertson, 30 December 1960.
59 RUSM 1/21, 15 June 1961, 20 June 1961, 28 August 1961.
60 MH 137/42, comments on proposals from East Anglian RHB, 1 June 1961, and Sheffield RHB, 5 June 1961.
61 MH 88/325, file note, 26 May 1961; note by Gedling, 29 May 1961.
62 MH 90/83, note of meeting between the Minister of Health and Chairmen of RHBs, 19 September 1961.
63 MH 166/323, Comments on Liverpool RHB plans, 6 October 1961.
64 MH 88/262, Emanuel–Wallis, 20 December 1961.
65 MH 88/262, note by Wallis, probably December 1961.

66 MH 137/42, Brooke–Powell, 16 November 1961 – emphasis added.
67 MH 137/171–4.
68 MH 156/72, 4 August 1961.
69 MH 134/40, Powell–Brandes, 8 July 1961.
70 CAB 134 / 1984, Home Affairs Committee, 19 December 1961.
71 MH 88/343, Templeman–Powell, 7 December 1961.
72 MH 90/83, Meeting between Powell and RHB Chairmen, 20 December 1960.
73 MH 90/83, 21 November 1961.
74 MH 88/262, Ministry – Newcastle RHB, 26.7.61.
75 T227/1313, Robertson–Douglas, 11 December 1961.
76 RUSM, letters, 1961; MH 90/83, meeting between Powell and RHB Chairmen, 20 December 1960.
77 MH 137/42, Fraser–Clarke, 23 October 1961; RUSM 1/21, 13 November 1961.
78 *H.C. Deb*, 4 June 1962, c. 54 (Kenneth Robinson), c. 142 (J. Dickson Mabon).
79 Newcastle RHB, 'Capital Development Programme, 1961–62 to 1970–71'.
80 MH 88/262, note of Ministry–RHB meeting, 19 August 1961.

7 From 'Plan' to 'Programme', 1962–73

 1 Geoffrey Johnson-Smith, H.C. Deb., c. 712–13.
 2 *BMJ*, 17 November 1962, 1319.
 3 *BMJ*, 1962, i, 709, 870, 1071, 1279; see also *The Times*, 17 September 1962, 26 September 1962, 29 September 1962, 3 October 1962.
 4 *BMJ*, 3 February 1962.
 5 Kenneth Robinson, H.C. Deb., v. 661, c. 48, 4 June 1962.
 6 *The Times*, 24 January 1962.
 7 T227/1313, Church–Douglas, 10 April 1962.
 8 MH 137/43, Harding–Gedling, 19 December 1962, Gedling–Russell-Smith, 24 December 1962.
 9 H.C. Deb., v. 686, c. 1468, 19 December 1963.
10 H. C. Deb., v. 696, c. 647–8, 764–9, 11 June 1964.
11 T227/1381, Clarke–Harding, 25 May 1964.
12 Quoted by Lord Balniel (Conservative MP for Hertford), H.C. Deb., v. 696, c. 740.
13 MH 90/88, Meeting of RHB Chairmen, 19 January 1965.
14 *BMJ*, 27 March 1965, 'Hospitals in the Air?', 807–8.
15 C(65)6, 'Hospital Capital Expenditure, 1965–6'; CC(65)3, 21 January 1965.
16 MH 160/168, office meeting, 26 October 1965.
17 PREM 13/2252, Robinson–Wilson, 11 May 1966.
18 TWAS, HA/NR/19/223, Newcastle RHB, *Review of the Hospital Plan and the Ten Year Capital Programme*, October 1965; *BMJ* 'Hospital Reappraisal', 4 June 1966.
19 *BMJ*, 11 June 1964, 1649; 6 July 1964, Supplement.
20 BMA Central Consultants and Specialists Committee, *The Realities of Hospital Finance*, *BMJ*, Supplement, 21 May 1966.
21 *Ibid.*; Ministry's response, *BMJ*, 24 September 1966, p. 760.
22 *BMJ*, Supplement, 16 July 1966.
23 T227/3026, HPC(67)11.
24 Author's calculations from DHSS, *Digest of Health Statistics* and *Health and Personal Social Services Statistics*.
25 Author's calculations from data in TWAS, HA/NR/21/14, RHB *Annual Accounts*; TWAS, 1913/9/2, SE Northumberland HMC, *Annual Accounts*.
26 *BMJ*, 1963, i, 533; *BHSSJ*, 24 May 1963.

27 T227/1381, Fraser–Clarke, 10 June 1964.

28 T227/3027, Widdup–Jordan-Moss, 5 November 1969, 18 December 1969.

29 Local support for the Report's recommendations was evident in, for example, the views of Henry Miller, an influential figure in the Freeman Road dispute (see Chapter 10), who argued for hospitals of around 2,000 beds (Miller 1973).

30 MH 150/57, Macdonald–Carswell, 8 November 1967.

31 MH 150/57, Wilson–Carswell, 6 November 1967.

32 MH 150/57, Mottershead–Godber, 8 December 1967; Mottershead–Carswell, 2 January 1968.

33 TWAS, HA/NR/19/223, Newcastle RHB – file note on modifications of hospital plans since Cmnd 3000, October 1970.

34 MH 166/444, Newcastle RHB – Functions of the District General Hospital: Report of the Senior Administrative Medical Officer and Secretary.

35 T227/3110 'Note of Meeting Between Treasury and DHSS Officials', 5 December 1969.

36 Select Committee on Estimates (1970), *Evidence*, Q.459–533, 2245–2254, 3371–3383.

37 Geoffrey Rippon, Minister of Public Building and Works, speaking in 1966 – quoted in Smyth 1985: 171.

38 *BHSSJ*, 28 February 1964, 12 June 1964.

39 *BMJ*, Supplement, 24 October 1964, p. 161.

40 *BMJ*, 1968, i, 364; *BHSSJ*, 21 November 1969.

41 For example, in letters to the *BMJ*: 1968, i, 364, 494, 620.

42 Select Committee on Estimates (1970), Evidence, Q.72.

43 TWAS, HA/NR/3/33, HA/NR/4/2, various dates.

44 This draws upon a paper to the RHB's CDSC: 'Ashington Hospital – Redevelopment', TWAS, HA/NR/4/2, CDSC, 6 March 1964.

45 TWAS, HA/NR/4/1, CDSC, 2 November 1962.

46 MH 160/167, Paget–Moyes, 21 May 1964.

47 TWAS, HA/NR/4/2, CDSC, 31 July 1964; for a Ministry view, MH 160/168, Moyes–Twohig, 7 December 1965.

48 MH 160/167, Dobbin–Moyes, 12 January 1965.

49 HA/NR/3/34, *Buildings Subcommittee*.

50 MH 160/168, Moyes–Twohig, 7 December 1965.

51 MH 166/610, Newcastle RHB, *Evidence to Select Committee on Estimates' Inquiry into the Hospital Building Programme*.

52 TWAS, NA/NR/19/223, Report of a meeting between officers of RHBs and the Ministry of Health, 30 June 1968.

53 TWAS, HA/NR/19/224,. Edgdell–Stewart, 14 December 1967.

54 Source of the following is author's calculations from RHB *Annual Accounts*.

55 It is an underestimate because the RHB Accounts do not include expenditure on the teaching hospital in Newcastle, which was a formally separate organisation. However, £2.17 million was spent on hospitals controlled by the Board of Governors between 1948 and 1965: Ministry of Health: *Progress Reports on Hospital Building*. It is not possible to express this figure at constant prices because this is a cumulative total, but as it equated to about 8 per cent of capital spending by the RHB, it would clearly inflate the share of resources going to Newcastle.

56 MH 160/166, Meeting between RHB and Ministry officials, 20 March 1963.

57 HA/NR/4/2, CDSC, 8 January 1965.

58 MH 160/167, Ministry file note, 12 January 1965.

59 MH 160/168, office meeting, 23 November 1965.

60 MH 160/168, Moyes–Twohig, 7 December 1965.

61 TWAS, HO/RVI/24, 25, 26.

62 A Labour Councillor in Newcastle; Chairman of the Northern Economic Planning Council.

63 *Newcastle Journal*, 28 July 1969.

64 Several high-level discussions are recorded in the RHB minutes: Board, 5 May 1967, 7 July 1967, 28 July 1967, 4 October 1968, 6 December 1968, 2 May 1969, 6 June 1969, 4 July 1969, 25 July 1969, 3 October 1969, 7 November 1969; Crossman (1976: 589, 656–9) describes his own role; Ministry of Health papers are in MH 112/34; contemporaneous press reports in the *Newcastle Journal* and the *Evening Chronicle* are also deployed.

65 MH 112/34, 'Brief on Newcastle's Hospital Services', September 1969.

66 MH 112/34, Henry Miller–Richard Crossman, 6 August 1969.

67 *Ibid.*

68 MH 160/178–9, various dates; HA/NR/4/2, CDSC, 8 January 1965.

69 TWAS, HA/NR/19/53, 'Notes of a Meeting with Washington NTDC', 3 August 1965.

70 TWAS, HA/NR/19/53, 'Comments on Washington NTDC Master Plan', 26 January 1967.

71 Dr M. Emrys-Roberts, letter to *The Times*, 26 September 1962. Emrys-Roberts later became a central figure in the cottage hospitals movement; see Emrys-Roberts 1991.

72 MH 156/72, Barber–Cashman, 25 November 1963.

73 MH 156/72, Gedling–Cashman, 3 December 1963.

74 MH 156/72, Powell–Fraser, 19 July 1963; Hutchinson–Williamson, 7 November 1963.

75 Estimated, because figures on total hospital numbers given in published sources do not give numbers of new hospitals opened.

76 Select Committee on Estimates (1970), DHSS memorandum of evidence.

77 Ministry of Health circulars RHB (49) 132 and HM (58) 29 gave details of relevant consultation procedures.

78 Ministry of Health circular HM (68) 31.

79 T227/3110, Crossman–RHB Chairmen, 17 November 1969.

80 T227/3110, Patterson–Widdup, 4 November 1969; Widdup–Jordan Moss, 6 November 1969.

81 MH 150/59, Thomson–Godber, n.d.

82 Kenneth Robinson, H.C. Deb., 661, c. 51, 4 June 1962.

83 HA/NR/19/222, 22 April 1963.

84 HA/NR/4/1, CDSC, 3 May 1963.

85 MH 166/444, Functions of the District General Hospital.

86 Select Committee on Estimates, 1970, *Evidence*, Q. 1204.

87 HA/NR/19/107, *Draft Answers to Parliamentary Questions*.

88 MH 166/586, 'Review of the Hospital Programme: Reallocation of Capital Monies', 15 March 1969.

89 See HA/NR/19/221–5 for files dealing with management of the RHB's capital programme.

90 *Hospital and Health Service Journal*, 59(5), 251–3.

91 *Hospital and Health Service Review*, 71(11), 1975, 379–81.

92 *The Hospital*, 58(11), 1962, 738.

8 A programme without a policy? hospital developments 1973–91

1 H. C. Deb., 5 July 1988, v. 136, c. 932 – emphasis added.

2 *Lancet*, ii, 20 December 1975, 1248–9.

3 Source: author's calculations from *Annual Abstract of Statistics*.
4 *Lancet*, i, 10 January 1976, 86–7.
5 *HSJ*, 23 October 1986, 26 March 1987.
6 *HSJ*, 19 March 1987, 26 March 1987, 30 April 1987, 22 October 1987.
7 Expenditure Committee, 1974, *Evidence*, Q29, 45, 94, 97, 98, 150, 151.
8 Expenditure Committee, 1977, *Evidence*, Q224–48.
9 Expenditure Committee, 1977, *Evidence*, Q237–8.
10 Committee of Public Accounts 1973, 1974, 1975, 1977
11 Committee of Public Accounts 1975, *Evidence*, Q1172, 1178–9.
12 Committee of Public Accounts 1975, para. 146; *Evidence*, Q1225; see also Smith 1984d: 1601.
13 'The Derriford Hilton', *Times Health Supplement*, 25 December 1981, p. 19.
14 *BMJ*, 1978, ii, 5–9.
15 Reported in *HSSJ*, 19 October 1979, 18 January 1980, 14 March 1980.
16 Quoted in *HSSJ*, 26 October 1979.
17 *Supply estimates*, Class XIII, 1992–3.
18 The affected developments are listed in *HSSJ*, 21 February 1981; the Committee of Public Accounts (1981) investigated the delays.
19 *Newcastle Journal*, 27 September 1981, 23 September 1981.
20 *BMJ*, 1975, i, 245–6; 1976, ii, 713.
21 *Hospitals and Health Service Review*, October 1974, July 1975.
22 *Newcastle Journal*, 1976–7, various dates.
23 *Newcastle Journal*, 13 June 1980, 14 April 1984.
24 *HSSJ*, 30 May 1980, 6 June 1980.
25 *BMJ*, 7 June 1980, 1335.
26 These figures are for total numbers by size category. They therefore are *net* figures: there will have been openings of some hospitals as well as closures while bed reductions at others may have brought them to below 250 beds.
27 *Newcastle Journal*, 28 February 1981, 24 July 1981.
28 *Newcastle Journal*, 26 January 1983.
29 *HSSJ*, 1980–1, various dates.
30 Committee of Public Accounts, 1980, Q1926, Sir Patrick Nairne, Permanent Secretary, DHSS.
31 Quoted in A. Dix, 'More Bricks than Kicks', *HSJ*, 10 December 1998, 24–7.
32 *BMJ*, 1976, i, 245–6; *Hospital and Health Services Review*, June 1976, 206–11; *HSSJ*, 4 May 1979.
33 Newcastle RHB, *Annual Accounts*.
34 Northern RHA, *Financial Reviews, passim*. The progress of some of the larger schemes has also been charted through the *Supply Estimates*.
35 Northern RHA, *Financial Reviews*; see also Northern RHA (1991).
36 *Newcastle Journal*, 31 July 1984.
37 The following discussion is based largely on unpublished health authority documents and press cuttings held in the Local History Collection, Newcastle City Library.
38 *Newcastle Journal*, 12 May 1986; *Evening Chronicle*, 13 May 1986.
39 *Newcastle Journal*, 13 May 1986, p. 1.
40 For similar – but much more detailed – studies, see Paton and Bach (1990), Pettigrew *et al.*, (1992), and also Davidson (1987) and Widgery (1979) on the social implications.
41 H. C. Deb., v. 976, c. 662, 19 December 1979.
42 H. C. Deb., v. 970, c. 1798, 18 July 1979.
43 See Health Services Board, *Annual Reports* (1978–1980) for details of the Board's activities. Over 1,000 pay-bed authorisations were revoked between 1977 and 1980.

44 HSJ, 26 November 1987.
45 There were several inquiries, during the 1980s, into the apparent failure of the Government to recover the full cost of private treatment; see Committee of Public Accounts (1985), which suggested that the NHS did not cost pay-beds adequately, to some extent bearing out the criticisms of the private sector's representatives.

9 Hospitals after the 1991 reforms: markets, hierarchies or networks?

1   HC Deb., v. 163, c. 694 – 5 – emphasis added.
2   'Bottomley Signals Fresh NHS Changes', *Guardian*, 27 June 1992.
3   The range of commentaries available is vast; they include Butler (1992), Paton (1992), Mohan (1995), Baggott (1998) and Webster (1998).
4   Source for this is health authority and trust annual reports. Note that the amount of detail given in these is variable, as is the geographical breakdown, so care must be taken in interpretation.
5   Health Committee 1991b: xviii.
6   *Guardian*, 19 December 1990, 'Bed Closures Force Health Cash U-turn', p. 2.
7   Health Committee 1993b, Evidence, Q5 – emphasis added.
8   *Ibid.*, Q12 – emphasis added.
9   'Mrs Bottomley and the London Lynch Mob', *BMJ*, 310, 962, 15 April 1995; 'Threat of Tory Revolt Averted', *BMJ*, 312, 1562, 22 June 1996; 'In Brief', *BMJ*, 313, 1504, 14 December 1996.
10 MH 166/44, 'Newcastle RHB: Policy Following the Bonham-Carter Report', 1969.
11 Some £5 million was spent on the General while it was under control of the RHB, more than any other hospital in the region except North Tees. Source: RHB *Annual Accounts*.
12 The following chronology is based largely on volumes 12 and 13 of press cuttings related to hospital services, compiled by Newcastle Central Library Local History Section; these volumes, which run to several thousand cuttings, are probably as comprehensive an archival record of recent changes in the region as exists, given recent archival cleansing in the NHS.
13 e.g. *Evening Chronicle*, 27 April 1993, 30 April 1993, 2 March 1994.
14 Newcastle and North Tyneside Health Authority, *Annual Reports*.
15 H.C. Deb., v. 163, c. 512, 7 December 1989.
16 The source for these figures is the Charities Aid Foundation's online publication, *Dimensions 2000 Online*, available at www.cafonline,org.
17 O. Dyer, 'Charities Demand Money Back in Guy's Changeover', *BMJ* (1994), 308, 935.
18 T. Shifrin, 'Bevan Can Wait', *Health Service Journal*, 25 May 2000, pp.14–15.
19 MH 99/37, Alexander to Nixon-Browne, 12 February 1957, 'Appeals for Funds by Hospital Authorities', n.d. but probably 1957; Guillebaud Committee (1956), paragraph 381.
20 Source is *Laing's Review of Independent Health Care* (annual).
21 For example, Health Committee 1998, evidence, Q20; Health Committee, 1999, Q446, 451, 471–2; Public Accounts Committee, 1999.
22 George Monbiot, *Guardian*, 7 June 2001; *Observer*, 8 July 2001.
23 Analyses of PFI business cases have concentrated on clinical staff. One reason for this is that 'ancillary' staff are transferred to the PFI consortium and the business cases produced for these developments give no details on staffing levels for this group.

24 *Guardian*, 23 July 2001.
25 *Newcastle Journal*, 31 July 2001.
26 A similar case was reported in the Health Service Journal (7 November 2000). Charitable support was being sought for a children's hospital in Manchester because purchaser commitments would not fund all the PFI payments, so charity was to close the gap.
27 *Newcastle Journal, Guardian,* May 2001.
28 Department of Health Press Release, 5 December 1997.

10 Conclusions

1 See www.foresight.gov.uk.
2 For a sample of exchanges along these lines which illustrates the main positions taken see Dunnigan *et al.* 1997, and the responses in the British Medical Journal, 1997, 314, 1619.
3 H.C. Deb., v. 661, c. 62–3, 4 June 1962.
4 Hughes (2001) discusses these issues in the context of the architectural aspects of hospital design and planning.
5 Quoted in *BMJ*, 1966, ii, *Supplement*, 136.
6 Ministry of Health, *Annual Report*, 1931–32, Cmd. 4113, 43.
7 This speech is available at www.fabian-society.org.uk. See also *Observer*, 6 January 2002.

Bibliography

Unpublished primary sources

This section gives guidance to the principal sources consulted but for reasons of space does not give details of individual pieces of material – for example, the summary of PRO material gives the government department and class of record (e.g. MH 80) but not individual pieces (e.g. MH 80/24). Endnote citations give full details of material directly referenced in the text.

Churchill Archives, Cambridge

CLRK Papers of Sir Richard Clarke
PTER Unpublished autobiography of John Pater
RUSM Letters of Dame Enid Russell Smith

Public Record Office

Ministry of Health (MH) papers

Class	Description
55	Public health series
58	General health questions
61	Commissioner for Special Areas: files of correspondence
66	Local Government Act 1929: public health survey
71	Various committees: correspondence, minutes and reports 1916–58
77	Post-war planning and NHS Act 1946
80	Parliamentary Bill papers
88	RHBs Registered files
89	General files: RHBs
99	Hospital services files
112	Regional offices: health services files
123	Specialist hospital services: registered files
134	Local health authority services: registered files
137	NHS: General Policy
148	Administration of Public and Environmental Health Services

150	Hospital medical, psychiatric and ancillary services
159	Health services and medical and nursing divisions: registered files
160	Hospitals: registered files
166	Hospital construction
170	Accountant General's Department: registered files

Treasury Papers (T)

Class	*Description*
227	Social services division: registered files
229	Central economic planning staff: registered files
291	Committee of enquiry on the Control of Public Expenditure

Tyne and Wear Archives, Newcastle-upon-Tyne (TWAS)

Records of the Newcastle RHB

HA/NR/1/1–12	Board Minutes
HA/NR/3/1–57	Planning Committee Minutes
HA/NR/4/1–5	Capital development subcommittee
HA/NR/19/1–297	Administration: main file series
HA/NR/20/1–8	Annual reports (to 1957)
HA/NR/21/1–27	Abstracts of accounts
HA/NR/22/1–13	Summaries of estimates
HA/NR/24/21–82	Treasurer's Files
HA/NR/33/1–25	Reports (miscellaneous)

Records of local authorities

MD/NC/98	Newcastle City Council – Health Committee
MD/NC/99	Newcastle City Council – Hospitals Joint Committee
CB/GA/18	Gateshead Borough Council – Health Committee
CB/SU/51	Sunderland Borough Council – Sanitary Committee

Records of individual hospitals

HO/RVI	Newcastle Royal Victoria Infirmary
HO/PM	Princess Mary Maternity Hospital, Newcastle
HO/PMH	Palmer Memorial Hospital, Jarrow
HO/FL	Fleming Memorial Hospital, Newcastle
1381	Sunderland Royal Infirmary
	Monkwearmouth and Southwick Hospital
	Sunderland Eye Infirmary
1130	Tynemouth Victoria Jubilee Infirmary

Durham County Record Office (DCRO)

| H/SWD | Lady Eden Cottage Hospital, Bishop Auckland |
| H/DU | Durham County Hospital |

Official publications

Barlow Report (1940) *Report of the Royal Commission on the Distribution of the Industrial Population* (Cmnd 6153), London: HMSO.

Beveridge, W. (1942) *Report on the Provision of Social Insurance, Medical and Allied Services* (Cmnd 6404), London: HMSO.

Board of Trade (1963) *The North East: a Programme for Regional Development and Growth* (Cmnd 2206), London: HMSO.

Central Health Services Council (CHSC) (1969) *The Functions of the District General Hospital*, London: HMSO.

Committee of Public Accounts (1973) *Fourth Report, Session 1972–73*, London: HMSO.

—— (1974) *Third Report, Session 1974*, HC-303, London: HMSO.

—— (1975) *Third Report, Session 1974–75*, HC-374, London: HMSO.

—— (1977) *Ninth Report, Session 1976–77*, HC-532, London: HMSO.

—— (1980) *Eleventh Report, Session 1979–80*, HC-498, London: HMSO.

—— (1981) *Seventeenth Report, Session 1980–81*, HC-225, London: HMSO.

—— (1985) *Thirty-third Report, Session 1984–85*, HC-543, London: HMSO.

—— (1988) *Fortieth Report, Session 1987–88: Estate Management in the NHS*, HC-481, London: HMSO.

—— (1990) *Eighteenth Report, Session 1989–90: Hospital Building in England*, HC-397, London: HMSO.

—— (1993) *Twenty-sixth Report, Session 1992–93: The Chelsea and Westminster Hospital*, HC-275, London: HMSO.

Consultative Council on Medical and Allied Services (CCMAS) (1920) *Interim Report on the Future Provision of Medical and Allied Services* (Dawson Report) (Cmnd 693), London: HMSO.

Department of Health (1997) *The New NHS: Modern, Dependable*, London: HMSO.

—— (2000a) *Shaping the Future NHS: Long-term Planning for Hospitals and Related Services* (Supporting Analysis), London: Department of Health.

—— (2000b) *The NHS Plan: a Plan for Investment, a Plan for Reform* (Cmnd 4818), London: TSO.

—— (2000c) *Department Investment Strategy*, London: Department of Health.

Department of Health for Scotland (1936) *Report of the Committee on Scottish Health Services* (Cathcart Report) (Cmnd 5204), Edinburgh: HMSO.

DHSS (1972) *Optimum Size of District General Hospitals*, DHSS Operations Research Service Note 114, London: DHSS.

—— (1974) *Community Hospitals: Their Role and Development in the NHS*, Circular HSC(IS)75, London: DHSS.

—— (1975) *Review of Health Services and Resources*, Circular DS 85/75, London: DHSS.

—— (1976a) *Priorities for Health and Personal Social Services in England: a Consultation Document*, London: HMSO.

—— (1976b) *Sharing Resources for Health in England: the Report of the Resource Allocation Working Party*, London: HMSO.

—— (1977) *Priorities for the Health and Personal Social Services*, London: DHSS.

—— (1979) *Review of Health Capital: a Discussion Document on the Role of Capital in the Provision of Health Services*, London: DHSS.

—— (1980a) *The Future Pattern of Hospital Services in England and Wales*, London: DHSS.

—— (1980b) *Inequalities in Health: Report of a Research Working Group*, London: DHSS.

—— (1980c) *Health Services Act, 1980: Private Medical Practice in NHS Hospitals and Control of Private Hospital Developments*, Circular HC (80), 10, London: DHSS.

—— (1981) *Contractual Arrangements with Independent Hospitals and Nursing Homes*, London: DHSS.

—— (1983a) *NHS Management Inquiry Report* (The Griffiths Report), London: DHSS.

—— (1983b) *Underused and Surplus Property in the National Health Service* (report of an inquiry chaired by Ceri Davies), London: HMSO.

—— (1988) *Review of the RAWP Formula: A Report by the NHS Management Board*, London: DHSS.

Guillebaud Committee (1956) *Report of the Committee of Enquiry into the Cost of the National Health Service* (Cmnd 9663), London: HMSO.

Health Committee (1991a) *Public Expenditure on Health Matters*, HC-408, London: HMSO.

—— (1991b) *Third Report, Session 1990–91: Public Expenditure on the Health and Personal Social Services*, HC-614, London: HMSO.

—— (1991c) *Public Expenditure on the Health and Personal Social Services: Minutes of Evidence*, HC-229i–vi, London: HMSO.

—— (1991d) *First Report, Session 1990–91: Public Expenditure on Health Services: Waiting Lists,* HC-429, London: HMSO.

—— (1992) *NHS Trusts: Minutes of Evidence*, HC-321, London: HMSO.

—— (1993a) *Public Expenditure on Health Matters*, HC-489, London: HMSO.

—— (1993b) *London's Health Service: Minutes of Evidence*, HC-370, London: HMSO.

—— (1993c) *First Special Report, Session 1992–93: Public Expenditure on Health Matters*, HC-902, London: HMSO.

—— (1998) *Public Expenditure on Health: Minutes of Evidence*, HC-988, London: HMSO.

—— (1999) *Public Expenditure on Health: Minutes of Evidence*, HC-469, London: HMSO.

Health Services Board (1978–80) *Annual Reports*, London: HMSO.

House of Commons (1970) *Hospital Building in Great Britain: Evidence Submitted to Sub-Committee B of the Select Committee on Estimates*, London: HMSO.

—— (1974) *Fourth Report of the Expenditure Committee, Session 1974: Expenditure Cuts in the Health and Personal Social Services*, London: HMSO.

—— (1977) *Ninth Report of the Expenditure Committee, Session 1976–77: Selected Public Expenditure Programmes*, London: HMSO.

—— (1979) *The Government's Expenditure Plans, 1980–81* (Cmnd 7746), London: HMSO.

—— (1980) *Third Report from the Social Services Committee: the Government's White Papers on Public Expenditure: the Social Services*, London: HMSO.

—— (1982) *Second Report from the Social Services Committee: Public Expenditure on the Social Services*, London: HMSO.

House of Lords (1890–92) *Reports of the Select Committee of the House of Lords on Metropolitan Hospital Accommodation* (3 vols), London: HMSO.

Ministry of Health (Annual) *Annual Reports*, London: HMSO.

—— (1921) *Final Report of the Voluntary Hospitals Committee* (Cmnd 1335), London: HMSO (Cave Committee).

—— (1925) *Final Report of the Voluntary Hospitals Commission*, London: HMSO (Onslow Commission).

—— (1944) *A National Health Service* (Cmnd 6502), London: HMSO.

—— (1946) *Hospital Surveys: North West England (vol. 9) and North East England (vol. 10)*, London: HMSO.

—— (1961–5, various dates) *Progress Reports on Hospital Building*, London: Ministry of Health.

—— (1962a) *A Hospital Plan for England and Wales* (Cmnd 1604), London: HMSO.

—— (1962b) *Health and Welfare: The Development of Community Care*, London: HMSO.

—— (1963) *A Hospital Plan for England and Wales* (Revision to 1972–3), London: HMSO.

—— (1964) *A Hospital Plan for England and Wales* (Revision to 1973–4), London: HMSO.

—— (1966) *The Hospital Building Programme* (Cmnd 3000), London: HMSO.

Ministry of Health/DHSS (1949 *et. seq.*) *Summarised Annual Accounts of Health Authorities in England and Wales*, London: HMSO.

Monopolies and Mergers Commission (1990) *The British United Provident Association Ltd and HCA United Kingdom Ltd: A Report on the Merger Situation* (Cmnd 996), London: HMSO.

National Audit Office (1987) *Use of Operating Theatres in the NHS*, HC-143, London: HMSO.

—— (1988) *Estate Management in the NHS*, HC-405, London: HMSO.

—— (1989) *Hospital Building in England*, HC-530, London: HMSO.

—— (1990) *The NHS and Independent Hospitals*, HC-106, London: HMSO.

—— (1991) *HIV and AIDS-Related Health Services*, HC-658, London: HMSO.

—— (1998) *Cost Over-runs, Funding Problems and Delays on Guy's Hospital Phase III Redevelopment*, HC-761, London: HMSO.

Office of National Statistics (ONS) (1997) *General Household Survey, 1995*.

Plowden Report (1961) *Control of Public Expenditure* (Cmnd 1432), London: HMSO.

Public Accounts Committee (PAC) (2000) *Twelfth Report, 1999–2000: The PFI Contract for the New Dartford and Gravesham Hospital*, HC-131, London: TSO.

Royal Commission on Local Government in the Tyneside Area (1936) *Report* (Cmnd 5402), London: HMSO.

Royal Commission on Medical Education (Chairman: Lord Todd) (1969) *Report* (Cmnd 3569), London: HMSO.

Royal Commission on the NHS (1979) *Report* (Cmnd 7615), London: HMSO.

Royal Commission on the Poor Laws (1909) *The Break-up of the Poor Law: Part 1 of the Minority Report of the Poor Law Commission*, London: HMSO.

Secretary of State for Health (1989) *Working for Patients* (Cmnd 555), London: HMSO.

Select Committee on Estimates (1957) *Sixth Report, Session 1956–57*, London: House of Commons.

Tomlinson, B. (1992) *Report of the Inquiry into London's Health Service, Medical Education and Research*, London: HMSO.

Treasury Select Committee (2000a) *Fourth Report, Session 1999–2000: The Private Finance Initiative*, HC-147, London: HMSO.

Secondary sources

Abel, A.L. and Lewin, W. (1959) 'Report on Hospital Building', *British Medical Journal* (Supplement), 109–14.

Abel-Smith, B. (1964) *The Hospitals 1800–1948*, London: Heinemann.

Abel-Smith, B. and Titmuss, R. (1956) *The Cost of the National Health Service*, Cambridge: Cambridge University Press.

Adam Smith Institute (1981) *Health and the Public Sector*, London: Adam Smith Institute.

—— (1984) *The Omega Health Papers*, London: Adam Smith Institute.

Airth, A.D. and Newall, D.J. (1962) *The Demand for Hospital Beds: Results from an Enquiry on Teesside*, Newcastle: King's College.

Aldridge, M. (1979) *The British New Towns: A Programme Without a Policy?*, London: Routledge and Kegan Paul.

Alford, R. (1975) *Health Care Politics: Ideological and Interest Group Barriers to Reform*, Chicago, IL: University of Chicago Press.

Allen, D. (1979) *Hospital Planning: The 1962 Hospital Plan for England and Wales: A Case Study in Decision-Making*, London: Pitman Medical.

—— (1981) 'An Analysis of Factors Affecting the 1962 Hospital Plan', *Social Policy and Administration*, 15: 3–18.

Appleby, J. *et al.* (1994) 'Monitoring Managed Competition', in R. Robinson and J. Le Grand (eds), *Evaluating the NHS Reforms*, London: King's Fund Institute, pp. 24–53.

Association of Community Health Councils for England and Wales (ACHCEW) (1987) *Mid Year Budget Cuts: Health Authorities in Crisis*, London: ACHCEW.

Audit Commission (1986) *Making a Reality of Community Care*, London: HMSO.

Baggott, R. (1998) *Health and Health Care in Britain*, Basingstoke: Macmillan.

Baldwin, P. (1994) *The Politics of Social Solidarity: Class Bases of the European Welfare State, 1875–1975*, Cambridge: Cambridge University Press.

Barker, C. (1997) 'Social Confrontation in Manchester's Quangoland: Local Protest Over the Proposed Closure of Booth Hall Children's Hospital', *North West Geographer*, 1: 18–28.

Barnett, C. (1995) *The Lost Victory*, Basingstoke: Macmillan.

Barnett, R. (1999) 'Hollowing Out the State? Some Observations on the Restructuring of Hospital Services in New Zealand', *Area*, 31: 259–70.

Barr, V. (1957) 'The Population Served by a Hospital Group', *Lancet*, ii: 1105–8.

Bartlett, W. and Le Grand, J. (eds) (1993) *Quasi-markets and Social Policy*, London: Macmillan.

Beech, R., Challah, S. and Ingram, R.H. (1987) 'Impact of Cuts in Acute Beds on Services for Patients', *British Medical Journal*, 294: 685–8.

Berliner, H. and Regan, C. (1987) 'Multinational Operations of US For-profit Hospital Chains: Trends and Implications', *American Journal of Public Health*, 77: 1280–4.

Bevan, A. (1952) *In Place of Fear*, London: Heinemann.

Booth, A. (1978) 'An Administrative Experiment in Employment Policy', *Public Administration*, 56: 139–57.

Bosanquet, N. (1999) *A Successful NHS: From aspiration to Delivery?*, London: Adam Smith Institute.

Bosanquet, N. and Townsend, P. (1980) *Labour and Equality: a Fabian Study of Labour in Power, 1974–79*, London: Heinemann.

Boyle, S. and Harrison, A. (2000) 'Private Finance and Service Development', in J. Appleby and A. Harrison (eds), *Health Care UK Autumn 2000*, London: King's Fund, pp. 55–63.

Bradbury, J. (1990) 'The 1929 Local Government Act', unpublished Ph.D. thesis, University of Bristol.

Bridgen, P. (2001) 'Hospitals, Geriatric medicine and the Long-term Care of Elderly People, 1946–78', *Social History of Medicine*, 14: 507–23.

Bridgen, P. and Lewis, J. (1999) *Elderly People and the Boundary Between Health and Social Care 1946–91: Whose Responsibility?*, London: Nuffield Trust.

Bridgen, P. and Lowe, R. (1998) *Welfare Policy under the Conservatives*, London: PRO Publications.

British Hospitals Association (1937) *Report of the Voluntary Hospitals Commission*, London: British Hospitals Association.

Brittan, S. (1969) *Steering the Economy: the Role of the Treasury*, London: Secker and Warburg.

Brown, M. (1996) 'Commentary: the Commercialisation of America's Health Care System', *Health Care Management Review*, 21: 13–18.

Burns, W. (1967) *Newcastle: A Study in Re-planning*, London: Leonard Hill.

Burrows, R. and Loader, B. (eds) (1994) *Towards a Post-Fordist Welfare State?*, London: Routledge.

Butler, J.R. (1992) *Patients, Policies and Politics: Before and After Working for Patients*, Buckingham: Open University Press.

Buxton, M.J. and Klein, R. (1978) *Allocating Health Resources: a Commentary on the Report of the Resource Allocation Working Party*, Research Paper 3, Royal Commission on the National Health Service, London: HMSO.

Calnan, M., Cant, S. and Gabe, J. (1993) *Going Private: Why People Pay For Their Health Care*, Buckingham: Open University Press.

Campbell, J. (1987) *Nye Bevan and the Mirage of British Socialism*, London: Weidenfeld and Nicolson.

Carney, J.G. and Hudson, R. (1978) 'Capital, Politics and Ideology: the North East of England, 1870–1946', *Antipode*, 10: 64–78.

Carr-Hill, R. (1990) 'RAWP is Dead – Long Live RAWP', in A. Culyer, A. Maynard and J. Poskett (eds), *Competition in Health Care: Reforming the NHS*, London: Macmillan.

Carter, J. (ed.) (1998) *Postmodernity and the Fragmentation of Welfare*, London: Routledge.

Castle, B. (1980) *The Castle Diaries, 1974–76*, London: Weidenfield and Nicolson.

Cawson, A. (1982) *Corporatism and Welfare*, London: Heinemann.

Cherry, S. (1980) 'The Hospitals and Population Growth', *Population Studies*, 34: 59–75.

—— (1997) 'Before the NHS: Financing the Voluntary Hospitals, 1900–1939', *Economic History Review*, L: 309–27.

Clark, G. and Root, A. (1999) 'Infrastructure Shortfall in the UK: the PFI and Government Policy', *Political Geography*, 18: 341–65.

Clarke, R. (1978) *Public Expenditure, Management and Control: the Development of the Public Expenditure Survey Committee*, Basingstoke: Macmillan.

Cooke, P. (1990) 'Modern Urban Theory in Question', *Transactions, Institute of British Geographers*, 15: 331–43.

Cowan, P. (1963) 'The Size of Hospitals', *Medical Care*, 1: 1–9.

—— (1965) 'Hospitals in Towns: Location and Siting', *Architectural Review*, xxxviii, 5: 417–21.

—— (1967) 'Hospital Systems and Systems of Hospitals', *Transactions of the Bartlett Society*, 5: 103–22.

—— (1969) 'Hospital Siting and Location in Relation to Urban Land Use and Development', unpublished Ph.D. Thesis, London University.

Crossman, R.M. (1972) *A Politician's View of Health Service Planning*, Glasgow: University of Glasgow Press.

—— (1976) *The Diaries of a Cabinet Minister* (3 vols), London: Hamish Hamilton and Jonathan Cape.

Daunton, M. (1996) 'Payment and Participation: Welfare and State-formation in Britain, 1900–51', *Past and Present*, 150: 169–216.

Davidson, N. (1987) *A Question of Care: The Changing Face of the National Health Service*, London: Michael Joseph.

Davies, B. (1968) *Social Needs and Resources in Local Service Administration*, London: Michael Joseph.

Davies, C. (1987) 'Things to Come: the NHS in the Next Decade', *Sociology of Health and Illness*, 9: 302–17.

Davies, J. and Lewin, W. (1960) 'Observations on Hospital Planning', *British Medical Journal*, 763–8.

Dawson, D. (1995) *Regulating Competition in the NHS*, DP-131: Centre for Health Economics, York: University of York.

—— (2001) 'The PFI: a Public Finance Illusion?', *Health Economics*, 10: 479–86.

Dawson, D. and Goddard, M. (2000) 'Long-term Contracts for Health Care Services: What Will They Achieve?', in P. Smith (ed.), *Reforming Markets in Health Care*, Buckingham: Open University Press, pp. 67–93.

Day, P. and Klein, R. (1989) 'The Politics of Modernisation: Britain's NHS in the 1980s', *The Milbank Quarterly*, 67, 1: 1–37.

—— (1991) 'Britain's Health Care Experiment', *Health Affairs*, 10: 39–59.

Doyal, L. (1979) *The Political Economy of Health*, London: Pluto.

Doyle, B. and Nixon, R. (2001) 'Voluntary Hospital Finance in North-east England: the Case of North Ormesby Hospital, Middlesbrough, 1900–1947', *Cleveland History*, forthcoming.

Dunn, C.L. (1952) *The Emergency Medical Services*, London: HMSO.

Dunnigan, M., Gaffney, D., Macfarlane, A., Majeed, A. and Pollock, A. (1997) 'What Happens When the Private Sector Plans Hospital Services for the NHS?', *British Medical Journal*, 314: 1266–71.

Durham CC (1951) *County Development Plan: Written Analysis*, Durham: Durham County Council.

Eckstein, H. (1958) *The English NHS: its origins, structure and achievements*, Cambridge, MA: Harvard University Press.

Edelman, M. (1971) *Politics as Symbolic Action*, Chicago, IL: Markham.

Ehrenreich, B. and Ehrenreich, J. (1972) *The American Health Empire: Power, Profits and Politics*, New York: Random House.

Elder, A.T. (1957) 'How Many Hospital Beds?', *British Medical Journal*, i: 753.

Elston, M. (1991) 'The Politics of Professional Power: Medicine in a Changing Health Service', in J. Gabe, M. Calnan and M. Bury (eds), *The Sociology of the Health Service*, London: Routledge.

Emrys-Roberts, M. (1991) *The Cottage Hospitals, 1859–1990*, Motcombe: Tern Publications.

Enthoven, A. (1985) *Reflections on the Management of the NHS*, London: Nuffield Provincial Hospitals Trust.

—— (1999) *In Pursuit of an Improving National Health Service*, London: Nuffield Trust.

Exworthy, M. (1998) 'Localism and the NHS Quasi-market', *Environment and Planning C*, 16: 449–62.

Exworthy, M., Mohan, J. and Powell, M. (1999) 'The NHS under Labour: Quasi-hierarchy, Quasi-market or Quasi-network?', *Public Money and Management*, 19: 15–22.

Eyles, J., Smith, D. and Woods, K. (1982) 'Spatial Resource Allocation and State Practice', *Regional Studies*, 16: 239–53.

Farrer-Brown, L. (1959) 'Hospitals for Today and Tomorrow', *British Medical Journal*, Supplement: 118–22.

Ferguson, B., Sheldon, T. and Posnett, J. (1997) *Concentration and Choice in the Provision of Hospital Services*, York: University of York.

Ferlie, E. (1994) 'The Creation and Evolution of Quasi-markets in the Public Sector: Early Evidence from the NHS', *Policy and Politics*, 22: 105–22.

Finlayson, G. (1994) *Citizen, State and Social Welfare in Britain, 1830–1990*, Oxford: Clarendon.

Fitzherbert, L. (1989) *Charity and the National Health*, London: Directory of Social Change.

Flora, P. and Heidenheimer, A.J. (eds) (1981) *The Development of Welfare States in Europe and America*, London: Transaction.

Foot, M. (1973) *Aneurin Bevan* (Vol. II: 1945–1960), Harmondsworth: Penguin.

Forsyth, G. and Logan, R. (1960) *Demand for Medical Care*, Oxford: Oxford University Press.

Forsyth, G., Thomas, R. and Jones, S. (1970) 'Planning in Practice: a Half-term Report', in G. McLachlan (ed.), *Problems and Progress in Medical Care*, London: NPHT/Oxford University Press, pp.3–26.

Fox, D. (1986) *Health Policies, Health Politics*, Princeton, NJ: Princeton University Press.

Fraser, B. (1964) 'Long-term Planning in the Hospital Service', *Public Administration*, 42: 101–12.

Fry, J. (1959) 'General Practitioners' Views of Hospital Planning', *British Medical Journal* (Supplement): 124–6.

Gaffney D. and Pollock, A. (1998) *Has the NHS Returned to Strategic Planning? The CPAG and the Second Wave of PFI*, London: Unison.

—— (1999a) 'Pump-priming the PFI: Why are Privately-financed Hospital Schemes being Subsidised?', *Public Money and Management*, 20: 1–8.

—— (1999b) *Downsizing for the 21st Century: the North Durham Acute Hospitals PFI Scheme*, London: UNISON.

Gaffney, D., Pollock, A., Price, D. and Shaoul, J. (1999a) 'NHS Capital Expenditure and the Private Finance Initiative', *British Medical Journal*, 319: 48–51.

—— (1999b) 'The Politics of the Private Finance Initiative and the New NHS', *British Medical Journal*, 319: 249–53.

Gamble, A. (1979) 'The Free Economy and the Strong State', *Socialist Register*, 1–25.

—— (1990) 'Theories of British Politics', *Political Studies*, 38: 404–20.

—— (1994) *Britain in Decline: Economic Policy, Political Strategy and the British State*, Basingstoke: Macmillan.

Garside, P. (1999) 'Evidence-based Mergers?', *British Medical Journal*, 318: 345–6.

Garside, P. and Hebbert, M. (eds) (1989) *British Regionalism, 1900–2000*, London: Mansell.

Giddens, A. (1990) *The Consequences of Modernity*, Cambridge: Polity.

Gilbert, E. (1939) 'Practical Regionalism in England and Wales', *Geographical Journal*, 94: 29–44.

—— (1948) 'The Boundaries of Local Government Areas', *Geographical Journal*, 111: 172–98.

Glennerster, H. (1995) *British Social Policy Since 1945*, Oxford: Blackwell.

Godber, G.E. (1958) 'Health Services, Past, Present and Future', *Lancet*, ii: 1–6.

—— (1959) 'The Physician's Part in Hospital Planning', *British Medical Journal* (Supplement): 115–18.

Goddard, M. and Ferguson, B. (1997) *Mergers in the NHS: Made in Heaven or Marriage of Convenience?*, London: Nuffield Provincial Hospitals Trust.

Gorsky, M. (2001) ' "Threshold of a New Era": The Development of an Integrated Hospital System in North-east Scotland, 1900–39', *Mimeo*, University of Wolver-hampton.

Gorsky, M. and Mohan, J.F. (2001) 'London's Voluntary Hospitals in the Inter-war Period: Growth, Transformation or Crisis?', *Nonprofit and Voluntary Sector Quarterly*, 30: 247–75.

Gorsky, M., Mohan, J.F. and Powell, M. (1999) 'British Voluntary Hospitals, 1871–1938: the Geography of Provision and Utilisation', *Journal of Historical Geography*, 25: 463–82.

—— (2002) 'The Financial Health of Hospitals in Inter-war Britain', *Economic History Review*, LV.

Gough, I. (1979) *The Political Economy of the Welfare State*, London: Macmillan.

Granshaw, L. (1989) 'Fame and Fortune by Means of Bricks and Mortar', in L. Granshaw and R. Porter (eds), *The Hospital in History*, London: Routledge, pp. 199–220.

Green, D. (1988) *Working-class Patients and the Medical Establishment: Self-help in Britain From the Mid-19th Century to 1948*, Aldershot: Gower.

—— (1993) *Reinventing Civil Society: the Rediscovery of Welfare Without Politics*, London: Institute of Economic Affairs.

—— (1996) 'Medical Care Without the State', in A. Seldon (ed.), *Re-privatising Welfare: After the Lost Century*, London: Institute of Economic Affairs.

—— (1998) 'Solidarity Without Public Sector Monopoly', in T. Ling (ed.), *Reforming Health Care by Consent*, Oxford: Radcliffe, pp. 53–63.

Griffith, B. (1999) 'Competition and Containment in Health Care', *New Left Review*, 236: 24–52.

Griffith, B., Iliffe, S. and Rayner, G. (1987) *Banking on Sickness: Commercial Medicine in Britain and the USA*, London: Lawrence and Wishart.

Griffith, B., Mohan, J. and Rayner, G. (1985) *Commercial Medicine in London*, London: GLC.

Hadfield, J. (1979) *Health in the Industrial North East, 1919–39*, Hull: Institute for Socioeconomics.

Hall, P. (1986) *Governing the Economy: the Politics of State Intervention in Britain and France*, Cambridge: Polity.

Hall, S. (1985) 'Authoritarian Populism: A Reply to Jessop *et al.*', *New Left Review*, 151: 115–24.

—— (1988) *The Hard Road to Renewal: Thatcherism and the Crisis of the Left*, London: Verso.

Ham, C. (1981) *Policy-making in the National Health Service*, London: Macmillan.

—— (1992) *Health Policy in Britain* (3rd Edition), London: Macmillan.

—— (1996) 'Contestability: a Middle Way for the NHS', *British Medical Journal*, 312: 70–1.

Hamilton, D. (1987) 'The Highlands and Islands Medical Services', in G. MacLachlan (ed.), *Improving the Common Weal*, Edinburgh: Edinburgh University Press, pp. 483–90.

Harris, B. (1991) 'Government and Charity in the Distressed Mining Areas of England and Wales, 1928–30', in J. Barry and C. Jones (eds), *Medicine and Charity before the Welfare State*, London: Croom Helm, pp. 206–24.

—— (1995) 'Responding to Adversity: Government–Charity Relations and the Relief of Unemployment in Inter-war Britain', *Contemporary Record*, 9: 529–61.

Harris, J. (1992) 'Political Thought and the Welfare State, 1870–1940: an Intellectual Framework for British Social Policy', *Past and Present*, 135: 116–41.

Harrison, A. (2000) 'The National Beds Inquiry: Did It Do the Right Job?', *Health Care UK*, Autumn: 3–6.

Harrison, A. and Prentice, S. (1998) *Acute Futures*, London: King's Fund.

Harrison, S. and Wood, B. (2000) 'Designing Health Service Organisation in the UK, 1968 to 1998', *Public Administration*, 77: 751–68.

Harrison, S. *et al.* (1980) *'The Future Pattern of Hospital Services': a Need for Parallel Policies*, Leeds: Nuffield Centre.

Hart, J.T. (1971) 'The Inverse Care Law', *Lancet*, i: 405–12.

Hassell, B. (1995) *Call to Account for Private Patient Activity in the NHS*, London: Independent Healthcare Association.

Hastings, S. (1941) *The Hospital Services*, Fabian Research Series 59, London: Fabian Society/Gollancz.

Hay, C. (1998) 'Globalisation, Welfare Retrenchment and the "Logic of No Alternative"', *Journal of Social Policy*, 27: 525–32.

Haynes, R. (1987) *The Geography of Health Services in Britain*, London: Croom Helm.

Haynes, R. and Bentham, G. (1979) *Community Hospitals and Rural Accessibility*, Farnborough: Saxon House.

Haywood, S. and Ranade, W. (1989) 'Privatising from Within: The NHS under Thatcher', *Local Government Studies*, 15: 19–34.

Heclo, H. and Wildavsky, A. (1981) *The Private Government of Public Money*, London: Macmillan.

Heffer, S. (1999) *Like the Roman: The Life of Enoch Powell*, London: HarperCollins.

Hensher, M. and Edwards, N. (1999) 'Hospital Provision, Activity and Productivity in England', *British Medical Journal*, 319: 911–14.

Higgins, J. (1988) *The Business of Medicine: Private Health Care in Britain*, Basingstoke: Macmillan.

—— (1993) *The Future of Small Hospitals in Britain*, Southampton: Institute for Health Policy Studies.

Hirst, P. (1994) *Associative Democracy*, Cambridge: Polity.

—— (1999) 'Associationalist Welfare: a Reply to Marc Stears', *Economy and Society*, 28: 590–7.

Hoggett, P. (1991) 'A New Management in the Public Sector?', *Policy and Politics*, 19: 243–56.

Hollingsworth, J.R. and Hollingsworth, E.J. (1985) 'Differences between Voluntary and Public Organisations: the Behaviour of Hospitals in England and Wales', *Journal of Health Policy, Politics and Law*, 10: 371–97.

Holly, K. (1997) 'NHS Charitable Trusts', in C. Pharaoh and M. Smerdon (eds), *Dimensions of the Voluntary Sector 1997*, West Malling: Charities Aid Foundation.

Honigsbaum, F. (1979) *The Division in British Medicine*, London: Kogan Page.

—— (1989) *Health, Happiness and Security: the Creation of the NHS*, London: Routledge.

Hudson, R. (1989) *Wrecking a Region*, London: Pion.

Hughes, J. (2001) 'The "Matchbox on a Muffin": the Design of Hospitals in the Early NHS', *Medical History*, 44: 21–56.

Hunter, T. (1963) 'The Role of the Hospital in a Sick Society', *The Hospital*, 59: 345–8.

Hutton, W. (1995) *The State We're In*, London: Jonathan Cape.

Iliffe, S. and Munro, J. (2000) 'New Labour and Britain's NHS: an Overview of Current Reforms', *International Journal of Health Services*, 30: 309–34.

Illich, I. (1973) *Medical Nemesis: The Expropriation of Health*, London: Calder and Boyars.

Jacobs, L. (1993) *The Health of Nations: Public Opinion and the Making of American and British Health Policy*, Ithaca, NY: Cornell University Press.

Jarman, B. (1993) 'Is London Overbedded?', *British Medical Journal*, 306: 979–82.

Jenkins, S. (1995) *Accountable to None: the Tory Nationalisation of Britain*, London: Hamish Hamilton.

Jessop, B. (1980) 'The Transformation of the State in Postwar Britain', in R. Scase (ed.), *The State in Western Europe*, London: Croom Helm, pp. 23–93.

—— (1991a) 'Thatcherism and Flexibility: the White Heat of a Postfordist Revolution', in B. Jessop *et al.* (eds), *The Politics of Flexibility*, Aldershot: Edward Elgar, pp. 135–61.

—— (1991b) 'The Welfare State in the Transition from Fordism to Postfordism', in B. Jessop *et al.* (eds), *The Politics of Flexibility*, Aldershot: Edward Elgar, pp. 82–105.

—— (1992) 'From Social Democracy to Thatcherism; Twenty-five Years of British Politics', in N. Abercrombie and A. Warde (eds), *Social Change in Contemporary Britain*, Cambridge: Polity, pp. 14–39.

—— (1993) 'Towards a Schumpeterian Workfare State? Preliminary Remarks on Postfordist Political Economy', *Studies in Political Economy*, 40: 7–39.

—— (1995) 'Towards a Schumpeterian Workfare Regime in Britain?', *Environment and Planning A*, 27: 1613–26.

—— (1998) 'The Rise of Governance and the Risks of Failure: the Case of Economic Development', *International Social Science Journal*, 155: 29–45.

Jessop, B., Bonnett, K., Bromley, S. and Ling, T. (1987) 'Popular Capitalism, Flexible Accumulation and Left Strategy', *New Left Review*, 165: 104–22.

—— (1988) *Thatcherism: A Tale of Two Nations*, Cambridge: Polity.

Jewkes, J. and Jewkes, S. (1961) *The Genesis of the British NHS*, Oxford: Basil Blackwell.

Johnson, N. (1987) *The Welfare State in Transition: The Theory and Practice of Welfare Pluralism*, Brighton: Wheatsheaf.

Johnson, P. (1986) 'Some Historical Dimensions of the Welfare State "Crisis"', *Journal of Social Policy*, 15, 4: 443–65.

—— (1996) 'Risk, Redistribution and Social Welfare in Britain from the Poor Law to Beveridge', in M. Daunton (ed.), *Charity, Self-interest and Welfare in the English Past*, London: UCL Press, pp. 225–48.

Joint Consultants' Committee (1999) *Organisation of Acute General Hospital Services*, London: BMA.

Jones, H. (1992) 'The Conservative Party and the Welfare State, 1942–55', Ph.D. thesis, University of London.

Kearns, A. (1992) 'Active Citizenship and Urban Governance', *Transactions, Institute of British Geographers*, 17: 20–34.

Kemp, R. (1964) 'The Golden Bed', *Lancet*, ii: 1025–7.

Kerr, D. (1998) 'The PFI Miracle', *Capital and Class*, 64: 17–27.

Kingman, S. (1994) 'Freeman Hospital: the Will to Survive', *British Medical Journal*, 309: 461–4.

King's Fund (1987) *Planned Health Services for Inner London: Back-to-Back Planning*, London: King Edward's Hospital Fund.

Kinnaird, J. (1987) 'The Hospitals', in G. MacLachlan (ed.), *Improving the Common Weal*, Edinburgh: Edinburgh University Press, pp. 215–75.

Klein, R. (1983) *The Politics of the NHS*, Harlow: Longmans.

—— (1984) 'The Politics of Ideology and the Reality of Politics: the Case of Britain's Health Service in the 1980s', *Milbank Memorial Fund Quarterly*, 62: 82–109.

—— (1985) 'Health Policy, 1979–83: the Retreat from Ideology?', in P.M. Jackson (ed.), *Implementing Government Policy Initiatives: The Thatcher Administration, 1979–83*, London: RIPA.

Kuttner, R. (1996) 'Columbia/HCA and the Resurgence of For-profit Hospital Business', *New England Journal of Medicine*, 335: 362–7, 446–51.

Laing, W. (annual) *Laing's Review of Independent Health Care*, London: Laing and Buisson.

Langman, M. (1987) 'Efficiency Savings or Financial Cuts: Morals from Birmingham', *British Medical Journal*, 295: 902–3.

Lattimer, M. (1996) *The Gift of Health*, London: Directory of Social Change.

Lattimer, M. and Holly, K. (1992) *Charity and NHS Reform*, London: Directory of Social Change.

Lee, R. (1988) 'Uneven Zenith: Towards a Geography of the High Period of Municipal Medicine in England and Wales', *Journal of Historical Geography*, 14: 260–80.

Le Grand, J. (1982) *The Strategy of Equality*, London: Allen and Unwin.

—— (1991) 'The Theory of Government Failure', *British Journal of Political Science*, 21: 423–42.

—— (1999) 'Competition, Cooperation, or Control? Tales from the British NHS', *Health Affairs*, 18: 27–39.

Le Grand, J. and Robinson, R. (eds) (1994) *Evaluating the NHS Reforms*, London: King's Fund Institute.

Letwin, D. and Redwood, J. (1988) *Britain's Biggest Enterprise: Ideas for Radical Reform of the NHS*, London: Centre for Policy Studies.

Levitt, R., Appleby, J. and Wall, A. (1999) *The Reorganised NHS*, Cheltenham: Nelson Thornes.

Leys, C. (1999) 'The NHS After Devolution', *British Medical Journal*, 318: 1155–6.

Light, D. (1997) 'From Managed Competition to Managed Cooperation: Theory and Lessons from the British Experience', *The Milbank Quarterly*, 75: 297–341.

Ling, T. (1998) *The British State since 1945*, Cambridge: Polity.

—— (2000) 'Unpacking Partnership: the Case of Health Care', in J. Clarke, *et al.* (eds), *New Managerialism, New Welfare?*, London: Sage, pp. 82–101.

Llewelyn-Davies, Weeks and Co. (1955) 'Planning to Meet Demand', in Llewelyn-Davies *et al.*, *Studies in the Function and Design of Hospitals*, London: Oxford University Press, pp. 149–86.

London Health Emergency (1980) *Downhill All the Way: the Crisis in London's Health Service*, London: LHE.

—— (1987) *Hitting the Skids: a Catalogue of Health Service Cuts in London*, London: LHE.

London Health Planning Consortium (1979) *Acute Hospital Services in London: a Profile*, London: HMSO.

—— (1980) *Towards a Balance: a Framework for Acute Hospital Services in London*, London: HMSO.

Lowe, R. (1989) 'Resignation at the Treasury: the Social Services Committee and the Failure to Reform the Welfare State, 1955–57', *Journal of Social Policy*, 18: 505–26.

—— (1997) 'Milestone or Millstone? The 1959–61 Plowden Committee and Its Impact on British Welfare Policy', *The Historical Journal*, 40: 463–91.

—— (1998) *The Welfare State in Britain since 1945*, 2nd edn, Basingstoke: Macmillan.

Lowe, R. and Rollings, N. (2000) 'Modernising Britain, 1957–64: A Classic Case of Centralisation and Fragmentation?', in R. Rhodes (ed.), *Transforming British Government: Vol. 1 Changing Institutions*, Basingstoke: Macmillan, pp. 99–118.

MacKenzie, T. (1946) *The Royal Northern Infirmary, Inverness: the Story of a Scottish Voluntary Hospital*, Inverness.

MacLachlan, G. (ed.) (1987) *Improving the Common Weal: Aspects of Scottish Health Services*, Edinburgh: Edinburgh University Press.

Macnicol, J. (1990) 'Review Essay: Democracy and Health Care', *Twentieth Century British History*, 4: 188–96.

Mallender, J. (2000) 'The National Beds Inquiry: Where Next?', *Health Care UK*, Autumn: 7–10.

Mansfield, J. (1991) 'From Competition to Cooperation: Coordination of Acute Hospital Services in Middlesbrough, 1920–1950, unpublished MA thesis, Teesside Polytechnic.

Manson, T. (1979) 'Health Policy and the Cuts', *Capital and Class*, 7: 35–45.

Marland, H. (1987) *Medicine and Society in Wakefield and Huddersfield, 1780–1870*, Cambridge: Cambridge University Press.

Mayhew, L. (1979) 'The Theory and Practice of Urban Hospital Location', unpublished Ph.D. thesis, London University.

—— (1986) *Urban Hospital Location*, London: Allen and Unwin.

Mays, N. and Bevan, G. (1987) *Resource Allocation in the Health Service: a Review of the Methods of the Resource Allocation Working Party*, London: Bedford Square Press (occasional papers in Social Administration No. 81).

Mayston, D. (1990) 'Managing Capital Resources in the NHS', in A. Culyer, A. Maynard and J. Posnett (eds), *Competition in Health Care: Reforming the NHS*, Basingstoke: Macmillan, pp. 138–67.

McKeown, T. (1959) 'Fundamental Problems in Hospital Planning', *British Medical Journal* (Supplement): 122–4.

Melling, J. (1991) 'Industrial Capitalism and the Welfare of the State', *Sociology*, 25, 2: 219–39.

Mess, H. (1928) *Industrial Tyneside: A Social Survey*, London: Ernest Benn.

Middlemas, K. (1986) *Power, Competition and the State: Vol. 1 Britain in Search of a Balance, 1940–61*, Basingstoke: Macmillan.

Middleton, R. (1996) *Government versus the Market: the Growth of the Public Sector, Economic Management and British Economic Performance, c. 1890–1979*, Cheltenham: Edward Elgar.

Miller, H. (1967) 'In Sickness and in Health: a Doctor's View of Medicine in Britain', *Encounter*, 28: 10–21.

—— (1973) *Medicine and Society*, Oxford: Oxford University Press.

Millman, M. (1974) 'The Influence of the Social Science Association on Hospital Planning in Victorian England', *Medical History*, 18: 122–37.

Mistry, P. (1997) *Rationalising Acute Care Services*, Oxford: Radcliffe.

Mohan, J.F. (1986) 'Private Medical Care and the British Conservative Government: What Price Independence?', *Journal of Social Policy*, 15: 337–60.

—— (1990) 'Spatial Implications of the NHS White Paper', *Regional Studies*, 24: 553–60.

—— (1991) 'The Internationalisation and Commercialisation of Health Care in Britain', *Environment and Planning A*, 23: 853–67.

—— (1995) *A National Health Service? The Restructuring of Health Care in Britain since 1979*, Basingstoke: Macmillan.

—— (1997) 'Neglected Roots of Regionalism? The Commissioners for the Special Areas and Grants to Hospitals in England', *Social History of Medicine*, 10: 243–62.

—— (1998) 'Uneven Development, Territorial Politics and the NHS Reforms', *Political Studies*, LXVII: 308–29.

—— (1999) *A United Kingdom? Economic, Social and Political Geographies*, London: Arnold.

—— (2001) 'The Adequacy of Pre-NHS Hospital Accommodation: an Analysis of Hospital Utilisation and Waiting Lists', *Mimeo*, Department of Geography, University of Portsmouth.

Mohan, J.F. and Gorsky, M. (2001) *Don't Look Back? Voluntary and Charitable Finance of Hospitals in Britain, Past and Present*, London: Office of Health Economics.

—— (2001b) '"The Caprice of Charity": A Geography of Voluntary Hospital Finance in Britain before the NHS', paper presented to Voluntary Action History Society Conference, Liverpool.

Monbiot, G. (2000) *Captive State: the Corporate Takeover of Britain*, London: Pan Books.

Moon, G. and Brown, T. (2001) 'Closing Bart's: Community and Resistance in UK Hospital Policy', *Environment and Planning D*, 19: 43–60.

Mooney, G., Luckin, B. and Tanner, A. (1999) 'Patient Pathways: Solving the Problem of Institutional Mortality in London during the later Nineteenth Century', *Social History of Medicine*, 12: 227–69.

Moran, M. (1992) 'The Health Care State in Europe', *Environment and Planning C*, 10: 77–90.

—— (1995) 'Explaining Change in the NHS: Corporatism, Closure and Democratic Capitalism', *Public Policy and Administration*, 10: 21–33.

Mulgan, G. (1991) 'Power to the Public', *Marxism Today*, May: 14–19.

Mullard, M. (1993) *The Politics of Public Expenditure*, London: Routledge.

Murdoch, J. (1997) 'The Shifting Territory of Government', *Area*, 29: 109–18.

Murray, R. (1991) 'The State after Henry', *Marxism Today*, May: 22–7.

Navarro, V. (1978) *Class Struggle, The State and Medicine*, London: Martin Robertson.

NEDO (National Economic Development Office) (1969) *The Organisation of Demand*, London: NEDO.

Newcastle DHA (1988) *Hospital Services Review*, Newcastle: Newcastle DHA.

Newcastle Health Authority (1988) *A Review of Newcastle's Hospital Services for the 21st Century*, Newcastle: Newcastle DHA.

—— (1993) *The Future of Health Care in Newcastle*, Newcastle: Newcastle DHA.

Newcastle Health Concern (1986) *Cause for Concern: the State of Newcastle's Health Service*, Newcastle: North East Trade Union Studies Information Unit.

NHSME (1993) *Managing the New NHS*, London: NHS Management Executive.

Northern RHA (1979) *Regional Strategic Plan, 1979–88*, Newcastle: Northern RHA.

—— (1986) *Regional Strategy, 1985–94 (revised 1986)*, Newcastle: Northern RHA.

—— (1991) *Building Health Care for the 21st Century*, Newcastle: Northern RHA.

—— (annual) *Financial Reviews*, Newcastle: Northern RHA.

Nuffield Provincial Hospitals Trust (NPHT) (1941) *Memorandum on the Coordination of Hospital Services*, Oxford: NPHT.

—— (1946) *The Hospital Surveys: the Domesday Book of the Hospital Service*, Oxford: NPHT.

Offe, C. (1984) *Contradictions of the Modern Welfare State*, London: Hutchinson.

Osborne, D. and Gaebler, T. (1992) *Reinventing Government: How the Entrepreneurial Spirit is Transforming the Public Sector*, New York: Plume.

Owen, D. (1976) *In Sickness and in Health*, London: Quartet Books.

Owen, J. (1990) 'Defending the County: the Reorganisation of Local Government in England', unpublished Ph.D. thesis, University of Bristol.

Panitch, L. and Leys, C. (2001) *The End of Parliamentary Socialism*, London: Verso.

Parston, G. (1980) *Planners, Politicians and Health Services*, London: Croom Helm.

Pater, J. (1981) *The Making of the National Health Service*, London: Kings Fund.

Paton, C. (1992) *Competition and Planning in the NHS*, London: Chapman and Hall.

—— (1993) 'Devolution and Centralism in the NHS', *Social Policy and Administration*, 27: 83–109.

—— (2000) 'New Labour, New Health Policy?', in A. Hann (ed.), *Analysing Health Policy*, Aldershot: Ashgate.

Paton, C. and Bach, S. (1990) *Case Studies in Health Policy and Management*, London: Nuffield Provincial Hospitals Trust.

Peden, G. (2000) *The Treasury and British Public Policy, 1906–1959*, Cambridge: Cambridge University Press.

Pepler, G. and Macfarlane, P.W. (1949) *The North-East Area Development Plan: Interim Report Presented to the Minister of Town and Country Planning*.

Pettigrew, A., Ferlie, E. and McKee, L. (1992) *Shaping Strategic Change*, London: Sage.

Pharaoh, C. and Mocroft, I. (2001) *Coming Full Circle: the Role of Charitable Funds in London's Health*, West Malling: Charities Aid Foundation.

Pickstone, J. (1985) *Medicine and Industrial Society*, Manchester: Manchester University Press.

Pierson, C. (1991) *Beyond the Welfare State?*, Cambridge: Polity.

—— (1998) 'Contemporary Challenges to Welfare State Development', *Political Studies*, XLVI: 777–94.

Pinker, R. (1966) *English Hospital Statistics, 1861–1938*, London: Heinemann.

Pliatzky, L. (1982) *Getting and Spending: Public Expenditure, Employment and Inflation*, Oxford: Blackwell.

Political and Economic Planning (PEP) (1937) *Report on the British Health Services*, London: PEP.

Pollitt, C. (1986) 'Performance Measurement in Public Services: Some Political Implications', *Parliamentary Affairs*, 39: 315–29.

Pollock, A. (2000) 'Editorial: Will Intermediate Care be the Undoing of the NHS?', *British Medical Journal*, 321: 393–4.

Pollock, A. and Dunnigan, M. (2000) 'Beds in the NHS', *British Medical Journal*, 320: 461–2.

Pollock, A., Price, D. and Dunnigan, M. (2000) *Deficits before Patients*, London: UCL.

Pollock, A., Dunnigan, M., Gaffney, D., Price, D. and Shaoul, J. (1999) 'Planning the "New" NHS: Downsizing for the 21st Century', *British Medical Journal*, 319: 179–84.

Porter, D. (1999) *Health, Civilization and the State*, London: Routledge.

Powell, M. (1992) 'Hospital Provision before the NHS: Territorial Justice or Inverse Care Law?', *Journal of Social Policy*, 21: 145–63.

—— (1995) 'The Strategy of Equality Revisited', *Journal of Social Policy*, 24: 163–85.

—— (1997) 'An Expanding Service: Municipal Acute Medicine in the 1930s', *Twentieth Century British History*, 8: 334–57.

Price, D., Gaffney, D. and Pollock, A. (1999) *'The Only Game in Town?' A report on the Cumberland Infirmary (Carlisle) PFI*, London: UNISON.

Prochaska, F. (1992) *Philanthropy and the Hospitals of London: the King's Fund, 1897–1990*, Oxford: Oxford University Press.

Rayner, G. (1986) 'Health Care as a Business: The Emergence of a Commercial Hospital Sector in Britain', *Policy and Politics*, 14: 439–59.

—— (1987) 'Lessons from America? Commercialization and Growth of Private Medicine in Britain', *International Journal of Health Services*, 17: 197–216.

Rhodes, R.A. (1992) 'Changing Intergovernmental Relations', in P. Cloke (ed.), *Policy and Change in Thatcher's Britain*, Oxford: Pergamon, pp. 55–76.

—— (1997) *Understanding Governance*, Buckingham: Open University Press.

Rivett, G. (1986) *The Development of the London Hospital System*, London: Kings Fund.

—— (1998) *From Cradle to Grave: Fifty Years of the NHS*, London: King's Fund.

Robinson, F. (1978) 'Peterlee: Aspects of New Town Development', unpublished Ph.D. thesis, Durham University.

Robinson, R. and Appleby, J. (1991) *Cutting Through the Confusion: a Review of Capital and Capital Charges in the NHS*, Birmingham: NAHAT.

Rodwin, V. (1984) *The Health Planning Predicament*, Berkeley, CA: University of California Press.

Rose, N. (1996) 'Governing "Advanced Liberal Democracies"', in A. Barry, T. Osbourne and N. Rose (eds), *Foucault and Political Reason*, London: UCL Press, pp. 37–64.

Rose, N. and Miller, P. (1992) 'Political Power Beyond the State: Problematics of Government', *British Journal of Sociology*, 43: 173–205.

Royston, G. *et al.* (1992) 'Modelling the Use of Health Services by Populations of Small Areas to Inform the Allocation of Central Resources to Larger Regions', *Socio-Economic Planning. Sciences*, 26 (3): 169–80.

Ruane, S. (2000) 'Acquiescence and Opposition: the PFI in the NHS', *Policy and Politics*, 28: 411–24.

—— (2001) 'A Clear Public Mission? Public-Private Partnerships and the Recommodification of the NHS', *Capital and Class*, 73: 1–6.

Salmon, J. (1995) 'A Perspective on the Corporate Transformation of Health Care', *International Journal of Health Services*, 25: 11–42.

Sayer, A. (1985) 'The Difference that Space Makes', in D. Gregory and J. Urry (eds), *Social Relations and Spatial Structures*, Basingstoke: Macmillan.

Scheffler, R. (1989) 'Adverse Selection: the Achilles' Heel of the NHS Reforms', *Lancet*, 99: 950–92.

Schumacher, E. (1975) *Small is Beautiful*, London: Blond and Briggs.

SE Thames RHA (1985) *Financing Community Hospitals: Possibilities for Liaison with the Private Health Sector*, Bexhill: SE Thames RHA.

Sheldon, T. *et al.* (1994) 'Allocating Resources to Health Authorities: Development of Method for Small Area Analysis of Use of Inpatient Services', *British Medical Journal*, 309: 1046–9.

Sheldrake, J. (1989) 'The LCC Hospital Service', in A. Saint (ed.), *Politics and the People of London*, London: Hambledon Press, pp. 188–97.

Shepherd, R. (1997) *Enoch Powell*, London: Pimlico.

Small, N. (1990) *Politics and Planning in the NHS*, Milton Keynes: Open University Press.

Smith, D. *et al.* (1995) 'Philanthropy and Hospital Financing', *Health Services Research*, 30: 615–35.

Smith, J. (1981) 'Conflict Without Change: The Case of London's Health Services', *The Political Quarterly*, 52: 426–40.

—— (1984a) 'Hospital Building in the NHS. Policy II: Reduced Expectations', *British Medical Journal*, 289: 1368–70.

—— (1984b) 'Hospital Building in the NHS. Policy I', *British Medical Journal*, 289: 1298–1300.

—— (1984c) 'Hospital Building in the NHS. Ideas and Designs II – Harness and Nucleus', *British Medical Journal*, 289: 1513–16.

—— (1984d) 'Hospital Building in the NHS. Things that Go Wrong', *British Medical Journal*, 289: 1599–1602.

Smith, M. (1998) 'Reconceptualising the British State: Theoretical and Empirical Challenges to Central Government', *Public Administration*, 76: 45–72.

Smith, T. (1998) 'The Social Transformation of Hospitals and the Rise of Medical Insurance in France, 1914–43', *The Historical Journal*, 41: 1055–87.

Smyth, H. (1985) *Property Companies and the Construction Industry in Britain*, Cambridge: Cambridge University Press.

Southall, H. (1988) 'The Origins of the Depressed Areas: Unemployment, Growth and Regional Structure in Britain before 1914', *Economic History Review*, XLI: 236–58.

Stears, M. (1999) 'Needs, Welfare and the Limits of Associationalism', *Economy and Society*, 28: 570–89.

Stevens, R. (1999) *In Sickness and in Wealth*, Baltimore, MD: Johns Hopkins University Press.

Stewart, J. (1997) ' "For a Healthy London": the Socialist Medical Association and the LCC in the 1930s', *Medical History*, 42: 417–36.

—— (1999) *'The Battle for Health': a Political History of the Socialist Medical Association*, Aldershot: Ashgate.

Sturdy, S. and Cooter, R. (1998) 'Science, Scientific Management, and the Transformation of Medicine in Britain, *c.* 1870–1950', *History of Science*, xxxvi: 421–66.

Sussex, J. (2001) *The Economics of the Private Finance Initiative*, London: Office of Health Economics.

Taylor, D. (1998) 'Social Identity and Social Policy: Engagements with Postmodern Theory', *Journal of Social Policy*, 27: 329–50.

Taylor, R. (1984) 'State Intervention in Postwar Western European Health Care: the Case of Prevention in Britain and Italy', in S. Bornstein, D. Held and J. Krieger (eds), *The State in Capitalist Europe*, London: Unwin, pp. 91–111.

Taylor, S. (1960) 'Hospitals of the Future', *British Medical Journal*, ii: 753.

Taylor-Gooby, P. (1997) 'In Defence of Second-best Theory: State, Class and Capital in Social Policy', *Journal of Social Policy*, 26: 171–92.

Terry, R. (1999) 'The Private Finance Initiative: Overdue Reform or Policy Breakthrough?', *Public Money and Management*, January–March: 9–16.

Thatcher, M. (1993) *The Downing Street Years*, London: Harper Collins.

Timmins, N. (1995) *The Five Giants: a Biography of the Welfare State*, London: HarperCollins.

Titmuss, R.M. (1950) *Problems of Social Policy*, London: Longman.

Tomlinson, J. (1995) 'Welfare and the Economy: the Economic Impact of the Welfare State, 1945–51', *Twentieth Century British History*, 6: 194–219.

—— (1998) 'Why so Austere? The British Welfare State of the 1990s', *Journal of Social Policy*, 27, 1: 63–78.

Townsend, A. (1986) 'Rationalisation and Change in the South Teesside Health Service', *Mimeo*, Durham: Geography Department, Durham University.

Townsend, P., Phillimore, P. and Beattie, A. (1992) *Deprivation and Ill-health: Inequality and the North*, London: Croon Helm.

Tucker, H. and Bosanquet, N. (1991) *Community Hospitals in the 1990s: a Case Study*, Chichester: Carden Press.

Tuohy, C. (1999) *Accidental Logics: the Dynamics of Change in the Health Care Arena in the US, Britain and Canada*, New York: Oxford University Press.

Turner, J. (1994–96) *Current Issues in Acute Care: Reconfiguring Acute Services I, II, III*, London: Institute for Health Service Management.

Vann-Wye, G. (1992) 'Hospitals in the UK: a History of Design Innovation', in R. Loveridge and K. Starkey (eds), *Continuity and Crisis in the NHS*, Milton Keynes: Open University Press, pp. 157–78.

Vetter, N. (1995) *Hospital – from Centre of Excellence to Community Support*, London: Chapman and Hall.

Waddington, K. (2000) *Charity and the London Hospitals, 1950–1898*, Woodbridge: Boydell.

Ward, S. (1984) 'List Q: a Missing Link in Interwar Public Investment', *Public Administration*, 62: 348–58.

—— (1988) *The Geography of Inter-war Britain: the State and Uneven Development*, London: Croom Helm.

Watkin, B. (1978) *The NHS: the First Phase, 1948–74 and After*, London: Allen and Unwin.

Webb, A. and Hanley, S. (1997) 'The Conflict in Transferring a Cystic Fibrosis Specialist Service Between Two Hospitals in Manchester', *British Medical Journal*, 315: 1009–11.

Webster, C. (1982) 'Healthy or Hungry Thirties?', *History Workshop Journal*, 13: 110–29.

—— (1985) 'Health, Wealth and Unemployment During the Depression', *Past and Present*, 109: 204–30.

—— (1988a) *The Health Services Since the War, Vol. I*, London: HMSO.

—— (1988b) 'Labour and the Origins of the NHS', in N. Rupke (ed.), *Science, Politics and the Public Good*, Basingstoke: Macmillan, pp. 184–202.

—— (1990) 'Conflict and Consensus: Explaining the British Health Service', *Twentieth Century British History*, 1: 115–51.

—— (1993) 'The Metamorphosis of Dawson of Penn', in D. Porter and R. Porter (eds), *Doctors, Politics and Society: Historical Essays*, Amsterdam: Rodopi, pp. 212–28.

—— (1994) 'Conservatives and Consensus: the Politics of the NHS, 1951–64', in A. Oakley and S. Williams (eds), *The Politics of the Welfare State*, London: UCL Press, pp. 54–74.

—— (1995) 'Overthrowing the Market in Health Care: the Achievements of the Early National Health Service', *Journal of the Royal College of General Practitioners*, 29: 502–7.

—— (1996) *The Health Services Since the War, Vol. II. Government and Health Care: the NHS, 1958–79*, London: HMSO.

—— (1998) 'Birth of the Dream: Bevan and the Architecture of the NHS', in G. Goodman (ed.), *The State of the Nation: the Political Legacy of Aneurin Bevan*, London: Gollancz, pp. 106–29.

Wells, A. (1951) 'The Hospital Service', *Public Administration*, 29: 39–49.

West, P. (1997) *Understanding the NHS Reforms: the Creation of Incentives?*, Buckingham: Open University Press.

—— (1998) *Future Hospital Services in the NHS: One Size Fits All?*, London: Nuffield Trust.

Whitney, R. (1988) *National Health Crisis: A Modern Solution?*, London: Shepheard-Walwyn.

Widgery, D. (1979) *Health in Danger: The Crisis in the NHS*, London: Macmillan.

—— (1988) The National Health: A Radical Perspective, London: Hogarth.

Williams, B.T. et al. (1984b) 'Analysis of the Work of Independent Acute Hospitals in England and Wales, 1981', British Medical Journal, 289: 446–8.

Williams, B et al. (2000) 'Private Funding of Elective Hospital Treatment in England and Wales, 1997–8', British Medical Journal, 320: 904–5.

Williams, I. (1989) The Alms Trade, London: Unwin Hyman.

Wistow, G. (1992) 'Health', in D. Marsh and R. Rhodes (eds), Implementing Thatcherite Policies, Milton Keynes: Open University Press, pp. 100–16.

Index